Resolving Dilemmas in Perimetry

Sagarika Patyal · Monica Gandhi
Editors

Resolving Dilemmas in Perimetry

Illustrated Manual of Visual Field Defects

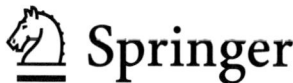

Editors
Sagarika Patyal
Centre for Sight, Dwarka
New Delhi
Delhi
India

Monica Gandhi
Dr. Shroff's Charity Eye Hospital
New Delhi
Delhi
India

ISBN 978-981-16-2603-6   ISBN 978-981-16-2601-2   (eBook)
https://doi.org/10.1007/978-981-16-2601-2

© The Editor(s) (if applicable) and The Author(s), under exclusive license to Springer Nature Singapore Pte Ltd. 2021
This work is subject to copyright. All rights are solely and exclusively licensed by the Publisher, whether the whole or part of the material is concerned, specifically the rights of translation, reprinting, reuse of illustrations, recitation, broadcasting, reproduction on microfilms or in any other physical way, and transmission or information storage and retrieval, electronic adaptation, computer software, or by similar or dissimilar methodology now known or hereafter developed.
The use of general descriptive names, registered names, trademarks, service marks, etc. in this publication does not imply, even in the absence of a specific statement, that such names are exempt from the relevant protective laws and regulations and therefore free for general use.
The publisher, the authors, and the editors are safe to assume that the advice and information in this book are believed to be true and accurate at the date of publication. Neither the publisher nor the authors or the editors give a warranty, expressed or implied, with respect to the material contained herein or for any errors or omissions that may have been made. The publisher remains neutral with regard to jurisdictional claims in published maps and institutional affiliations.

This Springer imprint is published by the registered company Springer Nature Singapore Pte Ltd. The registered company address is: 152 Beach Road, #21-01/04 Gateway East, Singapore 189721, Singapore

Dedicated to my husband

Lt Gen Shravan Kumar Patyal, PVSM, UYSM, SM, PhD

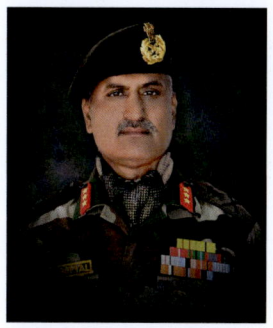

कर्मण्येवाधिकारस्ते मा फलेषु कदाचन ।
मा कर्मफलहेतुर्भूर्मा ते सङ्गोऽस्त्वकर्मणि ॥ ४७ ॥

You have a right to perform your prescribed duties, but you are not entitled to the fruits of your actions. Never consider yourself to be the cause of the results of your activities, nor be attached to inaction.

—Sagarika Patyal

Dedicated to my father

Mr S. C. Menocha

In loving memory of you Papa

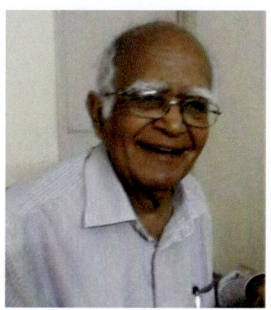

For all the support, strength, and endless love

—Monica Gandhi

Preface

We have found visual fields very intriguing and often challenging in a good way. They get us thinking on how we can look into the core of retinal sensitivities and interpret the disease process and make a scientific approach towards better management and patient care.

Perimetry has come a long way from its infancy and much has been written about this subject by renowned authors, practitioners, and academicians perimetry. Ophthalmologists, teachers, and students grapple with various parametric devices applying the information provided by a well done test to determine the medical ailment. However, there is a humongous area still unexplored and remains the reason to attempt this book. Dilemmas in interpretation of fields continue to puzzle us especially when two diseases coexist and despite a thorough clinical examination, we often need to think through the problem to fit the pieces of the jigsaw puzzle.

We hope that you have been equally fascinated by the visual fields and their analysis. Through this book we wish to share the intricacies and nuances of basic concepts, better execution, and interpretation of visual fields. A large number of thorough academicians, teachers, and clinicians were requested to put together their concepts, patient presentations which have baffled them and which may help others to be the "Sherlock Homes" for their patients' myriad complicated cases and help solve the dilemmas early and successfully.

This book, we hope, will help all across the spectrum—ophthalmologists, neurologists, academicians, and, most importantly, students. We have tried to make the text very lucid and reader friendly and have touched upon questions that have stimulated our inquisitiveness in the visual field analysis. So we hope that many unanswered questions will be understood with the illustrations that have been incorporated.

We would like your feedback and suggestions and do hope you will enjoy reading this book as much as we have compiling it together.

Best wishes

New Delhi, India Sagarika Patyal
New Delhi, India Monica Gandhi

Contents

1 **What Is Perimetry and How to Obtain the Best Results?**...... 1
Sagarika Patyal and Monica Gandhi

2 **Incorporating Perimetry in Managing Glaucoma**............ 5
Monica Gandhi and Sagarika Patyal

3 **Interpretation of a Humphrey Single Visual Field Printout**.... 21
Sagarika Patyal and Monica Gandhi

4 **Challenges in Interpreting Perimetry in Glaucoma** 31
Monica Gandhi and Sagarika Patyal

5 **Evaluating Progression on Perimetry**..................... 47
Medha Prabhudesai

6 **Interpretation of Octopus Visual Fields** 83
N. R. Rangaraj and P. Sathyan

7 **Progression Monitoring with an Octopus Perimeter**.......... 93
N. R. Rangaraj and P. Sathyan

8 **Structure–Function Relation in Humphrey Perimetry**........ 101
Col Madhu Bhadauria and Jyoti Bhat

9 **Structure–Function Relation in Octopus Perimetry** 123
N. R. Rangaraj and P. Sathyan

10 **Check–Recheck: Visual Field Dilemmas in Retinal Disorders** 133
Ritesh Narula and Chitralekha De

11 **Perimetry in Neurological Disorders**...................... 155
Sumit Monga

12 **Effect of Media Opacities on Perimetry: A Vexing Clinical Problem**............................... 173
Tulika Chauhan and Mithun Thulasidas

13 **Visual Field Defects with Tilted and Torted Optic Discs**....... 179
Sagarika Patyal

About the Editors

Sagarika Patyal is currently a Senior Consultant at Centre for Sight, New Delhi. Dr. Patyal completed her Diploma in Ophthalmology and MS from Army Hospital Delhi Cantt (Delhi University). She was trained in glaucoma from the Rajendra Prasad Center for Ophthalmic Sciences, AIIMS, New Delhi, and PGDGM from IGNOU University.

Dr. Patyal has rich teaching experience for both undergraduate and postgraduate curricula and has taught in Armed Forces Medical College, Pune, Army College of Medical Sciences Delhi, Army Hospital Research and Referral Center, and Base Hospital. She was also appointed as national faculty for glaucoma, MCI Inspector for MBBS, and assessor for DNB and referee for *Medical Journal of Armed Forces of India* (MJAFI) and other indexed journals. Her subjects of interests are cataract, glaucoma, ocular surface, cornea, high altitude ocular diseases, and trauma. She has been instrumental in establishing telemedicine nodes in high altitude (Siachen) to help soldiers stationed in the highest battleground in the world.

Dr. Patyal has more than 85 publications and presentations in international and national journals to her credit and has written chapters in books. She is member of All India Ophthalmological Society, Delhi Ophthalmological Society, Glaucoma Society of India, Pune Ophthalmological Society, Maharashtra Ophthalmic Society, Kolkata Association of Ophthalmologists, and All India Women's Ophthalmological Society.

She was honored with Chief of Army Staff Commendation 2004, Special Achiever's Award from Sunderji group of Institutes 2010, Chief of Army Staff Commendation 2011, AWWA Excellence Award for social work, Award for Best AFMRC project 2011 (Research), Army Commander's commendation 2013, Sena Medal 2014 for work done in the highest multispeciality hospital in the world, Leh, Visisht Sena Medal 2016, and Gold medal from IIRSI 2018.

Monica Gandhi is currently working as Associate Medical Director, Head—Digital Initiatives, and Senior Consultant in glaucoma and anterior segment services at Dr. Shroff's Charity Eye Hospital, New Delhi, India. She is an alumnus of Maulana Azad Medical College and Guru Nanak Eye Centre, under the University of Delhi. A former glaucoma fellow at the Glaucoma Imaging Centre under Prof. NN Sood, she has several publications and book chapters on glaucoma to her credit. She has delivered innumerable talks as invited faculty in various forums and has made a special contribution to perimetry workshops and lectures. Besides her keen interest in clinical and surgical training for fellows, she is also committed to mentoring fellows, DNB students, and trainees in their research work.

What Is Perimetry and How to Obtain the Best Results?

Sagarika Patyal and Monica Gandhi

Perimetry literally means outer boundary or border of a two-dimensional figure. In ophthalmology, it is a measurement of a person's field of vision which implies all objects seen at the same time by the eye while maintaining steady fixation in one direction [1]. The term "automated perimetry" implies quantification of a person's peripheral field of vision using standardised and efficient algorithms [2]. In the oft repeated words of Henry Moss Traquair, it is the "island of vision in a sea of darkness", being maximum in the fovea, represented by the top of the hill and gradually decreasing towards the periphery [3]. The extent of mono ocular field of vision is: central vision (30), central fixation and peripheral vision (60 superiorly and nasally, 100 temporally and 75 inferiorly) [1]. Field of vision can be divided into nasal and temporal hemifields by a vertical line bisecting the central fixation. The blind spot, situated in the temporal half of the field, is about 12–17 temporal to fixation and 1.5 inferiorly [1].

The measurement of perimetry is not new, as Hippocrates measured it in the fifth century BC. Ptolemy gave the first inkling of its circular shape to the world. The science of perimetry has seen many greats—Galen, Ulmus, Mariotte, Thomas Young, Purkinje, Boerhaave, Beer, Albrecht Von Graefe, Bjerrum, Henning Ronne, Harry Traquair, Hans Goldmann, John R Lynn, George W Tate, Franz Fankhauser, Anders Heijl, Douglas Anderson to name a few [2].

The basic method of detecting visual fields using a small target on a uniform background has remained the same but standardisation has improved due to technological advancement, statistical analysis improving reproducibility of defects and reliability. Presently, threshold testing is the most common tool used for perimetry, and standard automated perimetry tests the central field with a white stimulus on a white background [2].

Measuring visual fields qualitatively and quantitatively has been the subject of many researchers as it is an important diagnostic tool for diagnosing various diseases, assessing progression of damage by disease or effects of treatment, of the optic nerve, most commonly, glaucoma, of the optic pathway or of the retina. It is also used for quantifying ability or disability to drive and for determination of legal blindness [4].

To get the best perimetric results, the physician, technician, and patient must work in tandem. A physician's explanation to the patient of the importance of the test and how it will impact his diagnosis and treatment is the first step in this direction. So, a few extra minutes of chair time in

S. Patyal (✉)
Centre for Sight, Dwarka, New Delhi, Delhi, India

M. Gandhi
Dr. Shroff's Charity Eye Hospital, New Delhi, Delhi, India

explaining the test is always helpful. A thorough history, a comprehensive ocular examination and a dilated examination of the optic nerve and retina are mandatory requirements before a field examination is ordered. The doctor should be able to assess the patient's ability to perform the test while talking to him. His/Her systemic illnesses must be taken cognisance of, as a person with dementia/tremors/Parkinsonism will find it difficult to perform the test. A large number of patients are afraid of performing the test, so it helps to allay their fears and make it appear as simple as possible. On receiving the field reports, the patient should be explained the reasons for unreliability and how he/she can overcome them. If the patient is elderly and unable to concentrate, it is always better to schedule the tests in the morning when he/she is fresh and conduct one eye on one day and the other eye on the following day.

The next responsibility lies with the technician. It does wonders if the technician has performed the field test on himself/herself so that he/she is aware of the nuances of the test and is fully conversant with the equipment. The perimetrist must not be distracted by mobiles or conversations but must give his/her undivided attention to the patient while the test is being conducted. A video of the test, if shown at the waiting area, briefs the patient even before he/she steps into the room and decreases the explanation time of the technician. The perimeter should be placed in a quiet room with no distractions. It is preferable to keep a small table lamp to help the technician feed in the data into the perimeter so that overhead lights can be switched off. Data entry into the perimeter must be meticulous and exactly the same as earlier, if done before. Date of birth, especially year, must be verified from the patient and then entered into the menu.

The perimetrist should be attentive at all times, gently encourage the patient during the test (Fig. 1.1a) and see that the patient is sitting comfortably without bending his neck or arching his back. (Fig 1.1c, d).

The height of the perimeter and the patient chair must be appropriate and comfortable for the patient. Best Corrected Visual Acuity should be ascertained before inserting the wire-rimmed lenses (Fig 1.1d) onto the frame which should be placed close to the patient's eye without touching the eyelashes and should be well centred on the eye.

It is advisable to insert the spherical equivalent of astigmatic correction (if more than 2D) rather than insert two lenses [5].Smaller astigmatic errors do not affect the results [5].If the patient wears contact lens, he can continue to wear them during the test. The fellow eye should be closed comfortably with an eye shield. In the COVID era, it is advisable to apply a tape on the edge of the mask to the skin to prevent fogging of the lens. Additionally, the chin rest, forehead rest and buzzer should be cleaned after every patient.

Lid position must be checked to ensure that it is not occluding the pupil. If there is drooping of the lid, it should be adequately taped before beginning the test. Pupil size should be checked and, if miotic, must be dilated to at least 3 mm [6], and the same pupil size should be present for subsequent tests. The patient must be explained what he/she is expected to see and be given short demonstration of the same and be assured that there is no need to hurry as the instrument will adjust as per his/her response time. Blinking during the test and ability to pause the test when required allay the patients' fears of his/her ability to perform the test. Another frequent problem encountered by patients is lacrimation. This too must be addressed at the outset by explaining that the test can be paused to wipe the eyes and continued thereafter. Further, he/she should be assured that the test can be repeated and that he/she will be able to visualise only 50% of the lights, so he/she must not search for the lights but be mindful that lights will shine with varying intensity at any point in the four quadrants.

A well-done perimetric test depends not just upon the patient but upon the technician and doctor and goes a long way in ensuring correct diagnosis and treatment (Fig. 1.2).

Summary: Explanation by the ophthalmologist and perimetrist and gentle encouragement to a patient who has understood what is required for him to perform the test goes a long way in obtaining a reliable field test.

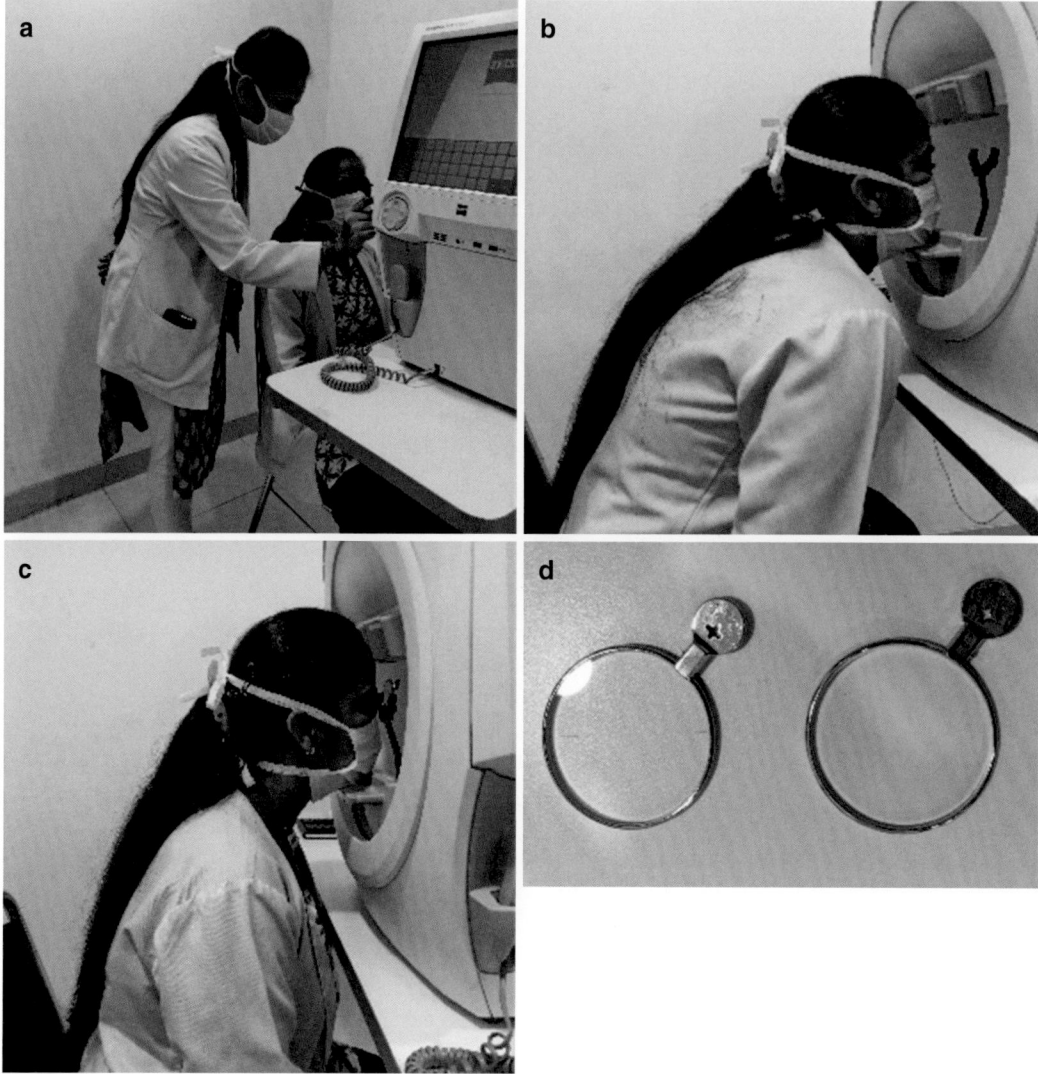

Fig. 1.1 (**a**) Perimetrist's clear explanation of procedure to patient. Courtesy: Raj Rani and Shivangi Rawat. (**b**) Incorrect posture. (**c**) Correct posture. (**d**) Wire-rimmed lens-Cylindrical and Spherical

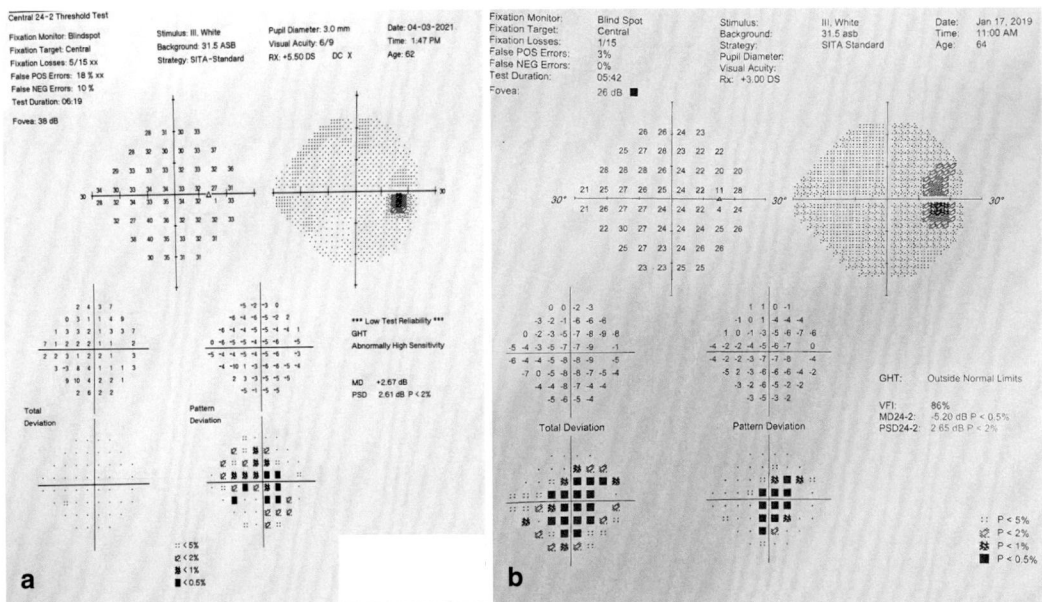

Fig. 1.2 Fields of the same patient. (**a**) All the reliability indices are flagged. (**b**) Improvement in reliability indices after proper counselling resulting in improvement in reliability indices

References

1. Spector RH. The pupils. In: Walker HK, Hall WD, Hurst JW, editors. Clinical methods: the history, physical, and laboratory examinations. 3rd ed. Boston: Butterworths; 1990.
2. Johnson CA, Wall M, Thompson HS. A history of perimetry and visual field testing. Optom Vis Sci. 2011;88:E1–15.
3. Grzybowski A, Traquair HM. Scottish ophthalmologist and perimetrist. Acta Ophthalmol. 1865–1954;2009(87):5455–9.
4. Less SY, Mesfin FB. Blindness (Updated 2020). In: StatPearls (Internet). Treasure Island, FL;2020. Available from: http://www.ncbi.nlm.nih.gov/books/NBK448182.
5. Anders H, Patella VM, Bengtsson B. The field analyser primer: effective perimetry. 4th ed. 2012.
6. Racette LF, Bebie H, Hollo G, Johnson C, Matsumoto C. External obstructions blocking stimuli from reaching the retina. In: AG H-S, editor. Visual field digest: a guide to perimetry and the octopus perimeter. 6th ed. Koniz: Haag-Striet AG; 2016. p. 44.

Incorporating Perimetry in Managing Glaucoma

Monica Gandhi and Sagarika Patyal

2.1 Introduction

Perimetry has stood the test of time in being a reliable test for devising a management plan for our glaucoma patients. There is no substitute for a clinical examination, but perimetry is complementary in understanding the visual field defects due to the neuropathy as a result of the retinal ganglion cells [1, 2].

There is evidence that structural damage may precede functional damage. In the ocular hypertension treatment study (OHTS) [3], disc damage was seen earlier than visual field abnormalities. Thus, there has been an increase in imaging the retinal nerve fiber layer defects (RNFLD) using optical coherence tomography, Heidelberg retinal tomography, and GDx nerve fiber analyzer; however, the validity of these in their role in management of glaucoma is not well established, and the information obtained is useful when used in association with other parameters that define glaucoma diagnosis and progression [4]. In comparison, visual field analysis is the reference standard used more universally.

M. Gandhi (✉)
Dr. Shroff's Charity Eye Hospital, New Delhi, Delhi, India

S. Patyal
Centre for Sight, Dwarka, New Delhi, Delhi, India

2.2 The Role of Perimetry in the Management of Glaucoma is Multifold

1. To compliment the clinical diagnosis—staging the disease and establishing a target IOP [5].
2. To follow up the patient and see that the management is helping in stabilizing the disease.
3. To identify progression of the disease.
4. To predict the course of disease progression in the future by plotting the rate of progression.
5. Traditionally, visual fields are the endpoints in various clinical trials.

2.2.1 To Help in Diagnosis of Glaucoma

The visual fields interpretation is a skill, based on a systemic approach to each part of the visual field analysis (VFA) printout. The clinical evaluation is of foremost importance.

As seen in Fig. 2.1, the visual field shows a field defect which meets the Hodapp–Parrish–Anderson criteria and reliability factors are good, but this does not mean it is glaucomatous till a clinical correlation is done. Looking at the optic nerve head in Fig. 2.2, a corresponding thinning of the neuroretinal rim and retinal nerve fiber layer defect is present, which is seen as the decreased sensitivity in

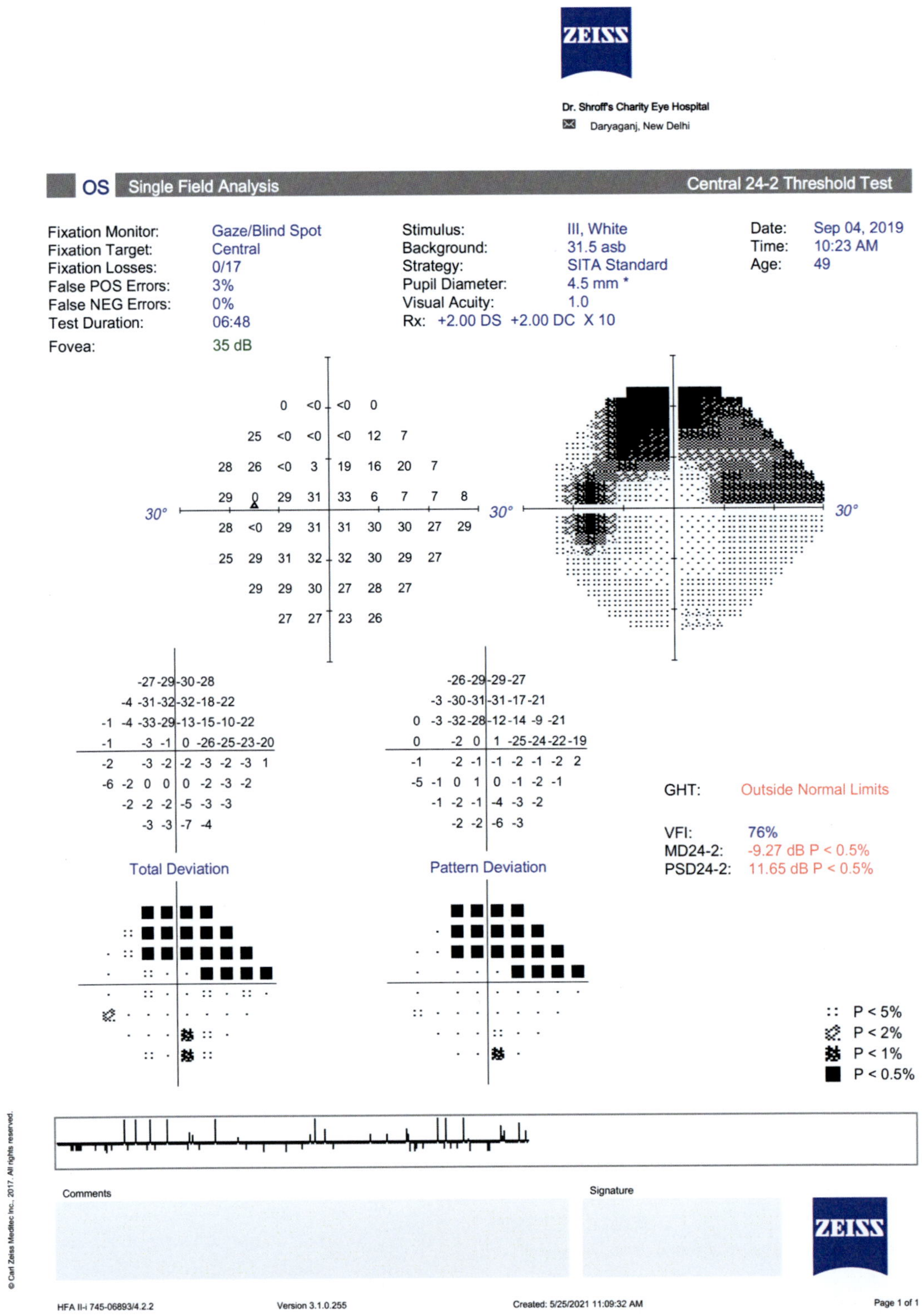

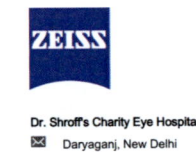

Fig. 2.1 A Central 24–2 SITA standard W on W test—Left eye of a 49-year-old patient. Vision 6/6 with corresponding foveal threshold. There is decreased sensitivity in the superior hemisphere, both in total and pattern deviation plots with MD and PSD < 0.5%, GHT outside normal limits. The VFA meets Hodapp–Parrish–Anderson criteria, however, a repeat field test is required to establish reproducibility

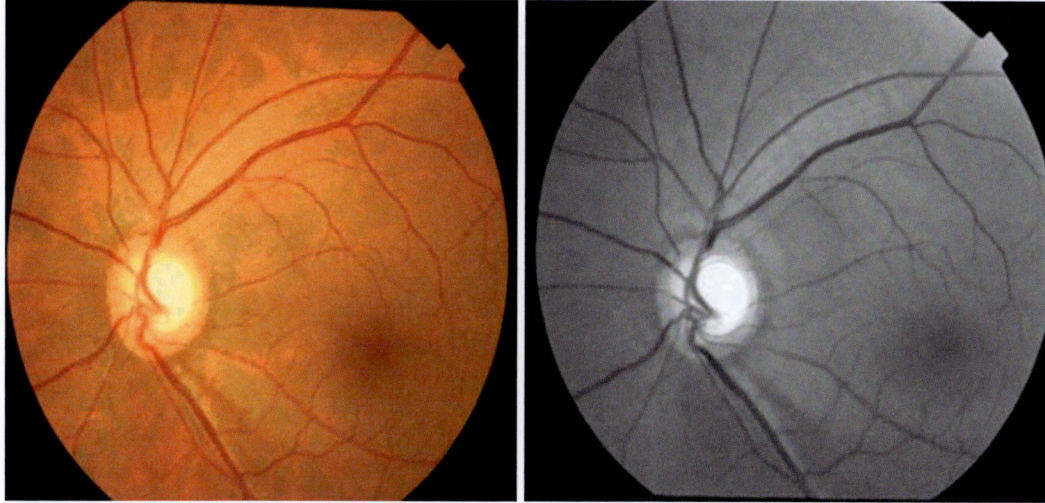

Fig. 2.2 Inferior rim equal to superior—ISNT (Inferior Superior Nasal Temporal) rule is not preserved, CD ratio 0.65:1. Note the bending of the inferior vessels, a notch is present. A wedge-shaped RNFL defect infero-temporally, which is more evident in the red-free photo

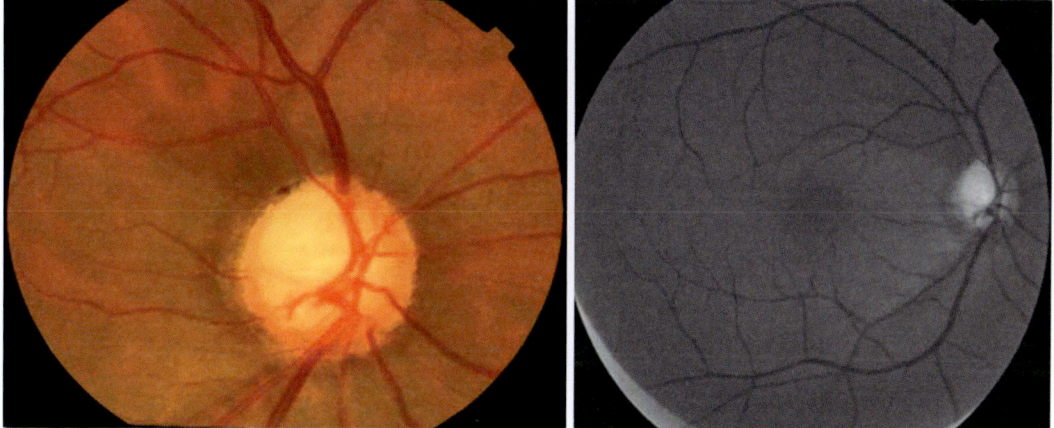

Fig. 2.3 Right eye with thin neuroretinal rim along with RNFLD superiorly. Small RNFLD is seen inferiorly also which is more evident in the red-free photograph

the superior hemisphere in the VFA. Thus, there is clinical and visual field correlation.

Even though there is correlation, this is not enough evidence to say that the defect is glaucomatous as similar visual field defects may be seen in neurological diseases, thus a good clinical history with examination of the other eye is important. Figure 2.3 and 2.4 show the disc and visual field of the right eye which also show the correlation but the inferior retinal nerve fiber layer defect (RNFLD) in the clinical picture is not seen as a corresponding visual field defect. Also, the fixation is threatened which is not evident in the macula or the visual acuity. The patient was started on anti-glaucoma management and followed-up regularly. A repeat field for reproducibility is desirable.

2.2.2 Staging the Disease Based on Visual Fields

There is no universally accepted staging method based on visual fields. Several systems in use are Hodapp–Parrish–Andersons criteria [6], glau-

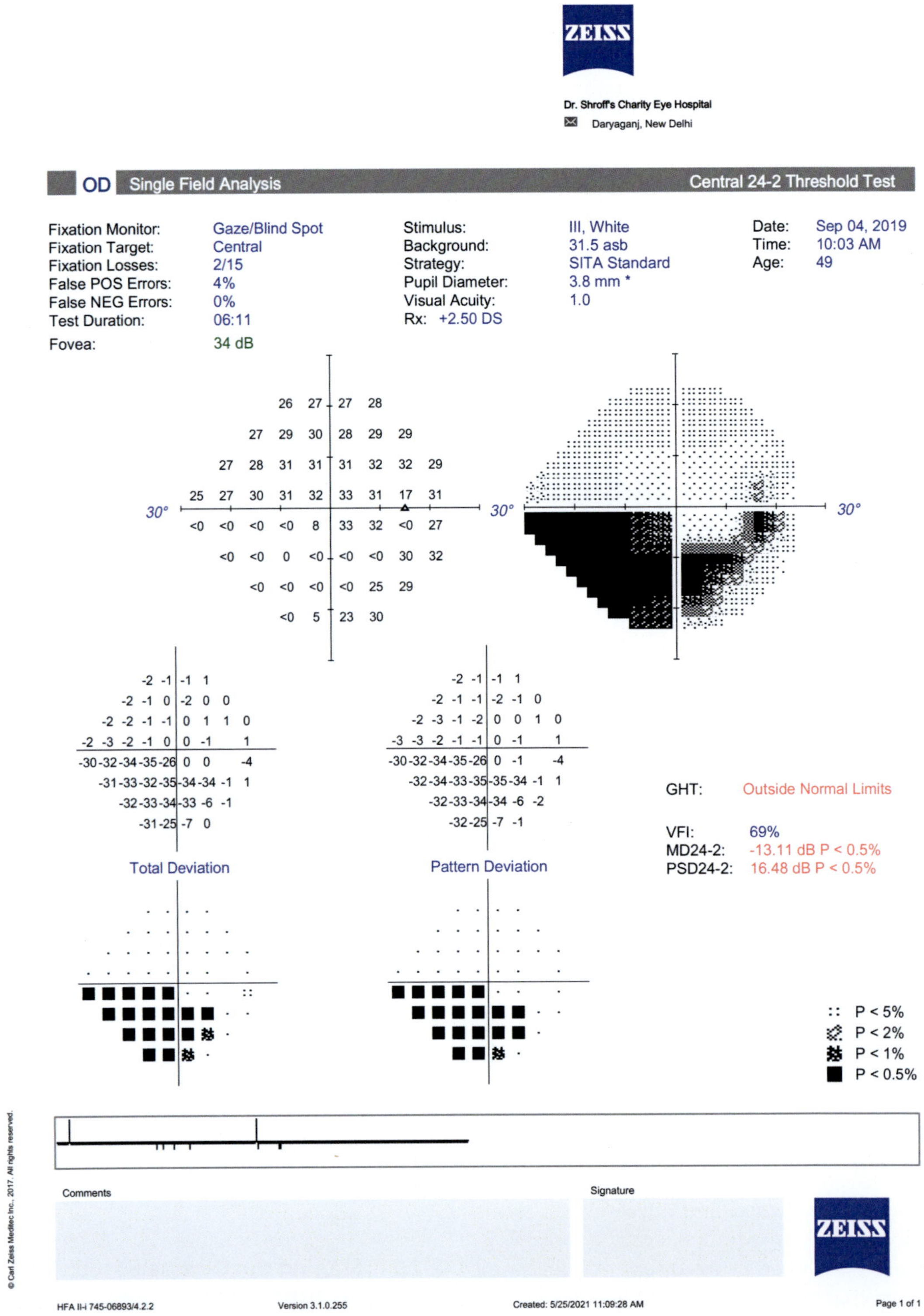

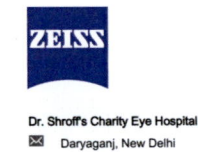

Fig. 2.4 Central 24-2 reliable field of the right eye. Decreased retinal sensitivity in the inferior hemisphere impinging on the fixation from below

coma severity staging system (GSS) [7], and enhanced GSS [8].

The criteria used are extent of damage, proximity to fixation, global indices, and percentage of significantly depressed loci. In EMGT and AGIS, the mean deviation loss at baseline was considered.

Criteria	Early	Moderate	Severe
MD	Less than −6 dB	Less than −12 dB	Greater than −12 dB
Points depressed on pattern deviation plot	Less than 25% below 5% and less than 10 points below 1%	Less than 50% depressed below 5% and less than 20 points below 1%	More than 50% below 5% and more than 20 points below 1%
Central 5%	All points have sensitivity of at least 15 dB	No points have sensitivity of 0 dB Only one hemisphere may have a point with sensitivity of <15 dB	At least one point has sensitivity of 0 dB Both hemispheres have points of sensitivity <15 dB

According to American Academy of Ophthalmology

1. Mild—where optic disc cupping is noted but no visual field changes.
2. Moderate—glaucomatous neuropathy with visual field loss, but not within the five degrees of fixation.
3. Severe—visual field loss in both hemispheres or within the five degrees of fixation.

Hodapp–Parrish–Anderson criteria:
1. Glaucoma hemifield test outside normal limits.
2. A cluster of three or more non-edge points in location typical for glaucoma, all of which are depressed on pattern deviation plot at $p < 5\%$ level and one of which is depressed at $p < 1\%$.
3. Corrected pattern standard deviation (CPSD) with $p < 5\%$.
4. All these on two consecutive reproducible fields.

2.2.3 Detecting and Monitoring Progression

Several studies have evaluated the detection of development and progression of glaucomatous vision loss measured with standard visual fields. OHTS [9] studied the effect of lowering of intraocular pressure and repeatability of abnormalities on three consecutive fields. In 35% of the eyes, the visual field defect was the first endpoint to be reached. Similar findings were seen in Diagnostic Innovations in Glaucoma Study (DIGS) [10] and EGPS [11]. In Early Manifest Glaucoma Trial (EMGT) [12], change in visual field as first endpoint was seen in 86% eyes. This high percentage, however, could be due to demographics, disease level, and criteria used.

Guided progression analysis is event-based analysis in Humphrey visual field analyzer, and it considers three consecutive tests and the progression as pattern deviation in three or more locations, as significant (Figs. 2.5 and 2.6). It helps in objectively analyzing progression and is seen to have a good agreement with glaucoma experts [13]. It is dependent on test–retest variability.

Trend-based analyzes of progression evaluates all tests available for statistical change over time using a linear regression method. It relates to magnitude of change over time not affected by previously established thresholds. This is estimated from the visual field index (VFI) [14] which is a global measure of visual function for calculating rate of progression and staging glaucomatous functional damage.

2.3 Limitations of Standard Automated Perimetry (SAP)

1. It evaluates the differential light sensitivity using a small, 0.47°, white stimulus of small duration of 200 ms. It checks the ability to identify the stimulus against a dim background constant illumination of 31.5 asb.
2. It is a nonselective test as all the primary retinal ganglion cells types respond to the stimuli.

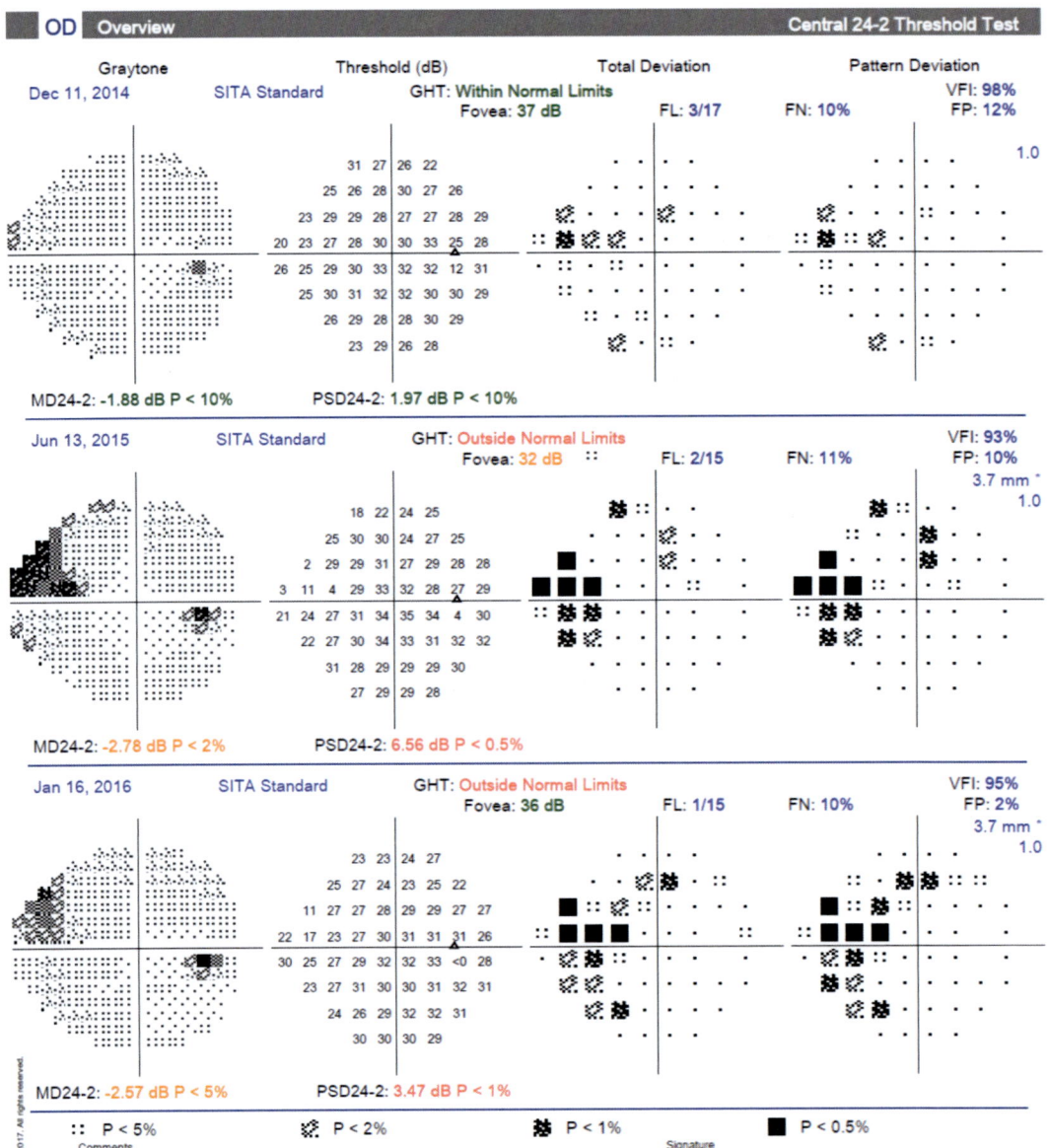

Fig. 2.5 Right eye overview

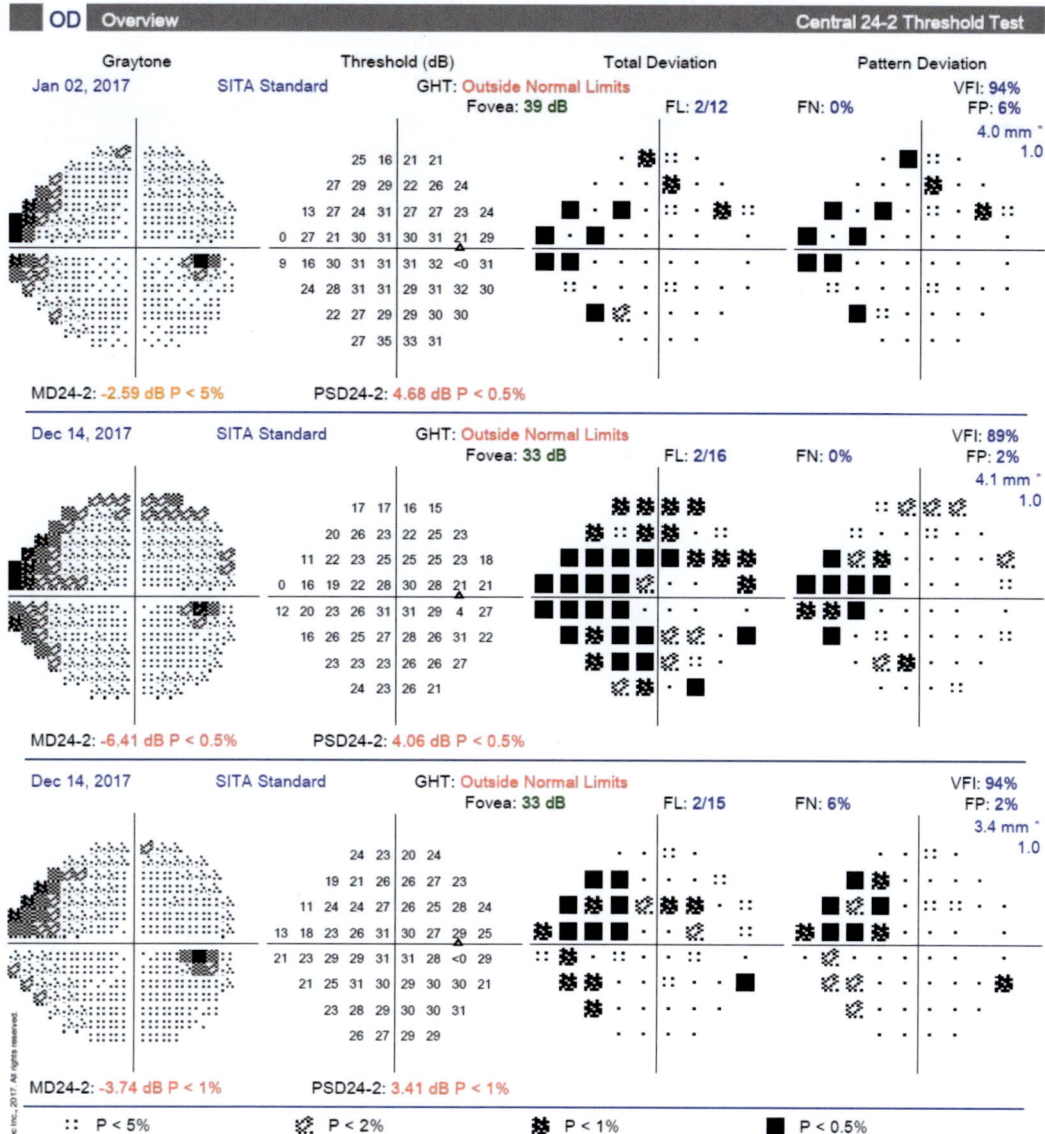

Fig. 2.5 (continued)

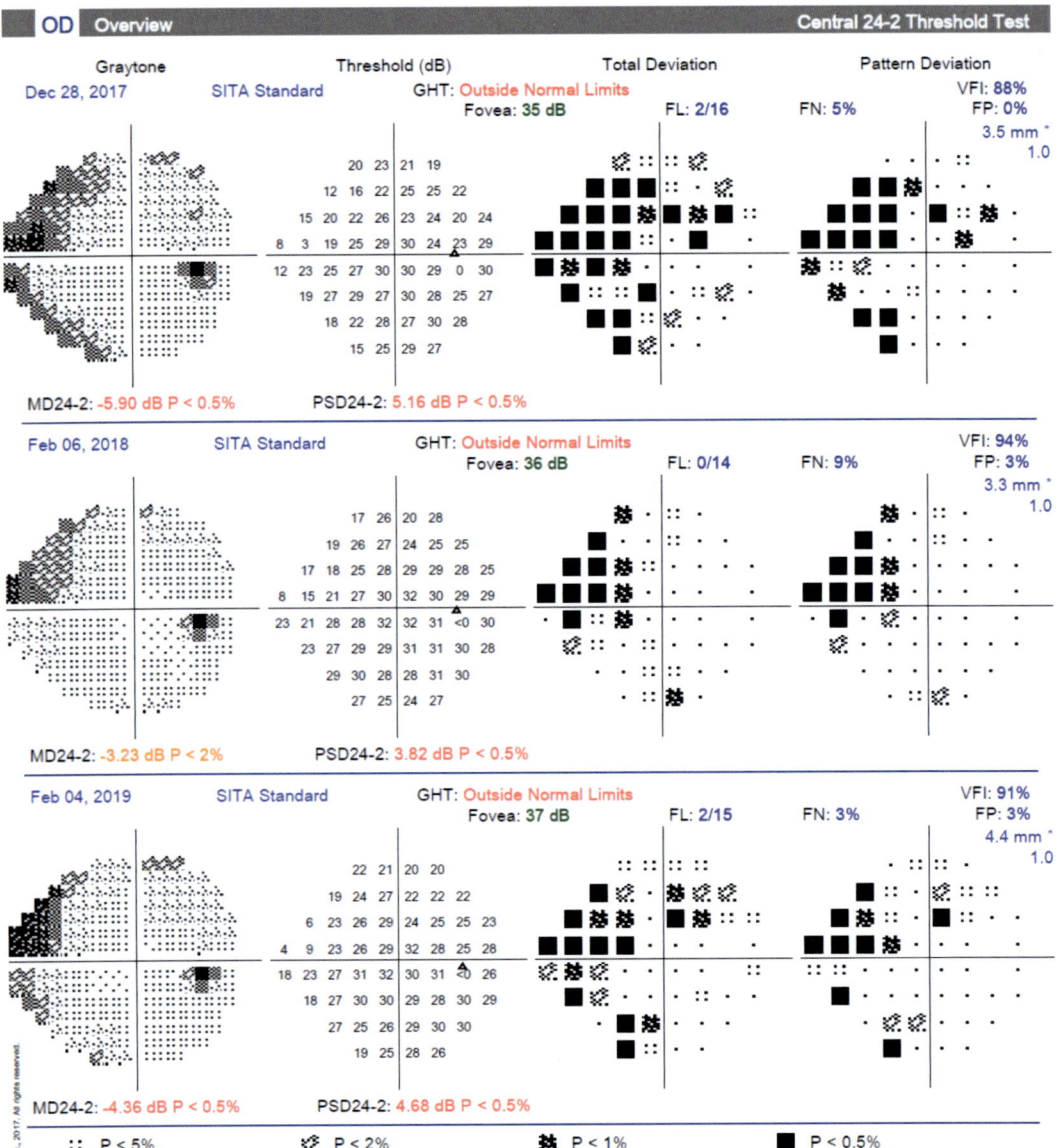

Fig. 2.5 (continued)

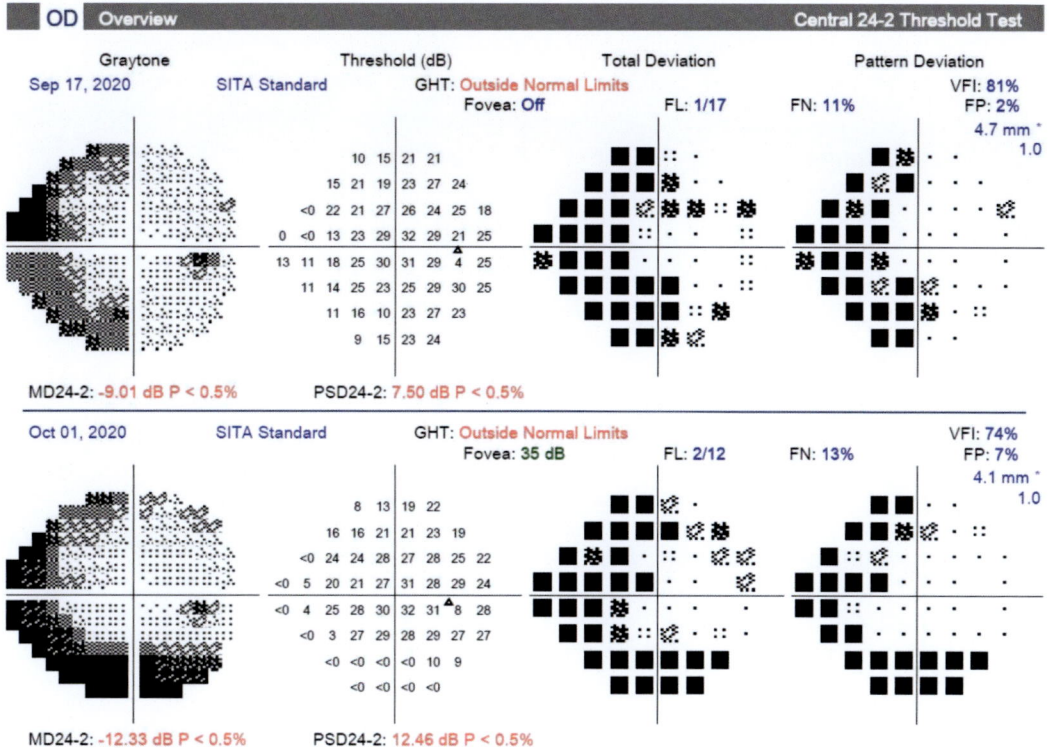

Fig. 2.5 (continued)

3. It may not provide adequate sensitivity to detect very early glaucomatous changes due to inherent redundancy of the visual system [15].
4. 25–50% ganglion cell loss may need to be present for SAP to detect functional deficit [16].
5. There is high test–retest variability and it has a learning curve which needs to be addressed before getting reliable baseline fields [17] (Figs. 2.7 and 2.8a and b). This has relevance in detecting progression also as it requires two to three consecutive reliable and repeatable fields for analysis In OHTS, many fields which showed abnormalities were not confirmed on repeat testing [18].
6. Since the logarithmic scale is used, visual field changes are minimized at high decibel levels and at low decibels are amplified. So, a significant loss of retinal ganglion cells in early disease can translate to a small decrease, relatively, in visual field function [19].
7. The test is considered time consuming and thus a shift from full threshold test to newer algorithms like Swedish interactive test algorithm (SITA) came into vogue. This too has evolved as SITA standard, SITA fast, and SITA faster. The use of different strategies and testing parameters helps in devising a better fit for the patient. Like visual field testing in 10° where a smaller field area with greater density of points may reveal glaucomatous defects which may not be apparent on 24–2 or 30–2 fields. Also the threat to fixation can be better studied. The patient with advanced glaucomatous defect may not be able to perform the test reliably especially with false-negative responses being high, but on a 10–2, one can get valuable information for both current plan and follow up. The use of size V is also applicable when the patient has low vision to appreciate the stimulus size

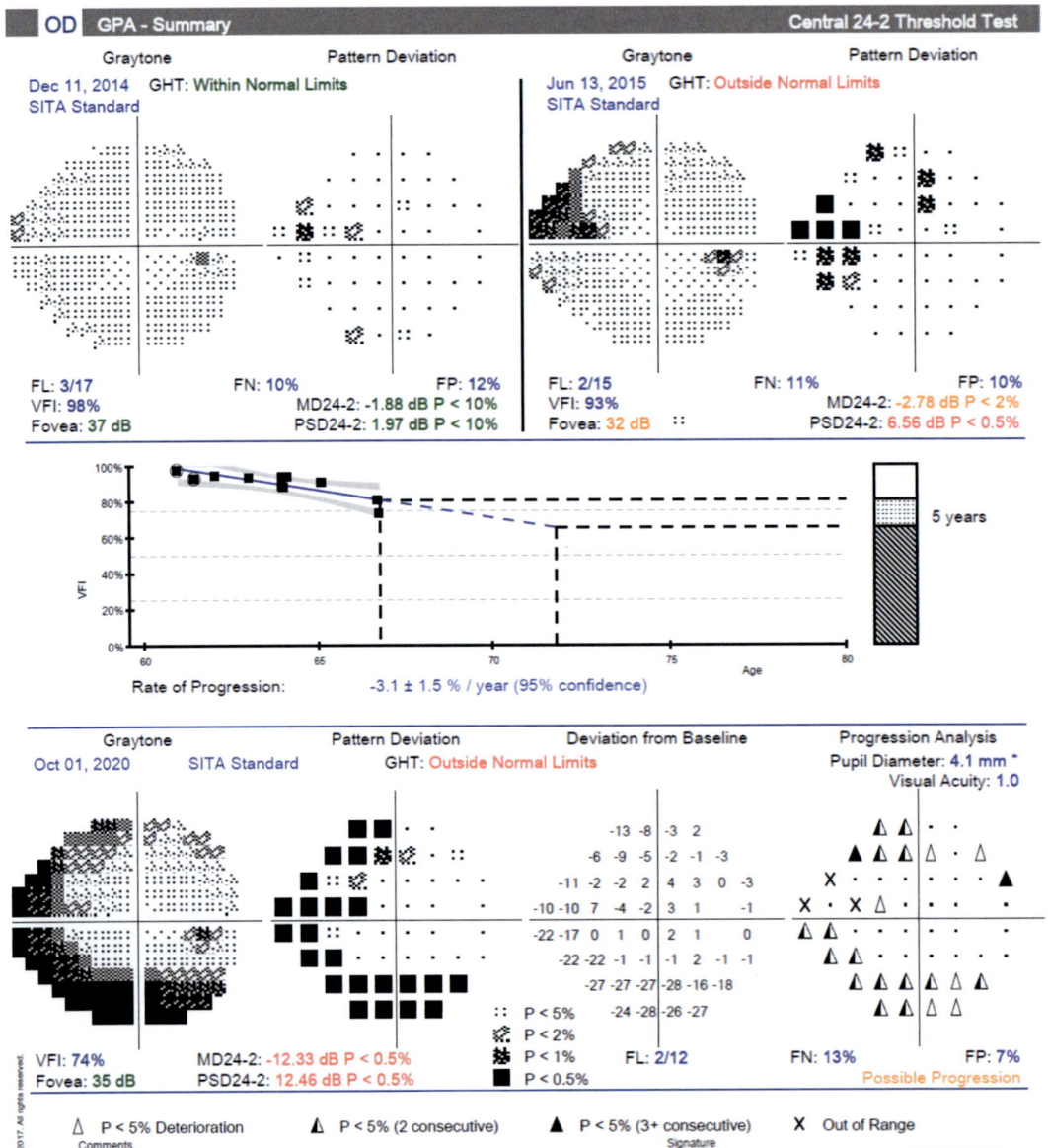

Fig. 2.6 GPA over the period with predicted rate of progression

III. However, normative data with this stimulus size is very limited.

2.4 Other Forms of Visual Field Testing

1. Short-wavelength automated perimetry (SWAP)—This uses a blue stimulus on a yellow background, and the stimulus is detected by short-wavelength cones and processed through blue-yellow ganglion cells and their axons to the koniocellular layer of lateral geniculate nucleus of the thalamus [20]. The testing time for SWAP is long and not comfortable for the patient due to the bright colors. Other limitations are larger individual variability, short- and long-term fluctuations, and performance of the test in case of media opacities.

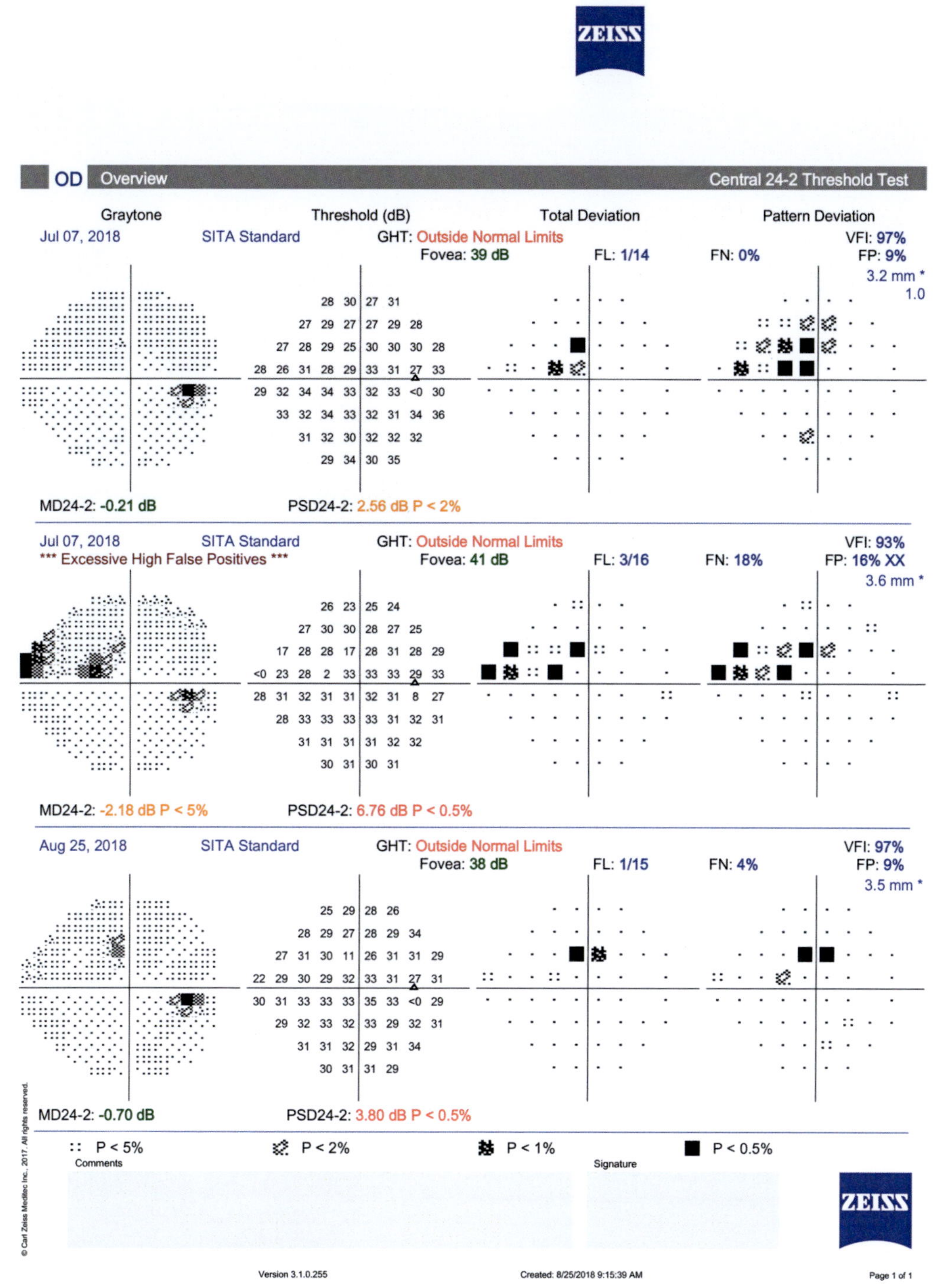

Fig. 2.7 This example shows the learning curve. The test needs to be repeated till clinical correlation, and reproducible defects are established to form a baseline

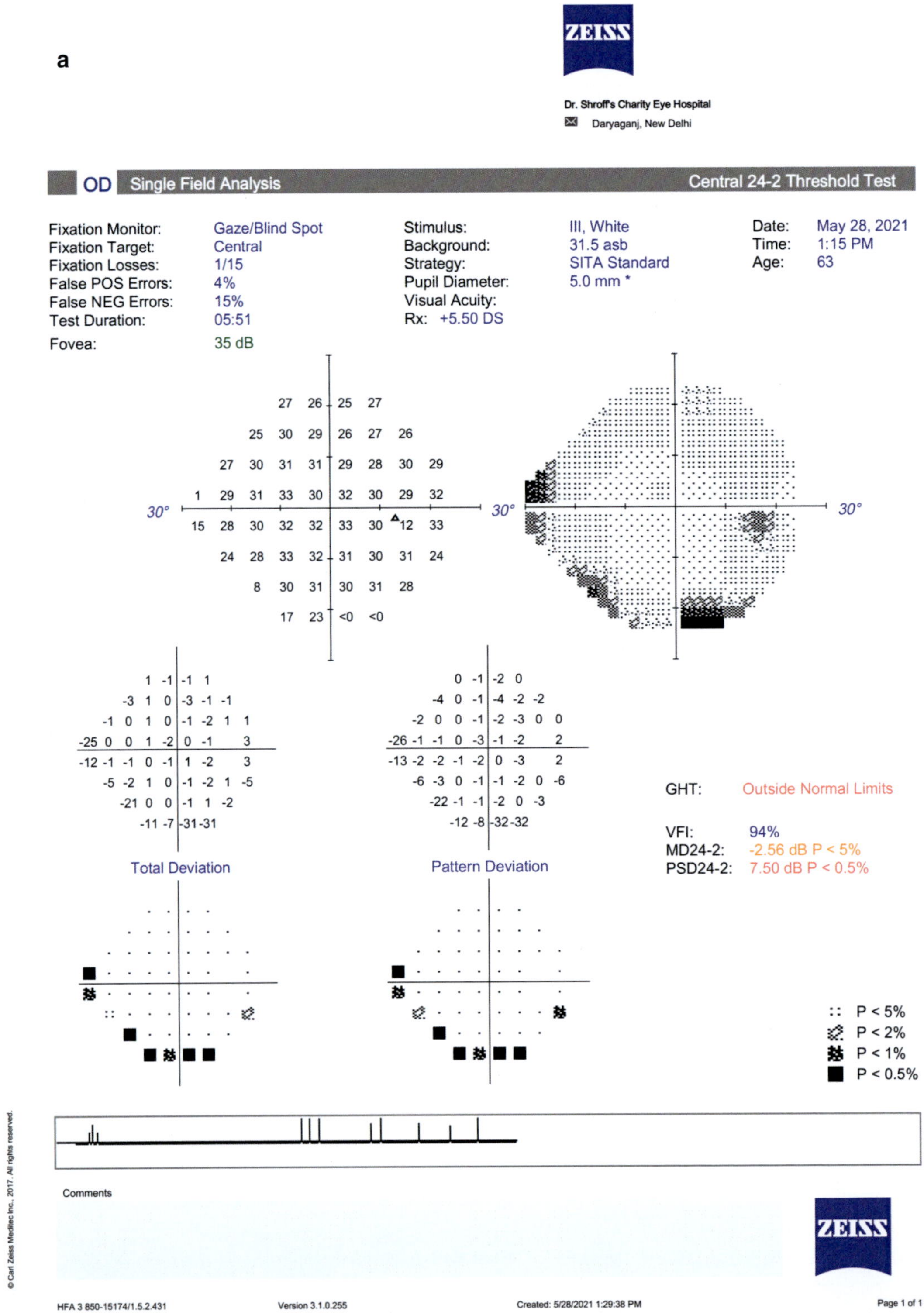

Fig. 2.8 (**a**) Shows learning curve (**b**) was done after repeating instructions and it helped to improve the performance of the test

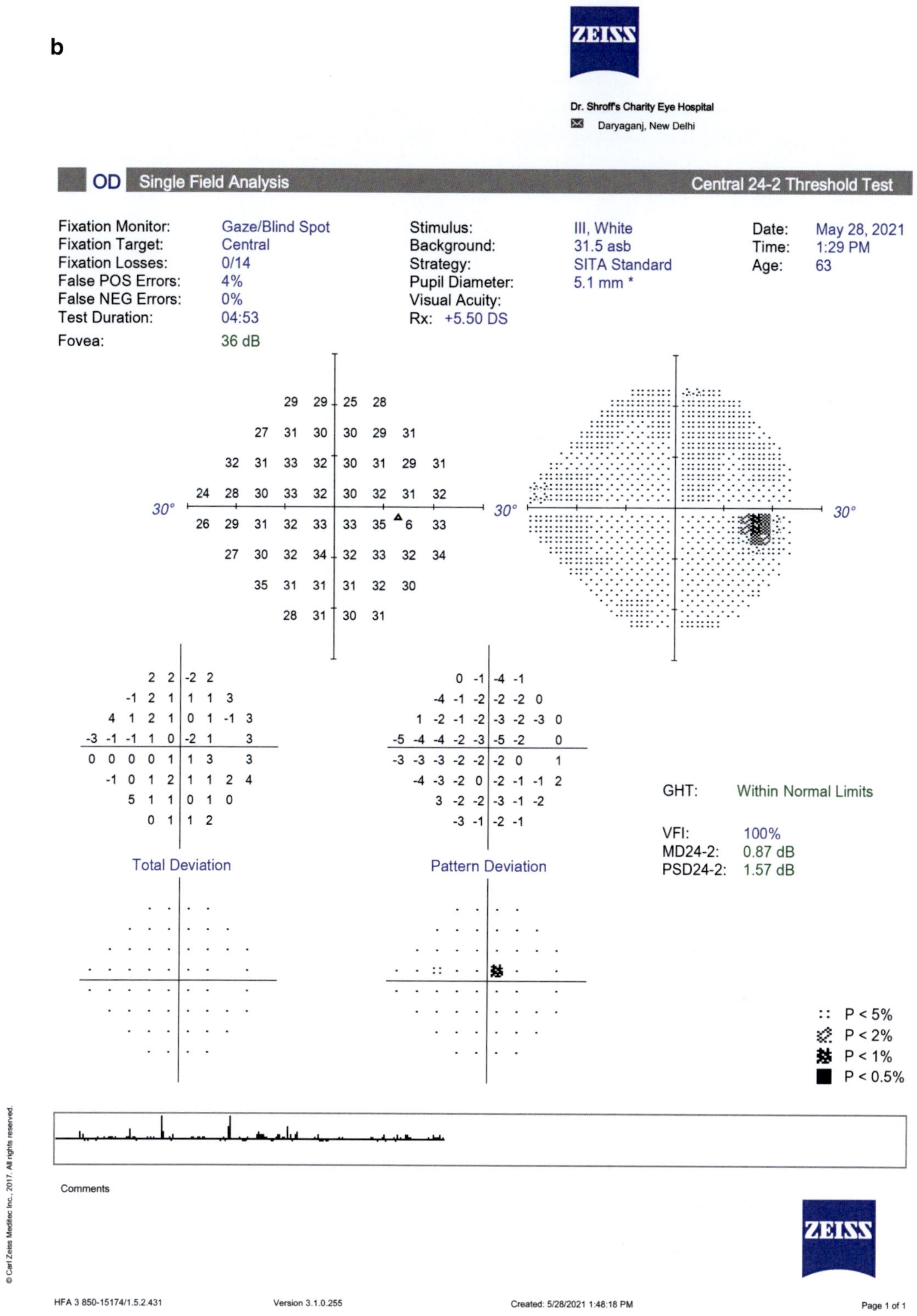

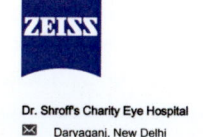

Fig. 2.8 (continued)

2. Frequency doubling technology perimetry (FDT)—Based on the frequency doubling illusion, viewing a grating with a low spatial frequency and high temporal rate. It measures the magnocellular retinal ganglion cells. It is used in screening for glaucoma also as it is faster. Second-generation FDT testing may have advantages over SAP, but lacks progression analysis component [21].
3. Pattern electroretinography —Measures the electrical activity delivered to the macula generated by the pattern stimuli. It has the potential to detect preperimetric glaucoma. Limitations are the requirement of a skilled examiner and clear media without opacities [22, 23].
4. Home testing—A motion displacement test as a screening visual field on a laptop. Portable head-mounted perimetry systems are also available. These are still being tested and require clinical validation. Cost is also a concern.
5. Combining structural and functional testing in a single platform and co-analyzing in hybrid instrument can help in better understanding and management [24].
6. Machine learning algorithms are being evaluated and may allow better early detection and prediction of progression. It will help in screening in areas where specialized skilled manpower is unavailable

2.5 Conclusion

Visual field analysis has undergone several modifications to make it more patient friendly and the interpretation more reliable. Different algorithms and analytical methods have been developed to assist and simplify detection of disease and progression of glaucoma. In spite of development of different instruments to detect early changes, visual fields are considered as gold standard and continue to play an important role in management of glaucoma.

References

1. Camp AS, Weinreb RN. Will perimetry be performed to monitor glaucoma in 2025? Ophthalmology. 2017;124(12S):S71–5.
2. Sharma P, Sample PA, Zangwill LM, Schuman JS. Diagnostic tools for glaucoma detection and management. Surv Ophthalmol. 2008;53(Suppl 1):S17–32.
3. Gordon MO, Beiser JA, Brandt JD, et al. The Ocular Hypertension Treatment Study: baseline factors that predict the onset of primary open-angle glaucoma. Arch Ophthalmol. 2002;120:714–20.
4. Lin SC, Singh K, Jampel HD, et al. Optic nerve head and retinal nerve fiber layer analysis: a report by the American Academy of Ophthalmology. Ophthalmology. 2007;114:1937–49.
5. Sihota R, Angmo D, Ramaswamy D, Dada T. Simplifying "target" intraocular pressure for different stages of primary open-angle glaucoma and primary angle-closure glaucoma. Indian J Ophthalmol. 2018;66(4):495–505.
6. Hodapp E, Parrish RK 2nd, Anderson DR. Clinical decisions in glaucoma. St. Louis: The C.V. Mosby Co; 1993. p. 52–61.
7. Mills RP, Budenz DL, Lee PP, Noecker RJ, Walt JG, Siegartel LR, et al. Categorizing the stage of glaucoma from pre-diagnosis to end-stage disease. Am J Ophthalmol. 2006;141:24–30.
8. Brusini P, Filacorda S. Enhanced glaucoma staging system (GSS 2) for classifying functional damage in glaucoma. J Glaucoma. 2006;15:40–6.
9. Gordon MO, Kass MA. The Ocular Hypertension Treatment Study: design and baseline description of the participants. Arch Ophthalmol. 1999;117:573–83.
10. Medeiros FA, Weinreb RN, Sample PA, et al. Validation of a predictive model to estimate the risk of conversion from ocular hypertension to glaucoma. Arch Ophthalmol. 2005;123:1351–60.
11. Gordon MO, Torri V, Miglior S, et al. Validated prediction model for the development of primary open-angle glaucoma in individuals with ocular hypertension. Ophthalmology. 2007;114:10–9.
12. Heijl A, Leske MC, Bengtsson B, et al. Measuring visual field progression in the Early Manifest Glaucoma Trial. Acta Ophthalmol Scand. 2003;81:286–93.
13. Tanna AP, Budenz DL, Bandi J, et al. Glaucoma progression analysis software compared with expert consensus opinion in the detection of visual field progression in glaucoma. Ophthalmology. 2012;119:468–73.
14. Bengtsson B, Heijl A. A visual field index for calculation of glaucoma rate of progression. Am J Ophthalmol. 2008;145:343–53.

15. Quigley HA, Dunkelberger GR, Green WR. Retinal ganglion cell atrophy correlated with automated perimetry in human eyes with glaucoma. Am J Ophthalmol. 1989;107:453–64.
16. Kerrigan-Baumrind LA, Quigley HA, Pease ME, et al. Number of ganglion cells in glaucoma eyes compared with threshold visual field tests in the same persons. Invest Ophthalmol Vis Sci. 2000;41:741–8.
17. Keltner JL, Johnson CA, Levine RA, et al. Normal visual field test results following glaucomatous visual field end points in the Ocular Hypertension Treatment Study. Arch Ophthalmol. 2005;123:1201–6.
18. Keltner JL, Johnson CA, Anderson DR, et al. The association between glaucomatous visual fields and optic nerve head features in the Ocular Hypertension Treatment Study. Ophthalmology. 2006;113:1603–12.
19. Medeiros FA, Zangwill LM, Bowd C, et al. The structure and function relationship in glaucoma: implications for detection of progression and measurement of rates of change. Invest Opthalmol Vis Sci. 2012;53:6939–46.
20. Martin P, White H, Goodchild AK, et al. Evidence that blue-on cells ae part of the third geniculocortical pathway in primates. Eur J Neurosci. 1997;9:1536–41.
21. Sample PA, Bosworth CF, Weinreb RN. The loss of visual function in glaucoma. Semin Ophthalmol. 2000;15:182–93.
22. Wilsey LJ, Fortune B. Electroretinography in glaucoma diagnosis. Curr Opin Ophthalmol. 2016;27:118–24.
23. Bode SFN, Jehle T, Bach M. Pattern electroretinogram in glaucoma suspects: new findings from a longitudinal study. Invest Ophthalmol Vis Sci. 2011;52:4300–6.
24. Medeiros F, Tatham A, Weinreb R. Strategies for improving early detection of glaucoma: the combined structure-function index. Clin Ophthalmol. 2014;8:611–21.

Interpretation of a Humphrey Single Visual Field Printout

Sagarika Patyal and Monica Gandhi

Perimetry or visual field testing is commonly performed on the Humphrey perimeter, the latest version of which is HFA3. Its enhanced features include SITA Faster (the newer SITA strategy), Mixed Guided Progression Analysis and addition of a new liquid trial lens which delivers the refractive correction of a patient by the press of a button (Zeiss website). The statistical software used for analysis is STATPAC.

A comprehensive ocular examination after obtaining a thorough history from a patient goes a long way in the correct interpretation of perimetry. A detailed optic disc examination through a dilated pupil can reveal an expected area of neuro-retinal thinning or a notch which can be verified in the field. Figure 3.1a shows a neuro-retinal thinning inferiorly, and Fig. 3.1b shows a corresponding field defect in the superior field.

3.1 Sequence for Interpretation of a Single Field

Patient demographics: Identification of patient by the name, the spelling of which should be identical; ID number and identification of the eye being tested must be checked (Fig. 3.2, Blue box 1).

Birthdate and age: The birth date must be recorded correctly and inserted similarly in the follow-up fields as all statistical analysis is made with the normative data which consists of age-matched controls in clusters of 10 years [1].

Testing algorithm: The same test should be used in subsequent tests unless there is a specific change in requirement (Fig. 3.2, Red box 2).

Fixation target (Central or Diamond): In the presence of a central scotoma, the patient will be able to fixate on a diamond rather than a central target, so a diamond should be chosen as the fixation target (Fig. 3.2, Red box 2).

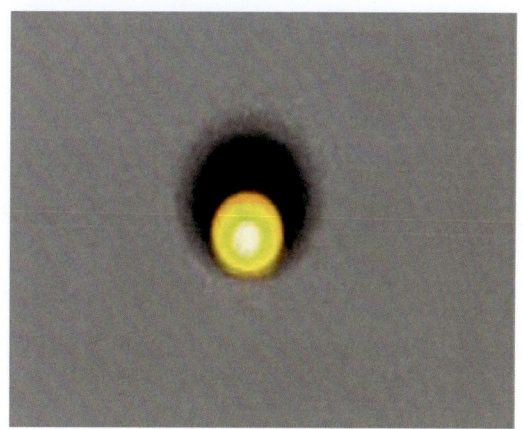

Central target

S. Patyal (✉)
Centre for Sight, Dwarka, New Delhi, Delhi, India

M. Gandhi
Dr. Shroff's Charity Eye Hospital, New Delhi, Delhi, India

© The Author(s), under exclusive license to Springer Nature Singapore Pte Ltd. 2021
S. Patyal, M. Gandhi (eds.), *Resolving Dilemmas in Perimetry*,
https://doi.org/10.1007/978-981-16-2601-2_3

Fig. 3.1 (**a**) Optic nerve head with thinning of inferior neuro-retinal rim. (**b**) Corresponding superotemporal visual field defect

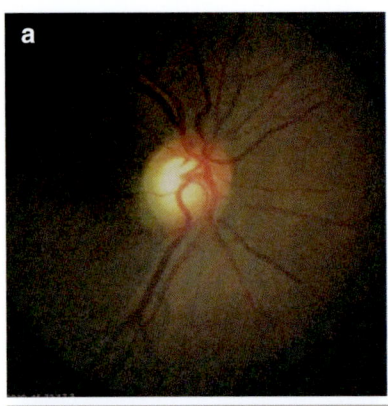

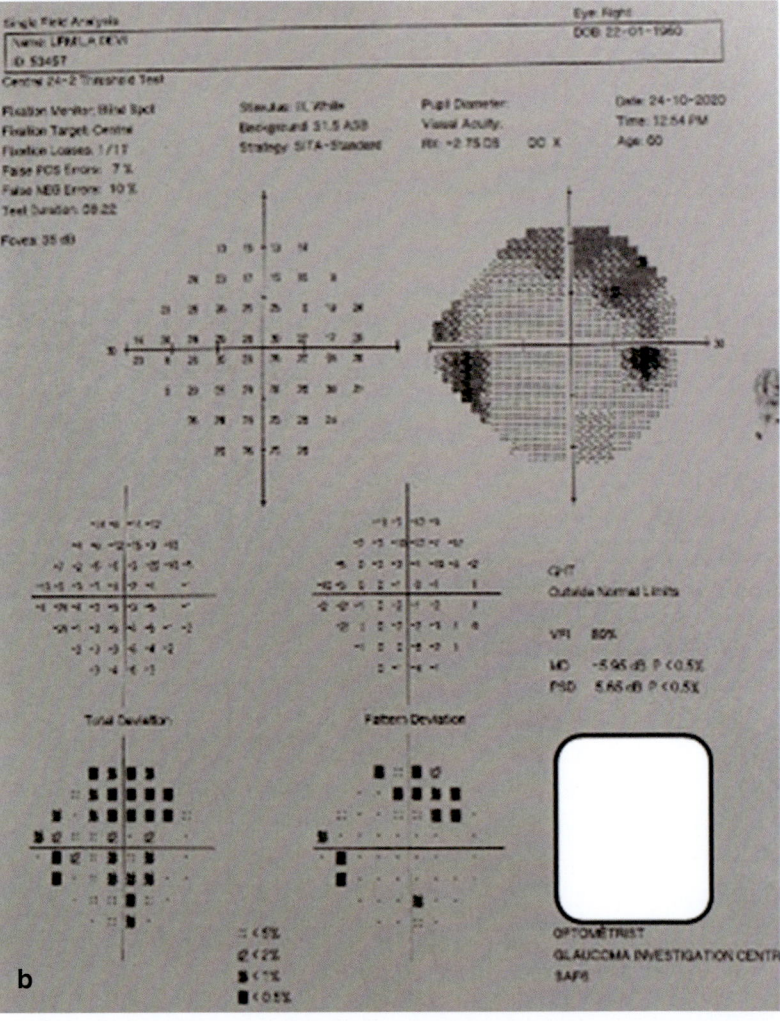

3 Interpretation of a Humphrey Single Visual Field Printout

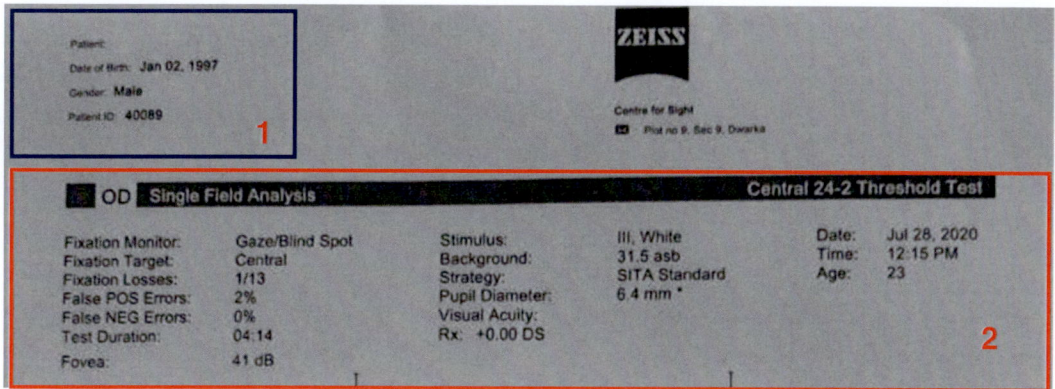

Fig. 3.2 (1) Patient demographics. (2) Reliability factors, fovea, strategy, stimulus, visual acuity with refractive correction, date, time, age of patient

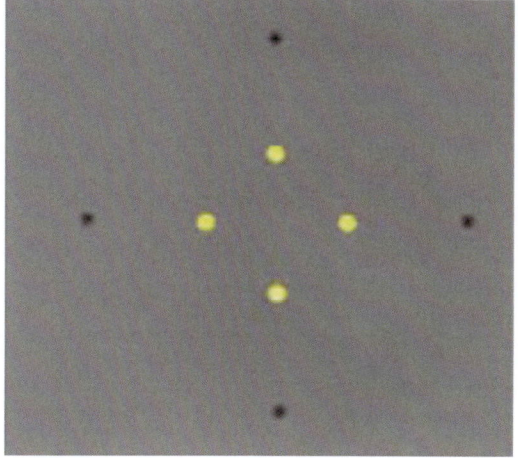

Yellow lights-small diamond. Black dots—large diamond

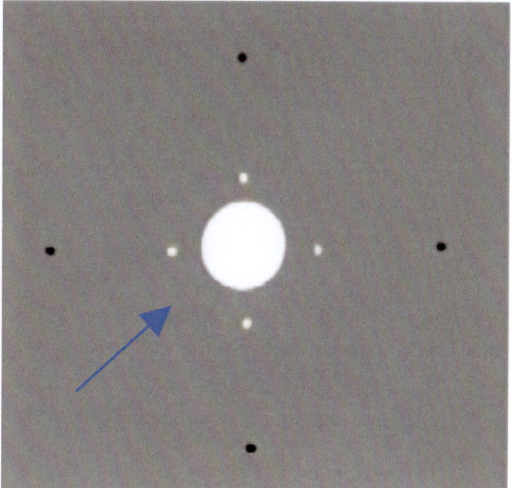

Size V stimulus

Stimulus size used for the test: Target sizes in all the models vary from I (0.25 mm^2) to V (64 mm^2). Target size III (4 mm^2) is the most commonly used stimulus size for patients with vision of at least 6/60 (20/200) for testing visual fields. In case of vision lesser than 20/200, size V may be used (Fig. 3.2, Red box 2) [1].

Pupil size: The size of the pupil should be the same for all tests so that comparison of follow-up tests is possible. Pupil size as small as 2 mm may cause false constriction of fields and should be dilated to at least 3 mm [2].

Dilated pupils affect perimetric results by causing variability and difference in visual field parameters in patients suffering from glaucoma [3]. In this example, the patient's pupil size is 6.4 mm and the field should be repeated with a 3–4 mm pupil (Fig. 3.2, Red box 2).

Visual acuity: The best corrected visual acuity must be checked prior to the field test, and appropriate correction must be included in the patient parameters. This is especially significant for individuals who have developed cataract with a change in visual acuity or for those who have undergone cataract surgery and now have improved visual acuity. The most appropriate method is to check refraction and correct vision before attempting perimetry (Fig. 3.2, Red box 2).

Time: Increased time taken for the test denotes patient fatiguability and occurs in increased global depression (Fig. 3.2, Red box 2).

Programs: The program must be chosen according to the indication for the field test (Fig. 3.2, Red box 2).

Various testing protocols are as follows (the first number denotes the extent of field measured from the temporal side):

24-2 measures 24° temporally and 30° nasally (Fig. 3.3a). A total of 54 points are tested, each point being 6° from the other with the grid spanning the horizontal and vertical meridians, 3° across the meridians. This is the most commonly used program as it shortens the time taken by the patient to perform the test and yet detects early glaucomatous field defects which commonly occur in the central region. 24-2 measures all the points including the two nasal points as in a 30-2 and eliminates the outermost ring of points of a 30-2.

24-2 C is the latest program available in the Humphrey perimeter which incorporates 10 additional test points, 5 in each hemifield which are not symmetrically distributed across the horizontal and vertical midlines. The sensitivity of this program is driven by SITA Faster [4].

30-2 measures 30° temporally and nasally, a total of 76 points are tested in this program, each point being 6° from the other [5].

10-2 measures 10° nasally and temporally with a total of 68 points being tested (Fig. 3.3b). It tests the central four points of

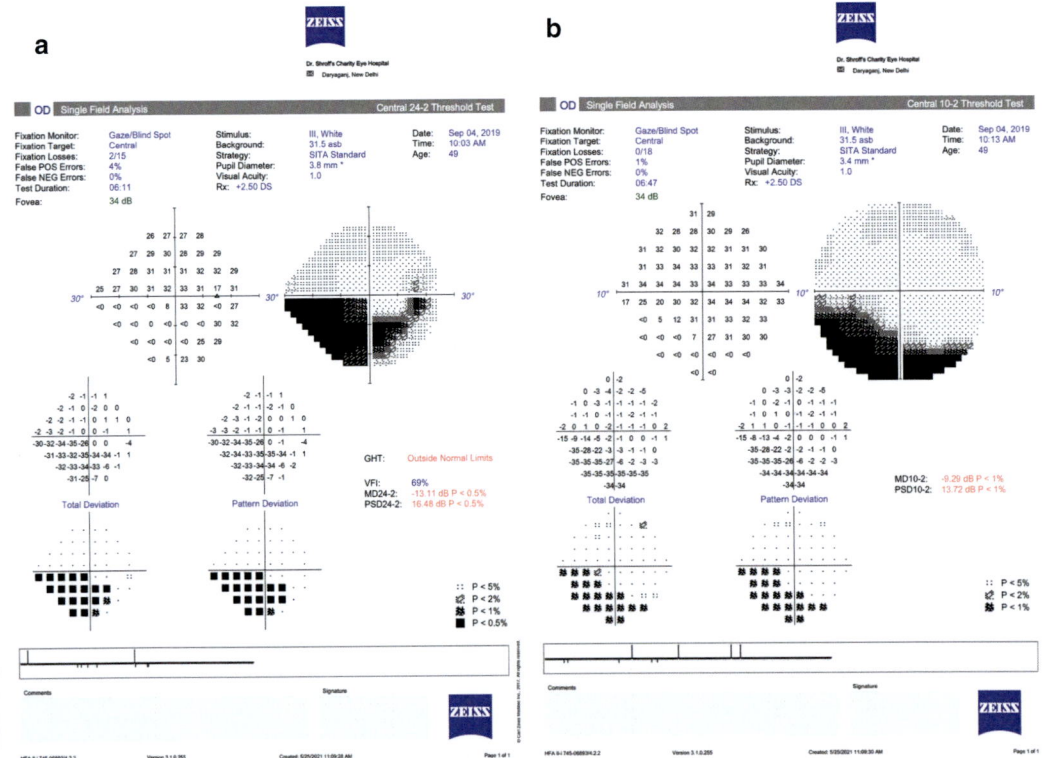

Fig. 3.3 (**a**) 30-2 SITA Standard visual field with affection of central points. (**b**) 10-2 SITA Standard of the same field. Courtesy: Raj Rani

the field; each point in this test is 2° away from the other. The main advantage of a 10-2 program is to follow-up the patients with severe disease but has limitations when used for diagnosing a disease.

Pearls 1: Size V stimulus (four times the diameter of size III) [6].

1. No normal database is available with size V stimulus.

2. Printout using size V stimulus is different from a STACPAC single field analysis printout. It contains the greyscale at the top, map of threshold sensitivity values at the bottom right and difference from the expected plot in the bottom left (defect depth grid, as in Fig. 3.4). The defect depth grid is derived by extrapolation from second-most sensitive of the four primary points and the point of fixation to obtain the central reference level which is then

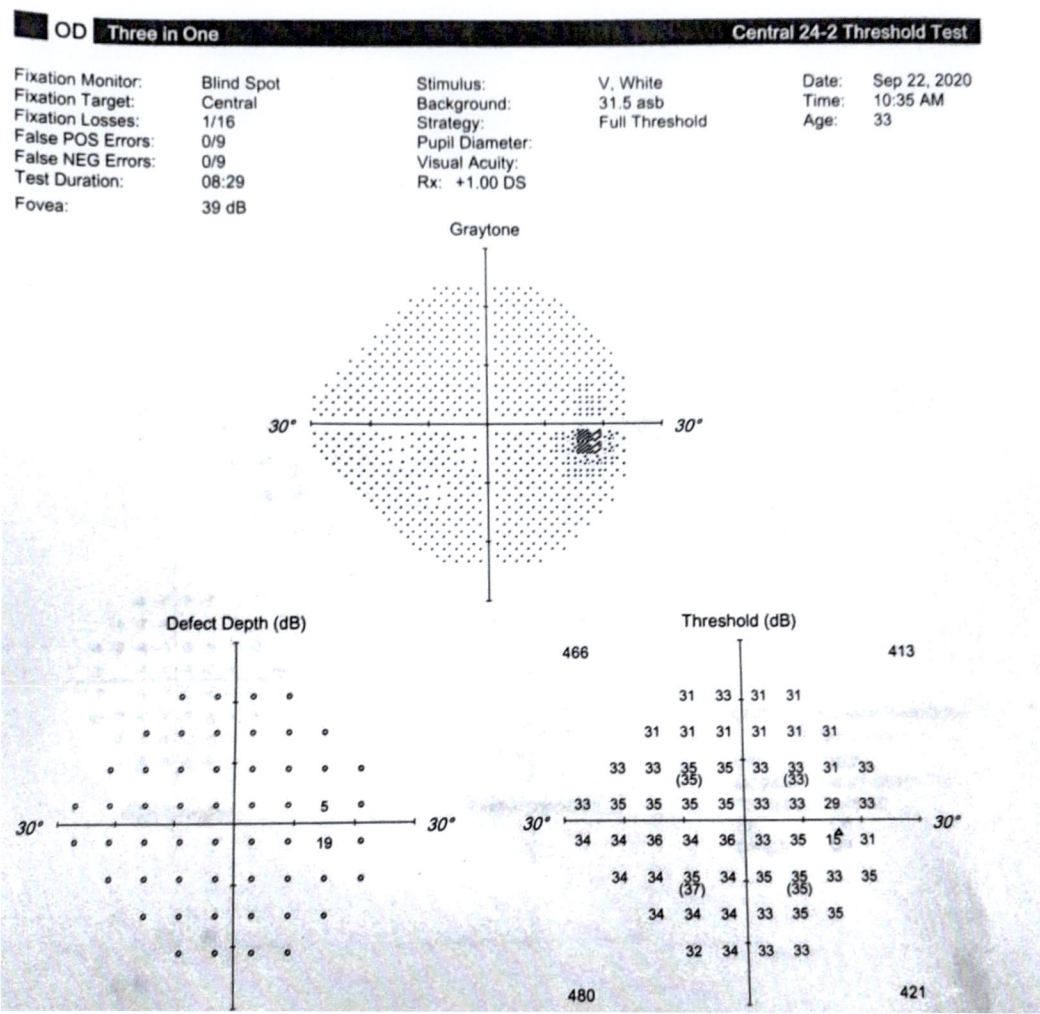

Fig. 3.4 Visual field using a size V stimulus in Full Threshold strategy with a greyscale, Defect depth and expected Threshold value (Courtesy: Shivangi Rawat)

used to calculate an expected threshold value at every point in the field based on its eccentricity from the point of fixation. The threshold values in the printout are the differences obtained between the expected value and the observed value.
3. It is best to perform a field with size III stimulus first to document normalcy or quantify the degree of abnormality and then perform the test with size V.

Fovea: The fovea should be tested for all patients. The fovea has the highest threshold and should match the visual acuity. Good visual acuity but poor foveal threshold points towards early foveal damage and in a patient with poor visual acuity but good foveal threshold, refraction should be rechecked.

The foveal threshold is tested by the patient gazing at the centre of the fixation diamond projected 10° below the normal fixation spot, i.e., the yellow light, which patients are made to fixate on. Normally a size III stimulus is projected onto the centre of the diamond for 0.2 s which remains for an additional 1.8 s before a response is recorded. A bracketing strategy of 4 dB increase of stimulus is made till the patient sees it after which the stimulus is decreased by 2 dB till it is no longer visible. The stimulus last seen by the patient is recorded as the Foveal threshold (Fig. 3.2, Red box 2).

Strategy: The strategies available in Humphrey field analyser are:

1. Supra threshold: A single suprathreshold stimulus is presented across the entire field, with a response as "seen" or "not seen". It is used as a screening tool.
2. Full threshold: Using the bracketing strategy, four primary points, one in each quadrant, nine degrees away from the horizontal and vertical meridians, are tested first with 25 dB. In order to save time, thresholds of adjacent points are extrapolated from neighbouring points. To further enable the test to become user friendly, after 10 responses, average response time is adjusted (average response time plus 0.85 s) as slow for slow responders and fast for fast responders.
3. Fastpac: Stimulus intensity changes in 3 dB steps and once the threshold is reached, reverse testing is not done.
4. Swedish interactive threshold algorithm (SITA): SITA was developed in the late 1980s to reduce the time taken for performing the test without compromising the accuracy and efficiency of the test. SITA was based on the Bayesian Prior model and iterative maximum posterior probability estimation of threshold values in real time. There are three versions: SITA Standard, SITA Fast and SITA Faster. In SITA Standard (SS) and SITA Fast (SF), four primary points, one in each quadrant, are tested with 25 dB, and several stimuli are shown before the endpoint is reached. SITA Fast may be done by perimetrically experienced patients. The newer strategy, SITA Faster, is used for the 24-2 program. It has been based on SITA FAST with seven modifications, i.e. test sequence beginning at the age-corrected normal threshold levels, only one staircase test reversal at each tested point, determining the endpoint for testing using iterative maximum posterior probability, no retesting at points at which the person had not responded to the maximum stimulus intensity, using gaze tracker to check for fixation, no false negative catch trials, elimination of 300 ms delay at the end of response time window at non-seeing points [7, 8].

Reliability factors which confirm the validity of the field: Fixation losses, false positive and false negative (Fig. 3.2, Red box 2).

False positive (FP) responses: Rates exceeding 15% indicate an unreliable test. The method of determination of FP varies in different strategies. In a Full threshold test, it is calculated from patient responses to non-visual clues (machine sounds or motion) despite no stimulus presentation. In SITA, it is calculated by responses made by the patient when none are expected. The term "Trigger Happy patients" applies to those who respond with no stimulus presentation and can be identified in the field by elevated FP score, white scotomas in the greyscale signifying areas of unusually high sensitivity, "abnormally high sensitivity" message in glaucoma hemifield test, points of statistically significant loss in pattern deviation probability plot than in total deviation (inverted cataract pattern) [9], and a strikingly positive mean deviation and threshold sensitivities above physiological limits.

False negative (FN) responses: This is failure to respond to visible stimuli. Rates exceeding 20% indicate an unreliable test. FN responses are measured by 9 dB greater stimuli, at ten points whose thresholds have been determined earlier. Higher FN responses may occur due to fatigue (also indicated by the increased time taken to perform the test) or inattention towards the end of the test or due to the inconsistency of visibility in a diseased area. A characteristic pattern seen in this type of response is the "cloverleaf pattern" where four primary points may show normal thresholds with a gradual decrease of sensitivities towards the periphery.

Fixation loss: Central fixation at the target is estimated by fixation losses and by the gaze tracker. The Heijl-Krakau method, in which stimuli are presented at the presumed location of the blind spot, is used to determine fixation losses, considered significant if in excess of 20%. Central fixation may also be artifactually defective if the nasal field of fellow eye is not occluded properly, in cases of high FP rate with patient responding even when stimuli are presented to the blind spot or when the blind spot is not in the expected position, due to changes in head tilt which rotates the blind spot in and out of the physiological position.

Background illumination: The standard illumination is 31.5 Apostilb (Fig. 3.2, Red box 2). This figure was used originally by the Goldmann perimeter and was adopted by the International Perimetric Society in 1979. It approximates the minimum amount of photopic vision, a function of the cones.

Threshold: It is that intensity of light which on presentation to a particular point can be seen 50% of the times. It is the minimum intensity of light seen by an individual. A normal threshold has been defined as "the mean threshold in normal people in a given age group at a given location in the visual field". Its unit is in decibels and ranges from 0 to 50 dB, 0 dB being maximum intensity and 50 dB being the least. This information is present in the raw data (Fig. 3.5). Threshold values are normally 30 dB, especially in the central area but values more than 40 dB imply patient response to anticipated stimuli.

Greyscale: This is a graphical representation of the raw data, in which values closer to 0 dB are marked in darker tones (decreased sensitivity). It should not be used to evaluate glaucoma but may be used by the examiner to determine the correct placement of the blind spot, for showing defects like partial ptosis, white scotomas and cloverleaf pattern. The greyscale can be used to explain the field loss to the patient (Fig. 3.6).

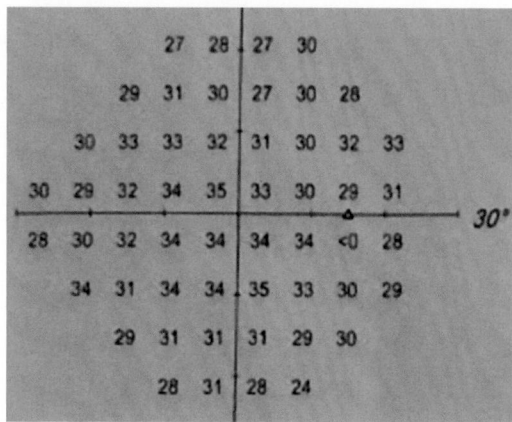

Fig. 3.5 Raw data

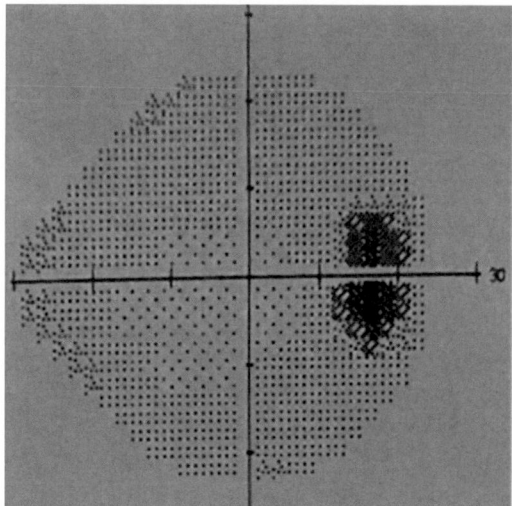

Fig. 3.6 Greyscale

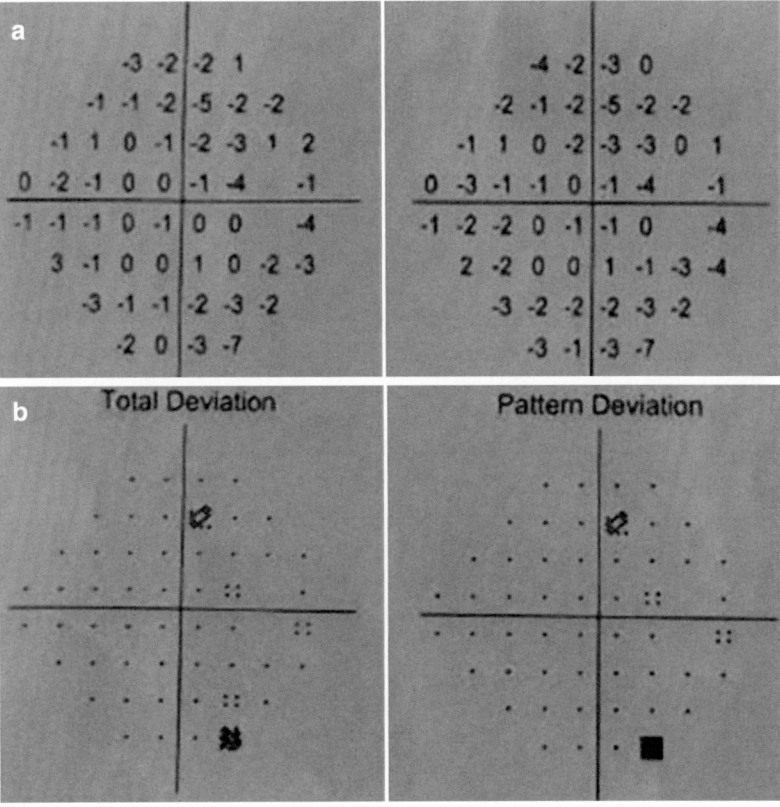

Fig. 3.7 (a) Numeric values of Total and Pattern deviations. (b) Probability plots of Total and Pattern Deviations

Total deviation: This is depicted in numerical (Fig. 3.7a) and probability values (Fig. 3.7b). The numerical values indicate the difference in the sensitivity of each point with normal of the same age. Deviations in the centre, even if less than 5 dB, are of greater significance than deviations of even 10 dB near the periphery. The statistical significance of the difference of each point which depends upon its location and strategy used is shown in the probability plot. This is shown in symbols, and darker symbols have greater significance as shown in the key in the bottom of the printout as 5%, 2%, 1% and 0.5%. A 5% symbol signifies that 95% of normals of the same age would have sensitivities greater than the recorded value.

Total deviation highlights overall depression of the visual field, which may be due to cataract, corneal opacities, miosis or refractive error, but does not bring out localised loss which is the hallmark of glaucoma.

Pattern deviation: This is also depicted in numerical values (Fig. 3.7a) and probability values (Fig. 3.7b) and shows a loss after adjusting for generalised depression or elevation of the hill of vision. These localised losses are highlighted using the same symbols as in total deviation. The probability plot is one area of the pattern deviation that must be observed carefully. Clusters of dark areas of probability lesser than 0.5% indicate localised loss and these clusters must be in typical locations or in patterns matched with clinical findings.

Global Indices (Fig. 3.8)

1. Glaucoma Hemifield test (GHT): It is a comparison of thresholds at five sets of points between the superior and inferior hemifields, the results being shown as GHT within normal limits, GHT Borderline and GHT outside normal limits. Two additional messages may be given depending upon the case: gen-

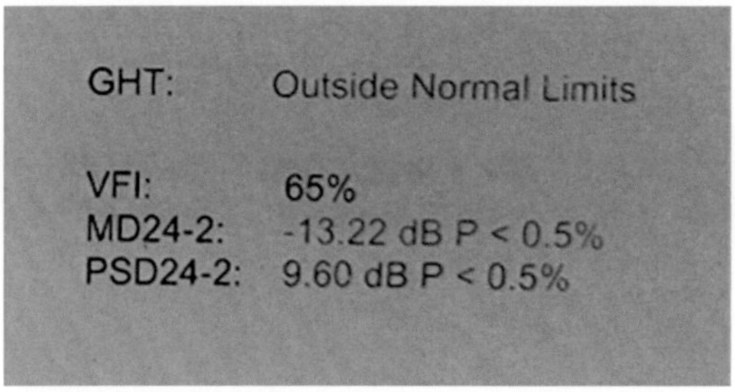

```
GHT:       Outside Normal Limits

VFI:       65%
MD24-2:    -13.22 dB P < 0.5%
PSD24-2:   9.60 dB P < 0.5%
```

Fig. 3.8 Global indices

eralised decrease in sensitivity or abnormally high sensitivity and low patient reliability.

2. Visual field index (VFI): Introduced by Bengtsson and Heijl, it is a single-digit number which summarises the patient's visual field status as a normal age-corrected sensitivity [10]. Derived from pattern deviation plot, it is centre weighted being 100% for a normal field and 0% for a blind field.
3. Mean deviation (MD): Signifies overall severity of field loss; it is the average of the total deviation plot. It may be a positive or a negative number. A positive number indicates a better than the normal field, and a negative number indicates lower than average normal sensitivity. The significance level of MD is compared to normal subjects in the perimeter database.
4. Pattern standard deviation (PSD): This value quantifies the amount of loss in glaucoma. It has a higher value in the localised loss but a lower value in the diffuse loss.

Gaze tracker: This is another method for determining fixation of the patient in which the position of the eye is recorded by a vertical bar or blank spaces. Upward spikes indicate fixation disparity with the length indicating a magnitude of disparity from 1° to a maximum of 10°. Short downward spike represents tracking failure, and a long one indicates eyelid closure. A record which shows excessive periods of poor fixation interspersed with correct fixation is associated with poor reliability.

3.2 Summary

Visual field analysis depends upon a sequential examination of various parts of the field in order to arrive at a diagnosis which is helpful to the clinician.

References

1. Kahook MY, Noecker RJ. How do you interpret a 24-2 humphrey visual field printout? Glaucoma Today. 2020. Available from https://glaucomatoday.com/articles/2007-nov-dec/GT1107_10-php.
2. Racette L, Fischer M, Bebie H, Hollo G, Johnson CA, Matsumoto C. External obstructions blocking stimuli from reaching the retina. In: AG H-S, editor. Visual field digest: a guide to perimetry and the octopus perimeter. 6th ed. Koniz, Switzerland: Haag-Striet AG; 2016. p. 44.
3. Salem DG, Mourad MS, Hamid MA. The effect of pupillary dilatation on visual field testing in glaucoma. J Egypt Ophthalmol Soc. 2020;113:54–68.
4. Phu J, Kalloniatis M. Ability of 24-2C and 24-2 grids to identify central visual field defects and structure-function concordance in glaucoma and suspects. Am J Ophthalmol. 2020;219:317–31.
5. Smita P, George R, Ariga M. Interpreting HFA single field reports. TNOA J Ophthalmic Sci Res. 2019;57:220–30.
6. Anderson DR, Patella VM. Automated static perimetry. 2nd ed. Mosby; 1999.
7. Heijl A, Patella VM, Chong LX, Iwase A, Leung CK, Tuulonen A, Lee GC, Callan T, Bengtsson B. A new SITA perimetric threshold testing algorithm: construction and a multicenter clinical study. Am J Ophthalmol. 2019;198:154–65.
8. Thulasidas M, Patyal S. Comparison of 24-2 faster, fast, and standard programs of Swedish interactive threshold algorithm of Humphrey field analyzer for perimetry in patients with manifest and suspect glaucoma. J Glaucoma. 2020;29:1070–6.
9. Heijl A, Patella VM, Bengtsson B. The field analyser primer: effective perimetry. 4th ed; 2012.
10. Nayak BK, Dharwadkar S. Interpretation of autoperimetry. J Clin Ophthalmol Res. 2014;2:31–59.

Challenges in Interpreting Perimetry in Glaucoma

Monica Gandhi and Sagarika Patyal

4.1 Introduction

Visual fields printout has a plethora of information, and this can help in the purpose for which it is done only if interpreted in a stepwise systemic manner. The Humphrey visual field has nine parts which have to be sequentially read and each can pose its own challenges.

In this chapter, we aim to bring out the methodology to read each part and look into the minute details which can make a difference.

4.1.1 Challenge 1: Is This the Printout of My Patient?

The first thing to check is that the printout belongs to the correct patient. There are different formats that every institution follows; like in Fig. 4.1, the first name is repeated in the second name also as sometimes it happens that the patient does not have a second name. But this is not a correct format as this is not universal. In Fig. 4.2, the surname is followed by the first name. The standardization is the choice of the institution but it should be uniformly followed else repeated fields will not be retrievable.

M. Gandhi (✉)
Dr. Shroff's Charity Eye Hospital, New Delhi, Delhi, India

S. Patyal
Centre for Sight, Dwarka, New Delhi, Delhi, India

The other qualifier is the patients' ID number which is again as per the record types used in a particular center. This is automatically entered in places where electronic medical records (EMR) are used which decreases the chances of human error. But when manually entered, extra care should be taken to avoid errors.

4.1.2 Challenge 2: Why Do I Need the Date of Birth to Be Accurate?

The essence of the test is to statistically compare the retinal sensitivity of our patient with the normative pooled data which is age matched, thus the age of our patient plays an important role and therefore it has to be correctly entered.

Figure 4.3 is the single-field printout of a 23-year-old patient showing decreased retinal sensitivity in the lower hemisphere both in total and pattern deviation plots. The test was repeated after 3 years, and there is apparent increase in the points affected in terms of number and depth of scotoma and can be interpreted as progression. However, for demonstration purposes, we changed the age to 61 years. Thus, now the actual 26-year-old patient is being statistically compared to a 61-year-old normal patient. The deviation thus is affected differently (Fig. 4.4).

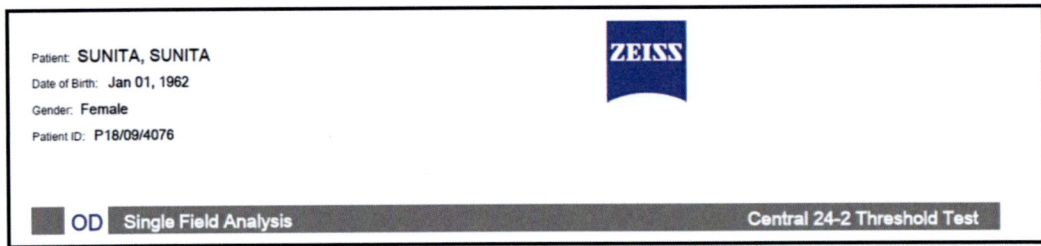

Fig. 4.1 One format of entering the name of the patient

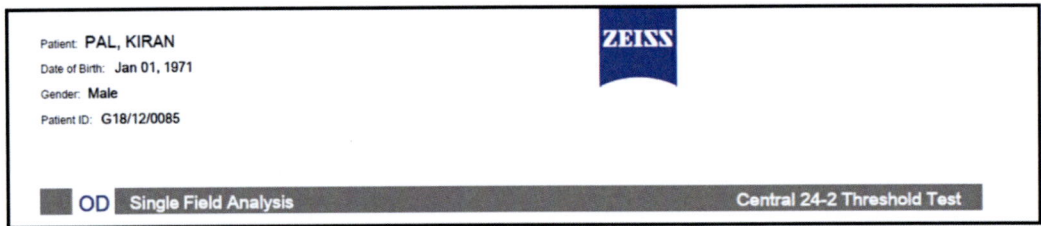

Fig. 4.2 A different format to enter the patients' name

4.1.3 Challenge 3. What Is the Fixation Loss Telling Me?

At the beginning of the test, the blind spot of the patient is mapped. For this, he is expected to look at the center of the fixation diamond projected about 10° below the normal fixation spot. A size III stimulus is projected for 0.2 s. The machine waits for 1.8 s for response.

Once this is done, the patient is asked to concentrate on the central target, and the test is started. During the test, the machine projects some stimuli on the mapped blind spot; if the buzzer is pressed, it is recorded as a fixation loss (Figs. 4.5 and 4.6). This is called the Heijl-Krakau method [1], and suprathreshold stimulus is presented at the blind spot. According to the manufacturer of Humphrey field analyzer, fixation losses exceeding 20% are considered unreliable [2].

This could happen due to a few reasons:

1. The blind spot was not mapped correctly.
2. The patient is not fixating on the central light target when the stimulus was projected.
3. The patient is "trigger happy," thus presses the buzzer irrespective of seeing the stimulus.
4. The other eye is not properly occluded so he can see the stimulus from that eye.
5. A head tilt can also produce a similar effect.

It is important that the perimetrist keeps a check on the eye position on the screen and encourages the patient to focus on the central target. In the latest machines of the Humphrey analyzer, it is possible to hover on the different positions of the test points to see the position of the patient's gaze.

4.1.4 Challenge 4: What Should I Do with a Field with High False Positives?

The machine, in a full threshold test, produces a sound but does not show a stimulus in an attempt to detect false positive responses which are recorded when the buzzer is pressed by the patient inspite of the fact that there was no stimulus projected. In the newer strategies like SITA, there are no explicit

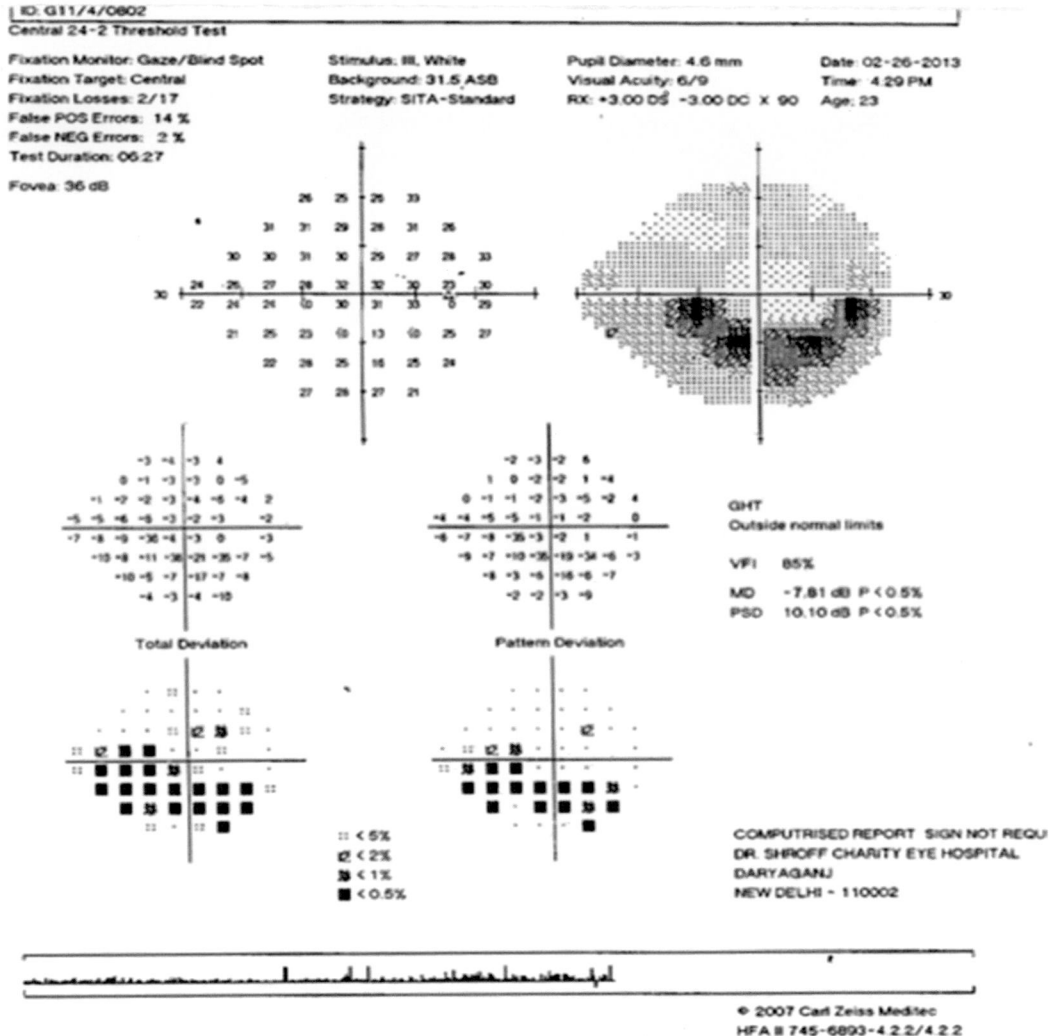

Fig. 4.3 Central 24-2 threshold test with SITA-standard strategy done for a 23-year-old patient in 2013

pauses by the machine. To decrease the test duration and improve patient test reliability, SITA algorithm eliminated false-positive catch trials by use of "listening windows" [3]. These are intervals between stimulus presentations where no response is expected. Minimum response time for a perimetric stimulus is 180 ms. [4] A response window is the time beginning at the minimum response time, adjusted according to the individual patient mean response time. A false-positive response is recorded if the response is detected at a time that it is not expected from an alert patient. And at the end, the percentage is reported of the overall errors.

The false-positive responses bring about a change in almost every part of the field. As seen in Fig. 4.7, the false positives are 33% and are marked with double crosses by the machine to show that it is unacceptable. The fixation losses are also double crossed. Since the patient is trigger happy, it is possible that the patient pressed the buzzer when the stimulus was projected on the blind spot not because he was not fixating on

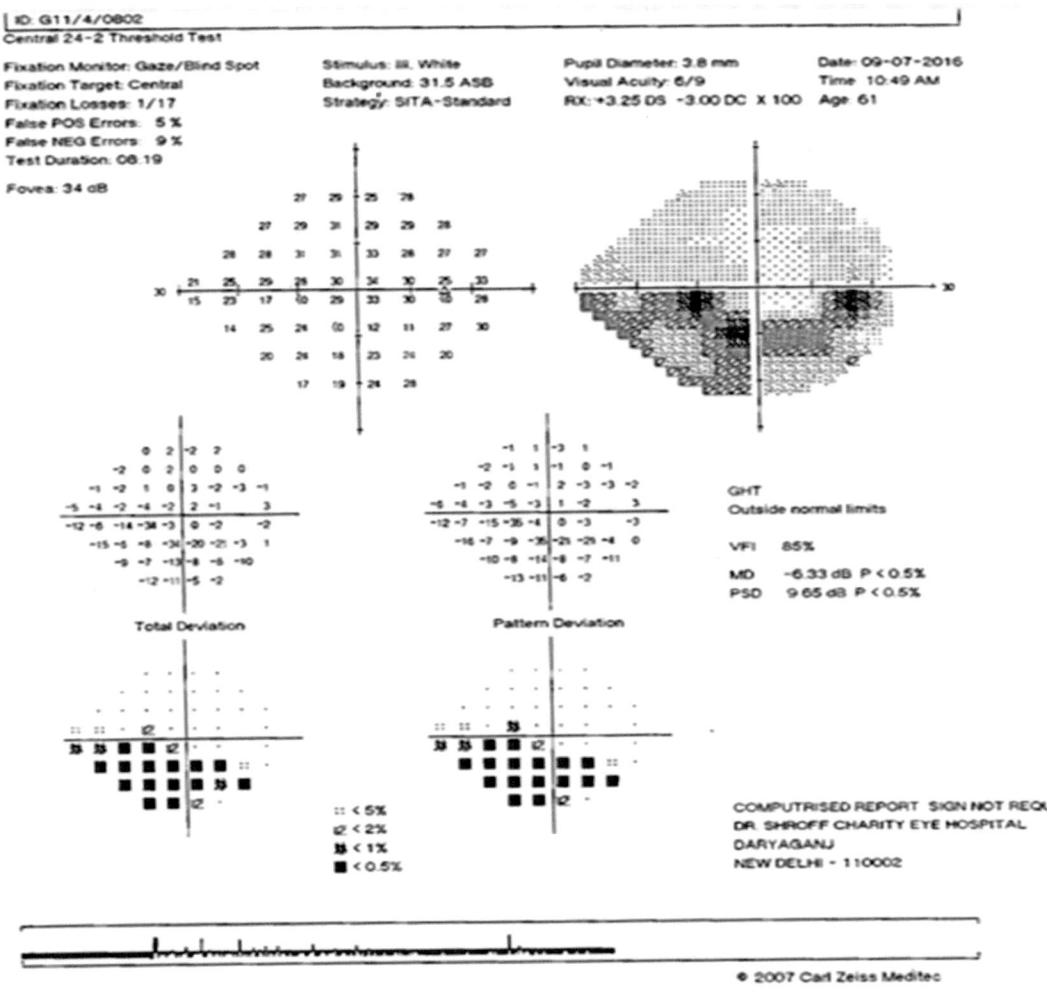

Fig. 4.4 Central 24-2 threshold test with SITA-standard strategy done for the same patient in 2016. For demonstration purposes, the age was changed to 61 years

the central target but because the buzzer was being pressed nonetheless.

The gray scale shows white scotomas. The patient is 68-year-old, and the raw data points are in late 20s and 30s. This high retinal sensitivity is not expected at this age. This is due to the fact that the buzzer is being pressed irrespective of the stimulus intensity. Since these values are more than expected in the normative age-matched patient, the total deviation plot has positive values leading to a positive mean deviation in the global indices.

An interesting phenomenon is noticed in the pattern deviation plot (PDP) which is very suggestive of a false-positive response. Even though there are no points of decreased retinal sensitivity in the total deviation plot (TDP), here in the PDP lower hemisphere one can observe decreased sensitivity. This can be explained by the derivation of pattern deviation plot from the total deviation plot. The seventh highest point of the TDP is calculated by the machine and is subtracted from all the points and this is the PDP. In this case, the seventh highest point is 2. Since the raw data

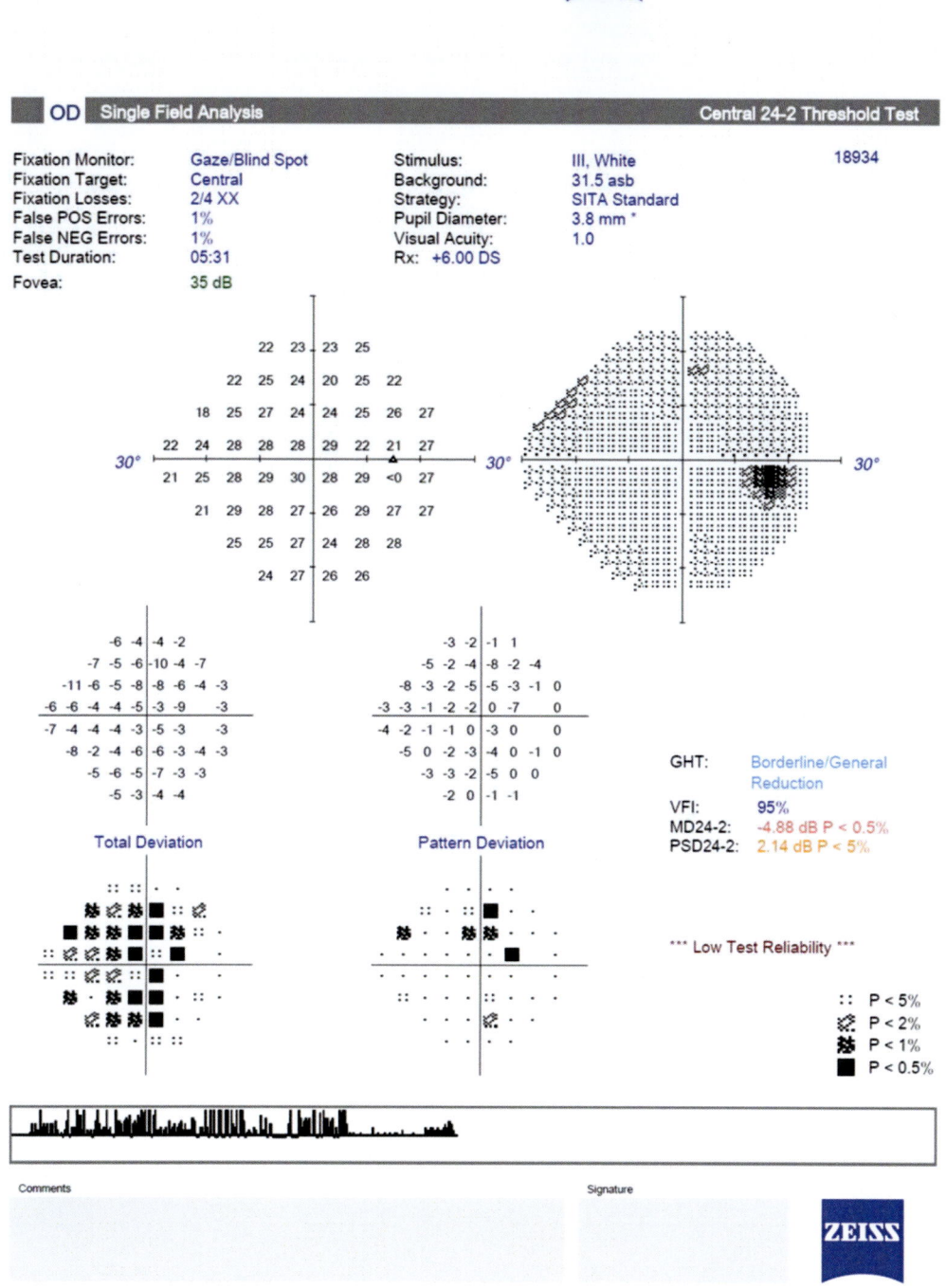

Fig. 4.5 This central 24-2 threshold test, SITA standard strategy done for a 51-year-old patient. The test duration is 5:31 min. The fixation losses are 2 out of 4, i.e., 50% which is unacceptable. The gaze monitor shows that the patient has not been fixating on the central target. Notice that the false positive and negative are very low. Total deviation plot shows generalized depression, and there are points of reduced sensitivity in the pattern deviation plot. The patient needs to be counseled to fixate properly to obtain a reliable field

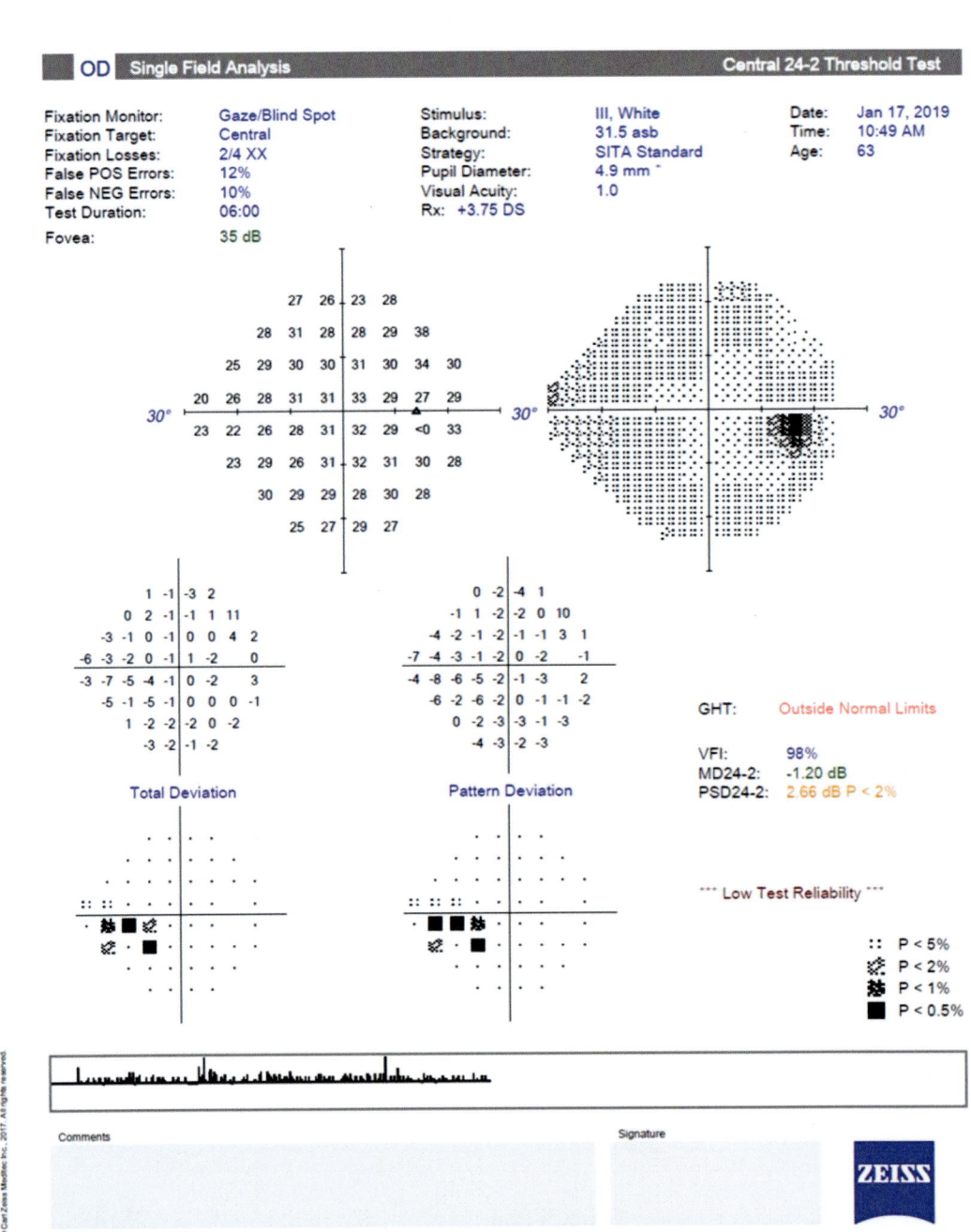

Fig. 4.6 This 63-year-patient has a good visual acuity, and the test was done in 6 min. The fixation losses are 2/4, but there are higher than normal false positive and negative responses. The gaze tracker is not as deviated as in the Fig. 4.5. In this case, it is more likely that the patient is trigger happy and not paying attention and the fixation loss is due to that. The test needs to be repeated after explaining the instructions again

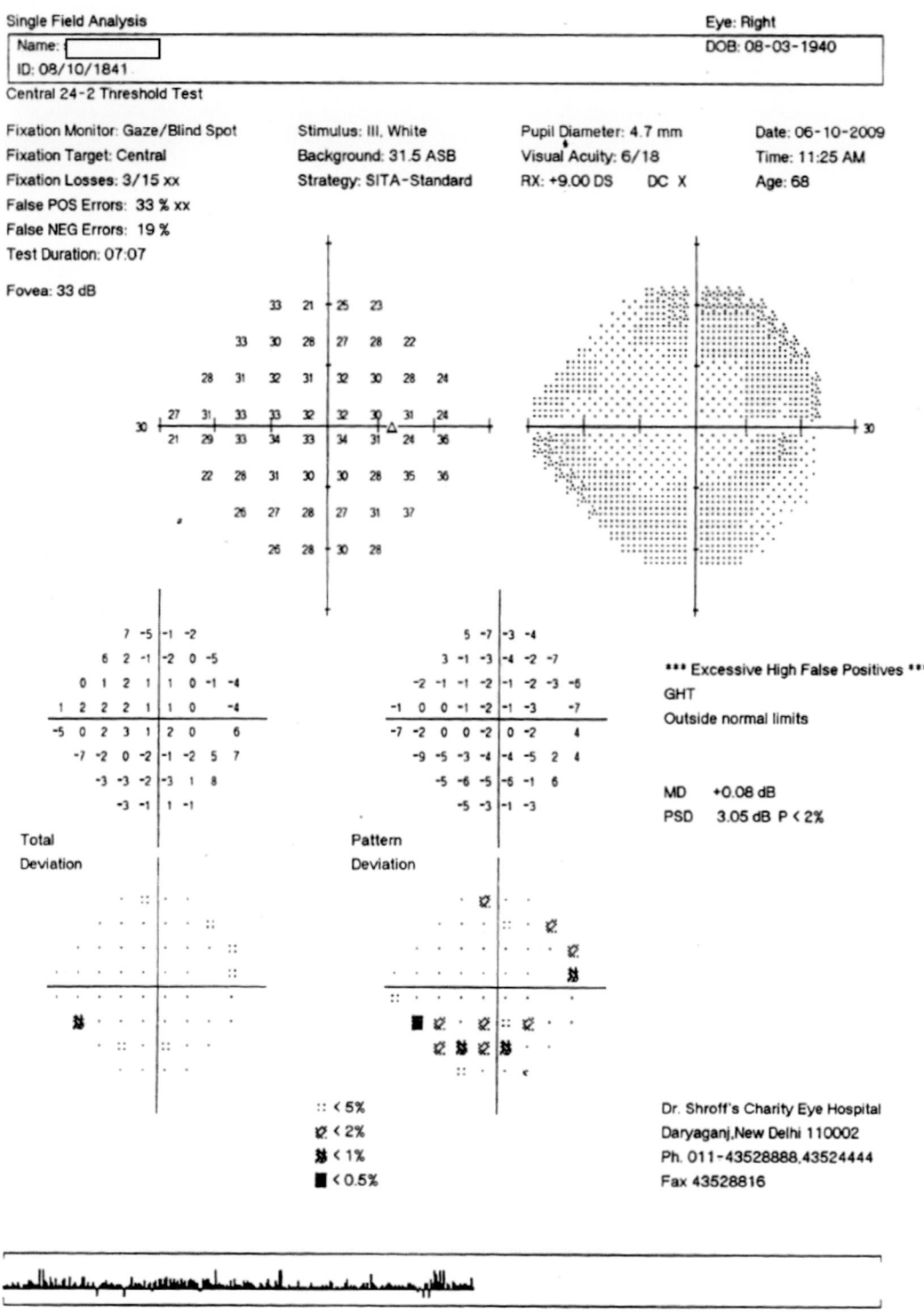

Fig. 4.7 Central 24-2 of right eye of a 68-year-old patient with "excessive high false positive". Note the difference in pattern and total deviation plots

numbers are not uniform and the lower hemisphere has lower values, PDP numbers after subtracting 2, fall below that expected in the normative data base and thus reflect as lowered sensitivity.

The GHT due to this difference in the superior and inferior mirror images shows "outside normal limits," and the field is flagged as "excessive high false positives."

False positives are a good indicator of the test reliability and patients' state of alertness. Without an accurate false-positive rate, it is difficult to establish the visual function in the visual fields and thus the fields should be repeated if needed. Although the manufacturer of the HVF machine recommend that 33% false positives are acceptable, any report exceeding 20% should be reevaluated and preferably repeated [2].

4.1.5 Challenge 5: What Is the Interpretation for High False Negative?

The machine shows a stimulus at a test point, and the patient can appreciate it and presses the buzzer. The machine tests a few points again with a stimulus which is 9 decibels brighter than the one projected earlier at that point. If the patient had seen a lower intensity stimulus, it is expected that this brighter one is seen too. But if the patient does not press the buzzer, it is recorded as false-negative response.

This can happen due to the following reasons:

1. The patient is tired. This is usually seen in the second eye being tested. The perimetrist should explain how the patient can pause the test by keeping the buzzer pressed on or can even be given an actual break and resume when patient is feeling less fatigued.
2. Sometimes the patient feels that the light was seen but it is too late to respond so they do not press the buzzer.
3. Inconsistency in responses due to not understanding the test.

4. In cases of advanced glaucoma, the responses can be variable particularly at the edge of the scotomas [5, 6]. These are beyond the patients' control. In these cases, changing from 24-2 test to a 10-2 gives better results which can be used for follow-up also.

According to Heijl et al., the current false-negative catch trial methods do not estimate the patient attentiveness, instead the frequency of the false-negative responses is associated with the amount of field loss [7]. Thus, improved patient instructions and monitored supervision may not improve test results (Fig. 4.8).

The test, when it starts, after the blind spot has been mapped, records the retinal sensitivity at 4 cardinal points which are located 9° away from the midline. The recorded sensitivity serves as a starting point of the stimulus to be projected on the adjacent points. Thus, the central points are tested earlier on in the test, and since the patient is alert, better sensitivities are recorded. As the test progresses, the peripheral points are tested, and if the patient becomes tired and does not respond, the sensitivities recorded are lesser and it produces this pattern of clover leaf scotomas (Fig. 4.8). False negative may also be seen in advanced glaucoma (Fig. 4.9).

4.1.6 Challenge 6: What Can I Pick Up from the Gray Scale?

The points being tested in the raw data are spaced 6° apart. The points in between do not get represented so the gray scale intrapolates these decibels lying in between the values of the surrounding points (Fig. 4.10). So it is just a representation which helps create a picture of continuity and is easier to explain to the patient. But since it is derived from raw data and not the statistical values of the normative data, it is not as useful clinically.

The pattern is chosen from the Fig. 4.11. It should be noted that the pattern for decibels 26 to 30 is the same and for 21 to 25 is the same. So if the sensitivity is 21 and the next point is 36, the

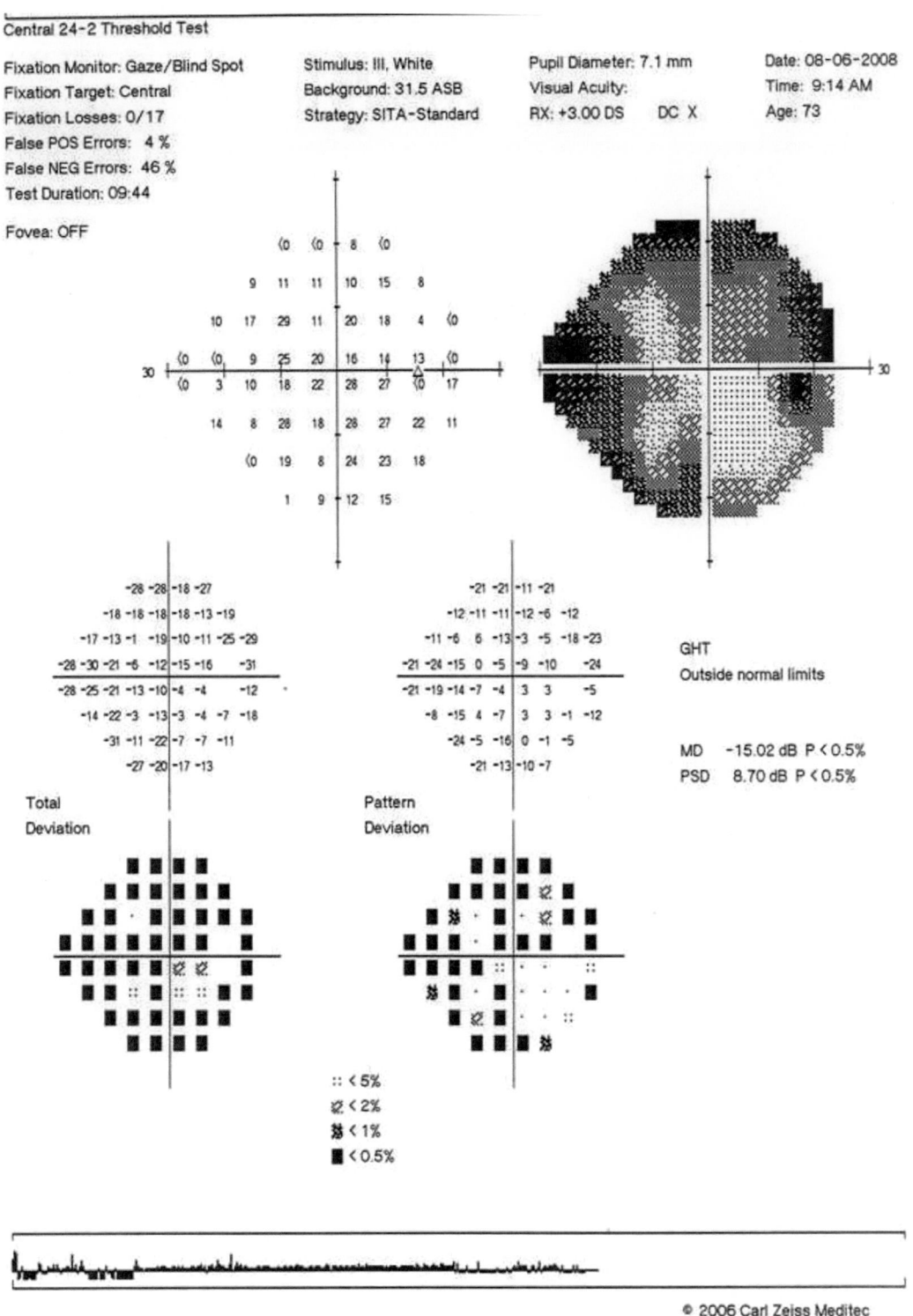

Fig. 4.8 73-year-old patient took 9:44 min for the test, and the false negative is 46% which is not acceptable. This could be as the patient is old and must have been fatigued. The gray scale shows the characteristic clover leaf pattern

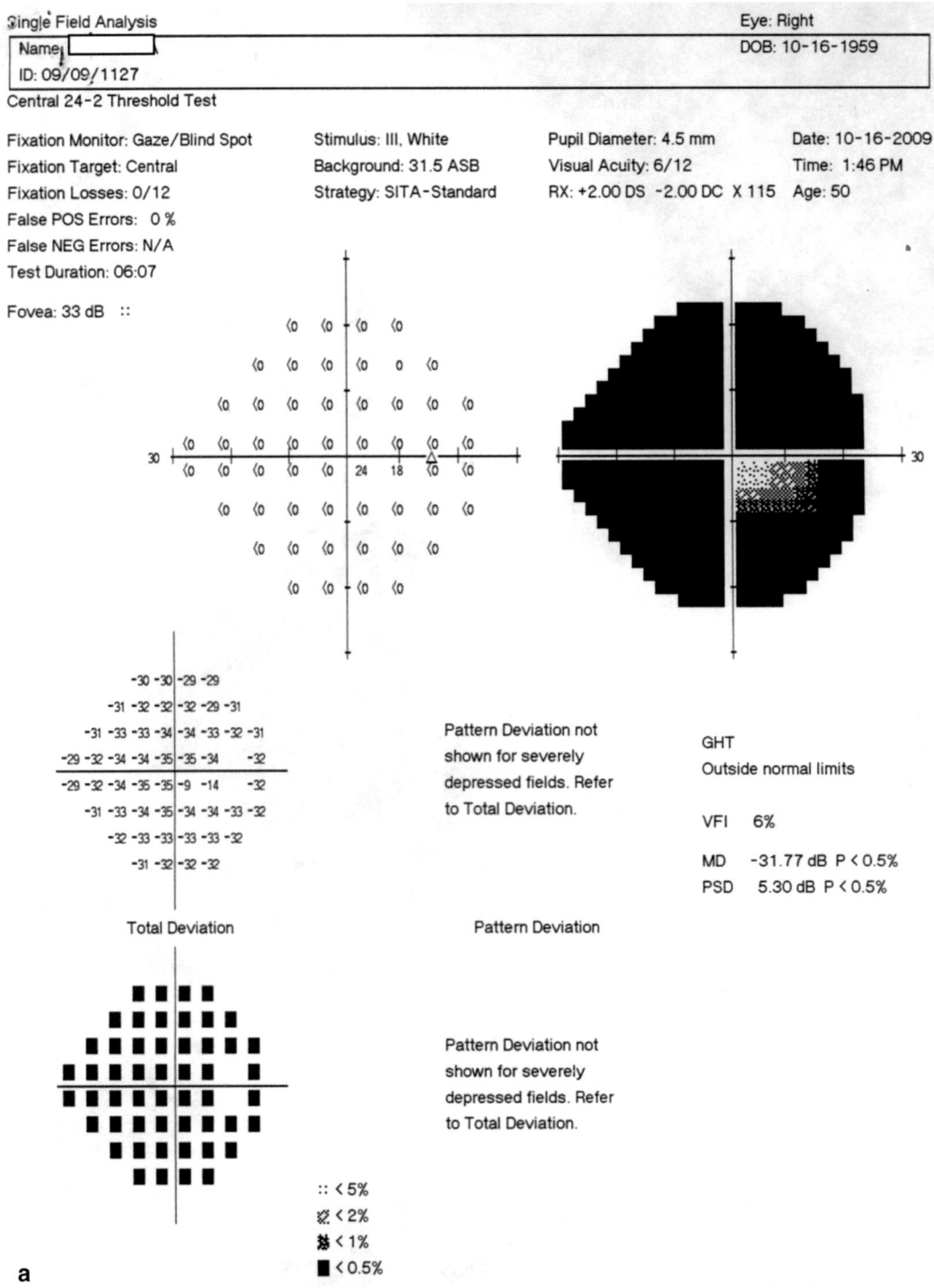

Fig. 4.9 (a) A 58-year-old took 6:07 min to complete the test but the test shows false negative to be beyond the limit and are not recorded. The raw data points are all zeros meaning that even the brightest stimulus was not visible. (b) The cause of this above visual field false negatives is the advanced glaucomatous optic neuropathy as seen in the optic disc photo. This patient needs to be followed up on 10-2 test

4 Challenges in Interpreting Perimetry in Glaucoma

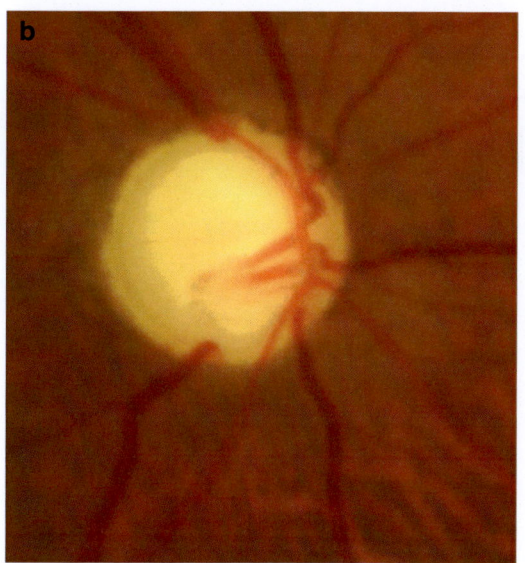

Fig. 4.9 (continued)

same pattern will emerge as compared to if the points are 25 and 26. So it does not have much clinical value.

4.1.7 Challenge 7: If the Total Deviation Plot Is Similar to the Pattern Deviation Plot. What Does it Mean?

The total deviation represents the deviation from the normative data and shows the generalized defect. The pattern deviation is derived from the total deviation by subtracting the seventh highest value to remove what is common to all and a pattern emerges which represents a localized defect, which is more useful in conditions like glaucoma.

Thus, if they are both same, it shows that the defects are both localized as in Fig. 4.12, or it could be that both are generalized defects.

4.1.8 Challenge 8: What Do the Probability Symbols Tell us?

There are four symbols at the bottom of the printout. Less than 5% symbol means that the probability that the retinal sensitivity at the said point is expected to be seen in <5% of the normal population (Fig. 4.13).

Less than 0.5% means that the probability of this is less than 5 in 1000 normal population, so if present it is more likely to be abnormal than normal.

4.1.9 Challenge 9: How Much Importance Do I Attach to the GHT?

Glaucoma hemifield test (GHT) is based on five zones in the superior hemisphere and their mirror images in the inferior hemisphere. These zones are based on patterns of retinal nerve fibers as seen in glaucomatous field loss, so it is not useful in other diseases. These zones are weighted based on percentile deviations in the pattern deviation plot. The GHT was designed to have a sensitivity of 94% but expected sensitivity depends on the stage of glaucoma in a given example.

GHT compares pattern deviation probability scores in five zones in the upper field with corresponding scores in mirror image of the zones in the lower hemisphere. The points are the same in 24-2 and 30-2 test patterns.

Five possible GHT messages are:

1. Outside normal limits: Sensitivities in one or more of the five upper zones are significantly different ($p < 0.01$) as compared to the corresponding zones in lower field.

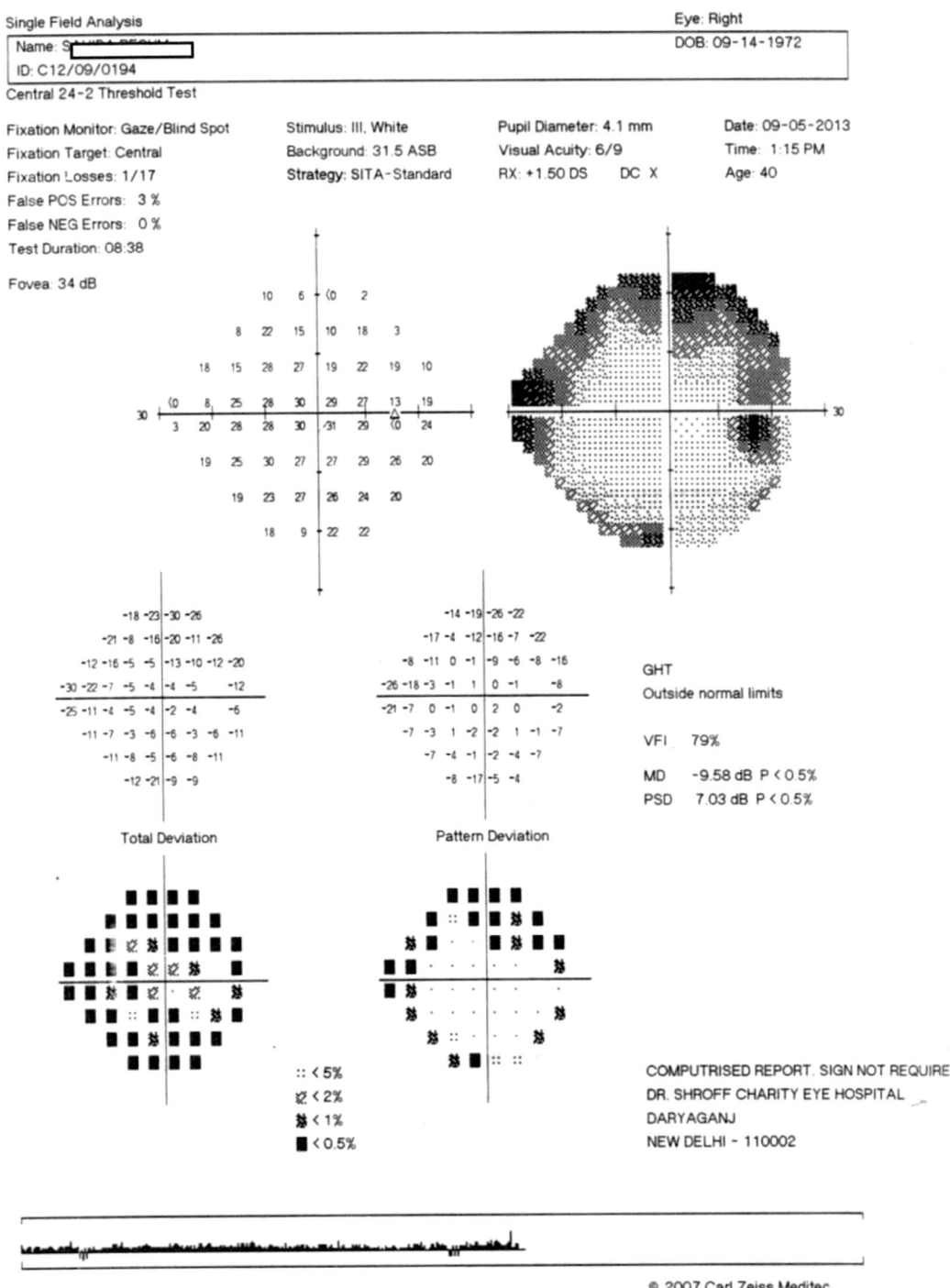

Fig. 4.10 Central 24-2 of right eye

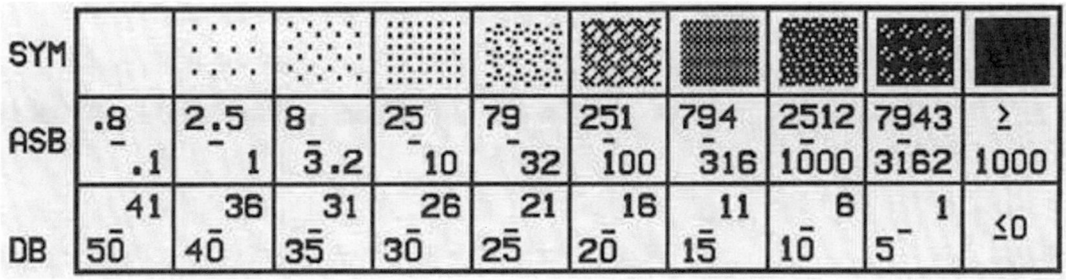

SYM										
ASB	.8 – .1	2.5 – 1	8 – 3.2	25 – 10	79 – 32	251 – 100	794 – 316	2512 – 1000	7943 – 3162	≥ 1000
DB	41 – 50	36 – 40	31 – 35	26 – 30	21 – 25	16 – 20	11 – 15	6 – 10	1 – 5	≤0

Fig. 4.11 Representative symbols of gray scale

2. Borderline: The sensitivity between the zone pair is greater than what is seen in normal subjects ($p < 0.03$), but difference does not reach what is seen on "outside normal limits."
3. General depression of sensitivity: Sensitivities are low and are seen in only 0.5% of normal subjects.
4. Abnormally high sensitivity: Test point locations are high as seen in only 0.05% normal subjects.
5. Within normal limits: This is seen when none of the above significant limits are reached.

4.1.10 Challenge 10: How Should the VFI Be Assessed?

The visual field index is a global index, developed by Bengtsson and Heijl, which is less affected by media opacities like cataract as compared to the mean deviation [8]. It is expressed as a percentage of the visual function and is 100% in a perfect age-adjusted perimetrically normal visual field and is 0% in a perimetrically blind field.

This is calculated from the pattern deviation probability plot by identifying the abnormal points and age-corrected sensitivity at each point from the total deviation numerical map. This is when the mean deviation is less than −20 dB. However, if the MD is worse than −20 dB, the calculation is done from total deviation probability plot. The central points are given more weightage.

MD is affected by media opacities and causes which lead to generalized depression, and the PSD though less affected by media opacities, falsely improves as the severity of visual field loss increases. And it was observed that the decrease in VFI when MD is worse than −20 dB can be highly variable, and this should be kept in mind when using the VFI in clinical and research purposes [9].

4.2 Practical Tips Which Can Help Standardize the Process

1. The entry for the patients' identification should be checked to ensure correct information.
2. The refraction should be checked and entered. The correct rimless lens provided with the machine are used. In case of high refractive power (myopia> −8Dsph, hypermetropia > +6Dsph), contact lenses can be used instead of the rimless lenses.
3. Choose the correct test strategy as per the requirement. It is easier to compare similar strategies so the same strategy must be repeated if the patient is being tested subsequently.
4. Make sure that the patient understands the procedure and is comfortably seated. Explain that every light stimulus is not expected to be seen, and they can pause the test if feeling tired. And they can communicate with the perimetist in case of any discomfort.

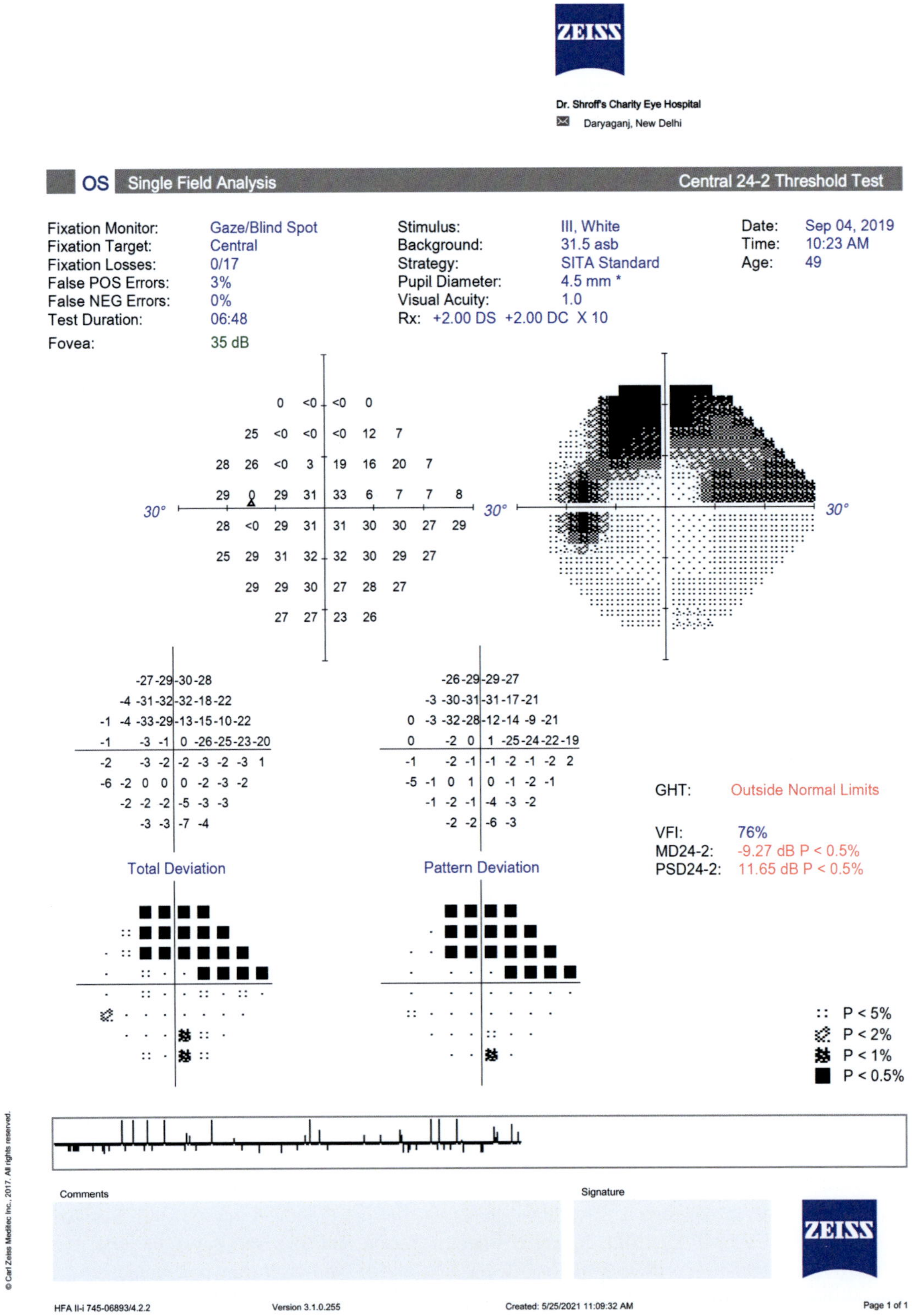

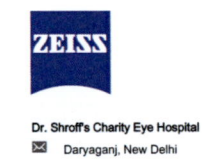

Fig. 4.12 Central 24-2 of the left eye with similar points of decrease sensitivities in the total and pattern deviation plots

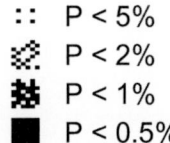

P < 5%
P < 2%
P < 1%
P < 0.5%

Fig. 4.13 The probability symbols

5. The perimetrist should be present during the test, encouraging the patient and if need be, stopping the test and reexplaining. Humanoid robots and computer speakers have been used to replace human interaction during perimetry and have been preferred by patients and have helped improve compliance [10].
6. Foveal threshold and blind spot mapping to be done meticulously and make sure that the fixation is not turned off during the test.

4.3 Factors Affecting the Variability of the Visual Field Tests [11]

1. Stage of the disease [12].
2. Patient motivation.
3. Technician skill and patience.
4. Appropriate refraction [13].
5. Clear instructions before and during the test with reassurance and encouragement [14].
6. Patient monitoring during the test.
7. Cognitive function and circadian rhythms—this decreases over age and also time of the day and elderly may find it difficult to perform the test in the later part of the day [15]. Lowest sensitivity was found after lunch and highest during early morning [16].

4.4 Summary

A comfortable well-instructed patient and a skillful perimetrist with patience can make a big difference in getting a good visual field. This, followed by a systematic step-by-step evaluation of the parts of the field printout understanding the nuances, can help in developing a scientific management plan for the patient.

References

1. Olsson J, Bengtsson B, Heijl A, Rootzén H. An improved method to estimate frequency of false positive answers in computerized perimetry. Acta Ophthalmol Scand. 1997;75:181–3.
2. Humphrey field analyzer II user's guide. San Leandro, CA: Humphrey Instruments Inc.;1994.
3. Bengtsson B, Olsson J, Heijl A, Rootzén H. A new generation of algorithms for computerized threshold perimetry, SITA. Acta Ophthalmol Scand. 1997;75:368–75.
4. Greve EL. Single and multiple stimulus static perimetry in glaucoma; the two phases of perimetry. Doc Ophthalmol. 1973;36:1–355.
5. Katz J, Sommer A. Reliability indexes of automated perimetric tests. Arch Ophthalmol. 1988;106:1252–4.
6. Anderson DR, Patella VM. Automated static perimetry, vol. 93. 2nd ed. St. Louis: Mosby; 1999. p. 105,339.
7. Bengtsson B, Heijl A. False-negative responses in glaucoma perimetry: indicators of patient performance or test reliability? Am J Ophthalmol. 2000;130(5):689.
8. Bengtsson B, Heijl A. A visual field index for calculation of glaucoma rate of progression. Am J Ophthalmol. 2008;145:343–53.
9. Rao HL, Senthil S, Choudhari NS, Mandal AK, Garudadri CS. Behavior of visual field index in advanced glaucoma. Invest Ophthalmol Vis Sci. 2013;54:307–12.
10. McKendrick AM, Zeman A, Liu P, Aktepe D, Aden I, Bhagat D, Do K, Nguyen HD, Turpin A. Robot assistants for perimetry: a study of patient experience and performance. Transl Vis Sci Technol. 2019;8(3):59.
11. Blumenthal EZ, Sample PA, Berry CC, et al. Evaluating several sources of variability for standard and SWAP visual fields in glaucoma patients, suspects, and normals. Ophthalmology. 2003;110:1895–902.
12. Bengtsson B, Heijl A. False-negative responses in glaucoma perimetry: indicators of patient performance or test reliability? Invest Ophthalmol Vis Sci. 2000;41:2201–4.
13. Mutlukan E. The effect of refractive blur on the detection sensitivity to light offsets in the central visual field. Acta Ophthalmol. 1994;72:189–94.
14. Kutzko KE, Brito CF, Wall M. Effect of instructions on conventional automated perimetry. Invest Ophthalmol Vis Sci. 2000;41:2006–13.
15. Blatter K, Cajochen C. Circadian rhythms in cognitive performance: methodological constraints, protocols, theoreticalunderpinnings. Physiol Behav. 2007;90:196–208.
16. JunoyMontolio FG, Wesselink C, Gordijn M, Jansonius NM. Factors that influence standard automated perimetry test results in glaucoma: test reliability, technician experience, time of day, and season. Invest Ophthalmol Vis Sci. 2012;53(11):7010–7.

5 Evaluating Progression on Perimetry

Medha Prabhudesai

Abbreviations

dB	Decibel
GPA	Guided progression analysis
HFA	Humphrey field analyser
IOP	Intraocular pressure
MD	Mean deviation
Nd YAG laser	Neodymium yttrium aluminium garnet laser
NRR	Neuroretinal rim
OCT	Optical coherence tomography
OD	Oculus dexter—right eye
OHT	Ocular hypertension
ONH	Optic nerve head
OS	Oculus sinister—left eye
OU	Oculus uterque—both eyes
POAG	Primary open angle glaucoma
PSC	Posterior subcapsular
PSD	Pattern standard deviation
RGC	Retinal ganglion cell
RNFL	Retinal nerve fibre layer
ROP	Rate of progression
VF	Visual field
VFI	Visual field index

5.1 Progression

It is difficult to assess progression, only by looking at multiple visual field printouts. We can track the MD or PSD, to see if individual values have worse or remained the same. This can be a time-consuming process.

There can be visual field variability initially which is seen as variability in decibel values (short-term fluctuations/long-term fluctuations). Later, the depressed points become constant [1, 2].

5.2 Patterns of Progression

1. Diffuse decrease in sensitivity.
2. Deepening of existing defect.
3. Expansion of existing defect.
4. Appearance of a new defect.

Usually progression occurs by expansion or deepening of the defect more commonly, than a new defect [3].

M. Prabhudesai (✉)
Insight Vision Foundation, Pune, Maharashtra, India

Department of Ophthalmology, Bharati Vidyapeeth Medical College, Pune, Maharashtra, India

S. Patyal, M. Gandhi (eds.), *Resolving Dilemmas in Perimetry*,
https://doi.org/10.1007/978-981-16-2601-2_5

5.3 Criteria for Progression Are as Follows

- Three points in an abnormal region decreased by 10 dB or two new points near a defect reduced by 10 dB.
- Two points in central 15° or three outside 15° down by 10 dB.
- Statistical comparisons ($p < 5\%$) [4, 5].

5.4 Importance of Finding Out Progression

- To decide stability or worsening of the eye.
- To change the patient's treatment and management plan.

If worsening is seen, it is important to know if the change is due to glaucoma or any other pathology.

5.5 The Guided Progression Analysis (GPA) Software on HFA

For management of glaucoma, it is important to look at event and trend analysis. The guided progression analysis is a combination of both event-based and trend-based analysis. We require both to confirm progression and for accurate tracking of progression [6]. Event analysis shows statistically significant change of a point or group of points, and trend analysis quantifies the rate change over time and future projection of progression.

Zeiss Humphrey perimeter has a glaucoma progression analysis software (GPA) which analyses consecutive perimetry tests and helps in tracking progression and future prediction of progression if the rate remains unaltered.

5.5.1 Event Analysis

This evaluates change from baseline. Progression is evaluated based on the occurrence of changes for two or more consecutive fields. However, it does not provide any information on the rate at which the glaucoma is progressing [6, 7].

In GPA, individual test locations are flagged as possible progression, likely progression or no progression from baseline if statistically they have progressed by $P < 5\%$ on consecutive fields [6].

5.5.2 Trend Analysis

This estimates the rate of change as well as identifies progression. The trend lines are a statistical regression line analysis of the VFI value that reflects the overall field sensitivity. When followed over time, it gives values as well as statistical significance of the rate of change [6, 7].

5.6 Rate of Progression

Change from baseline is more sensitive than rate of change; however, rate of change is essential for judging whether a patient is at risk for vision loss during his or her lifetime. Estimating the rate of progression, by individual fields, is always difficult and time consuming. There is no universally agreed upon standardized set of criteria for judging progression [2].

Some patients can be slow progressors, while some are fast progressors [7]. Rate of progression is highly individual among patients, and not all patients progress at vision-threatening rate. Still, it is important to know the rate at which field is progressing, as past rates of progression are future predictors of progression [8].

There is a need to modify treatment options accordingly. Faster rates of progression can affect quality of life of the patient. Rate of progression may change after medical or surgical intervention to control IOP. A new baseline needs to be established after an intervention [9, 10].

5.7 The Guided Progression Analysis (GPA; Carl Zeiss Meditec, Inc., Dublin, CA)

GPA™ software differentiates statistically significant progression of visual field loss from random variability. The analysis is based upon detailed empirical knowledge of the variability found at various stages of glaucomatous visual field loss through information acquired in extensive multicenter clinical trials worldwide [6].

GPA uses the Visual Field Index™ (VFI) for calculation of glaucoma rate of progression. It is a measurement of visual field status expressed as a percent of a normal age-adjusted visual field [11]. VFI is optimized for progression analysis. VFI is center-weighted to correlate with retinal ganglion cell density and visual function. It is less influenced by cataract and other media changes compared with earlier indices [11, 1].

For GPA, always same test strategy and pattern should be used to allow easier comparison and monitoring for progression. Each test strategy uses its own normative database. Tests should be repeated if not reliable, to establish better baseline measurements or to confirm possible progression.

- First two visual field tests are identified as baseline.
- Subsequent visual field tests are then compared with the averaged baseline using the pattern deviation values. The frequency of follow-up VFs should be based on the risk of progression based on extent of damage.
- When follow-up values decline to a degree larger than the variability of an age- and defect-matched population of stable glaucoma patients, the point is identified.
- If the change persists on consecutive repeat testing, points are marked as possibly (two consecutive fields) or likely (three or more consecutive fields) [12].
- *GPA Alert:* The GPA alert is a message that indicates whether GPA progression criteria was present. It is indicative of the eye as a whole, not only to specific progressing points in the visual field. The GPA alert assists in recognizing deterioration in consecutive tests [12]. (Table 5.1).
- Accurate progression analysis of VF changes is essential to monitor patients with glaucoma. The VFI is a staging index for the total amount

Table 5.1 GPA alert

Possible progression	Three or more points show deterioration in at least two consecutive tests
Likely progression	Three or more points show deterioration in at least three consecutive tests
No progression detected	Neither of the above conditions applies

a'No progression detected' has been removed from HFA 3

of field loss. Values range from 100% (normal) to 0% (perimetrically blind). This percentage value can be tracked over a series of tests and can used as an indicator for assessing progression over time. It is reported to be less sensitive to changes of nuclear sclerosis [1].

- *VFI Bar*: A graphical estimate of the patient's remaining useful field, at the current VFI value. It also gives 2- to 5-year projection of the VFI regression line if the current trend continues. Five-year projection of VF loss is an important tool to judge patients, who are worsening rapidly. These progression plots have largest impact on patient management for glaucoma. They significantly improve ability to identify future worsening over years.
- *Progression Analysis Probability Plot*: The progression analysis probability plot gives the statistical significance of the decibel changes shown in the deviation from baseline plot. It compares the changes between the baseline and follow-up exams to the inter-test variability typical of stable glaucoma patients and then shows a plot of point locations, which have changed significantly. Points that have changed by more than the expected variability are identified with a simple and intuitive set of symbols (Table 5.2).
- For data that is out of range, GPA cannot determine whether or not the encountered deviation at that point is significant. This occurs mainly with field defects that were already quite deep at baseline, such that even the maximum available stimulus brightness is

within the range of normal variability, but can also occur when the measured threshold is higher than the baseline [12].

Table 5.2 Symbols for progression analysis probability plot

•	A single, solid dot	Point not changing by a significant amount
Δ	An open triangle	Progression at 95% significance level ($p < 0.05$)
◮	A half filled triangle	Significant deterioration at that point in two consecutive tests
▲	A solid triangle	Significant deterioration at that point in three consecutive tests
X	An X	The data at that point was out of range for analysis

5.8 Reading the GPA Printout

This can be divided into three parts:

5.8.1 First Part

5.8.1.1 Baseline Tests (Fig. 5.1)

5.8.2 Second Part: I

5.8.2.1 Progression Analysis (Fig. 5.2)

5.8.3 Second Part: II

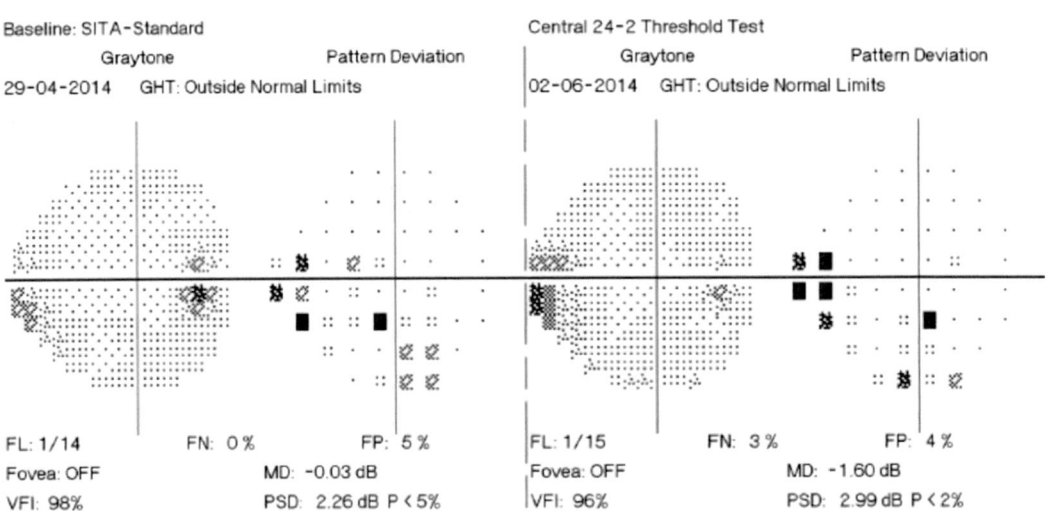

Fig. 5.1 This consists of first two visual field tests and labeled as baseline. This displays protocol used for the test, date, graytone, pattern deviation, glaucoma hemifield test, reliability indices, and global indices for both baseline tests

5 Evaluating Progression on Perimetry

5.8.3.1 Progression Bands (Fig. 5.3)

5.8.4 Third Part

5.8.4.1 Recent Visual Field Report with Progression Analysis (Fig. 5.4)

5.9 Progression Artifacts

As with routine visual field testing, artifacts due to eyelid and brow ptosis, rim artifacts, incorrect refractive error correction, or patient fatigue can give rise to false analysis of visual field progression.

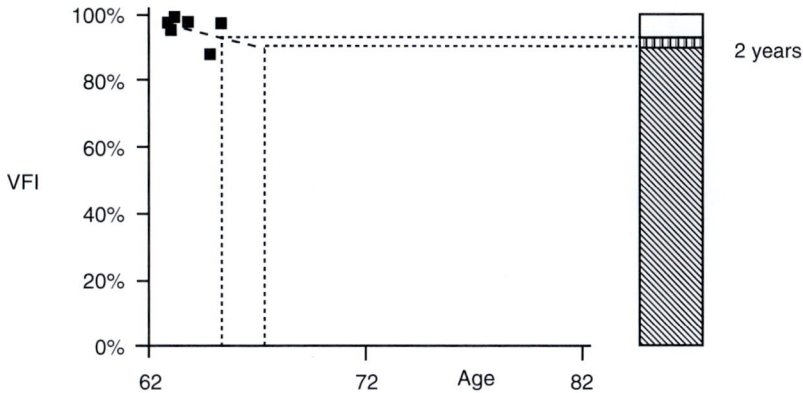

Rate of Progression: -1.7 ± 4.8 % /year (95% confidence)
Slope not significant

Fig. 5.2 *VFI Rate of Progression Analysis*: This gives trend analysis of the patient's overall visual field history. A line with a negative slope indicates worsening of the VF defect. *VFI Bar*: A box is given on the right side, which gives a graphical estimate of the patient's remaining useful field at the current VFI value. It also gives 2–5 years projection of the VFI regression line if the current trend continues. Rate of progression is given below the graph. A comment is given, if the slope is significant or not. (*In HFA 3 this comment is removed)

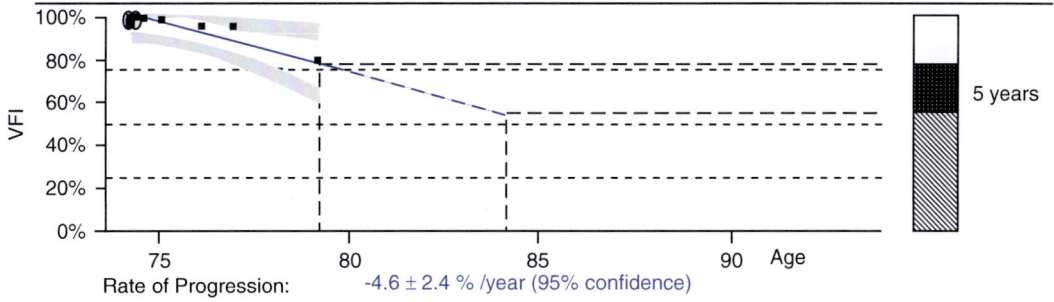

Rate of Progression: -4.6 ± 2.4 % /year (95% confidence)

Fig. 5.3 HFA 3 gives additional feature of progression bands. The gray bands indicate the statistical significance of the regression analysis. The upper/top band represents 97.5% significance for the upper edge and 90% significance for the lower edge. The edges of the lower/bottom band represent 10% significance upper edge and 2.5% significance lower edge

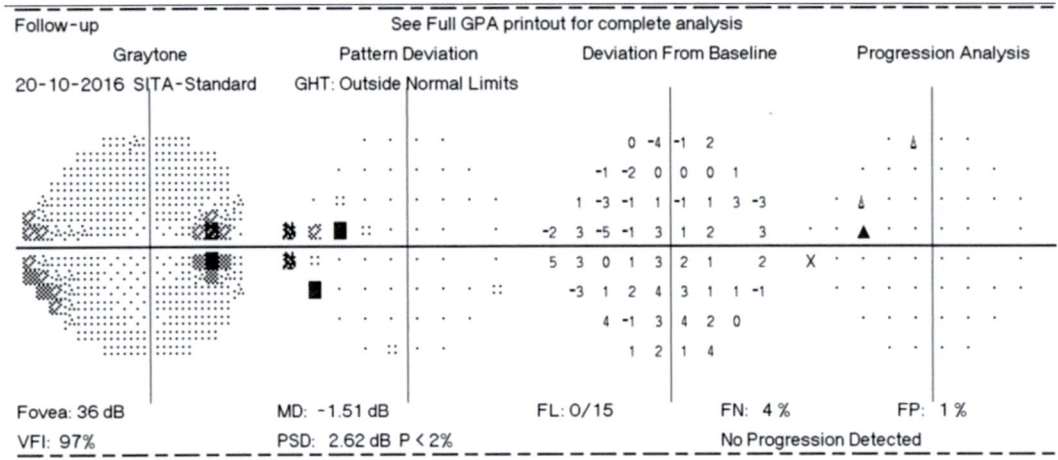

Fig. 5.4 Conclusive report of most recent or selected visual field includes VFI, MD, PSD, and global indices. It provides deviation in decibel values from baseline along with "progression analysis probability plot" and the "GPA alert." *In HFA 3 "no progression detected" comment from GPA alert is removed

5.10 Case 1

A patient with OHT, deep cups, disc asymmetry, and family history of POAG.

OD GPA between 45 and 51 years (2013–2019).

5.10.1 OD ONH Color Photo

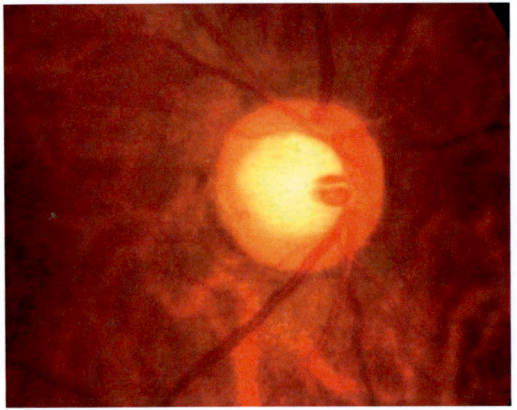

5.10.2 OS ONH Color Photo

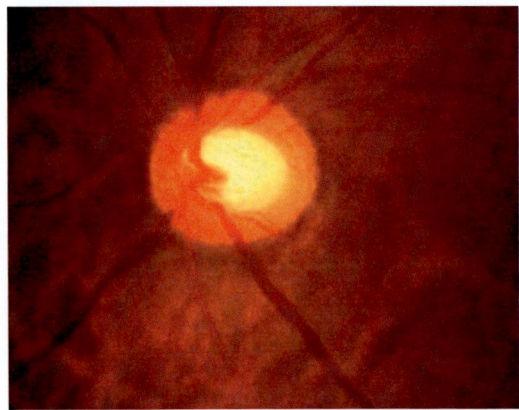

5.10.3 OD GPA

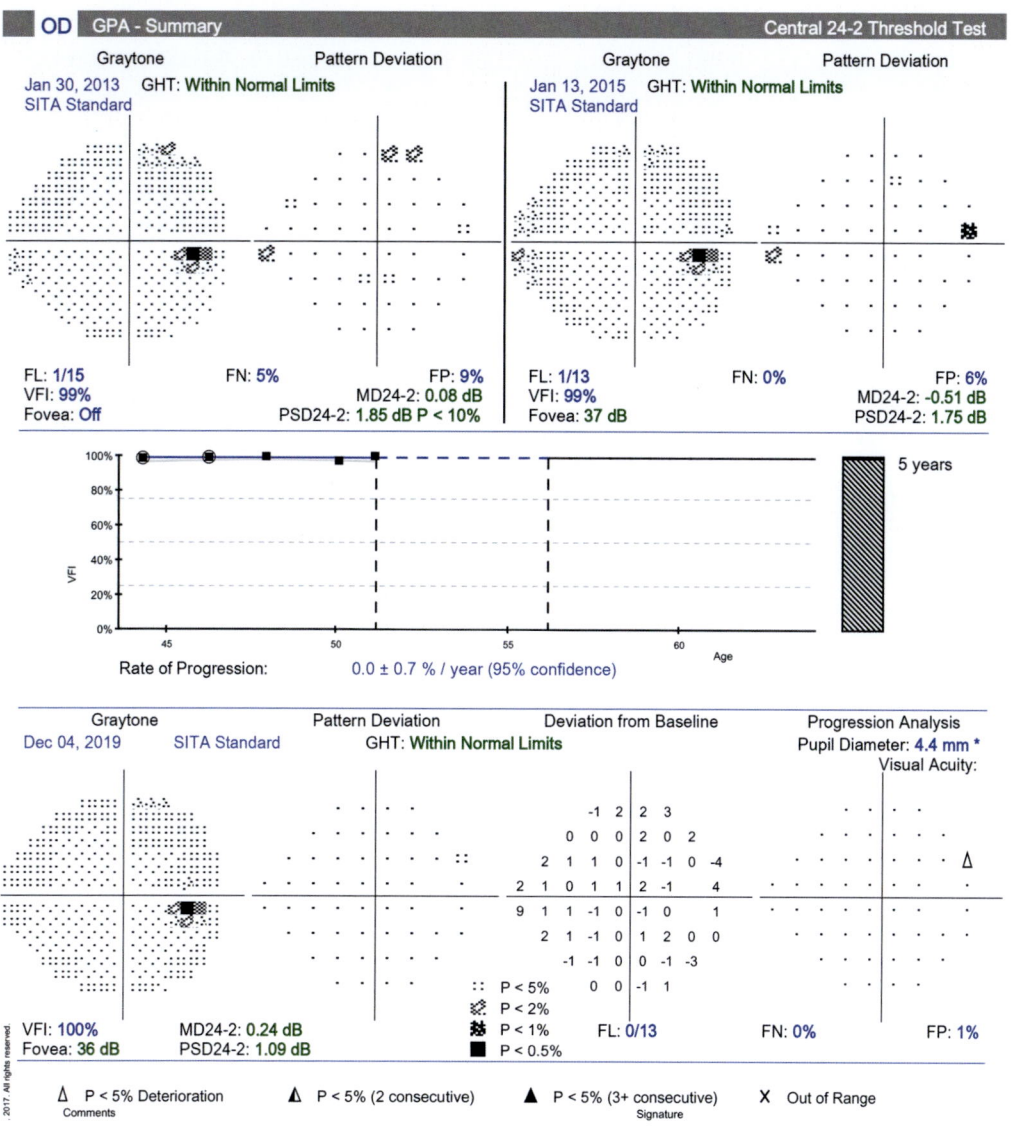

5.10.4 OS GPA

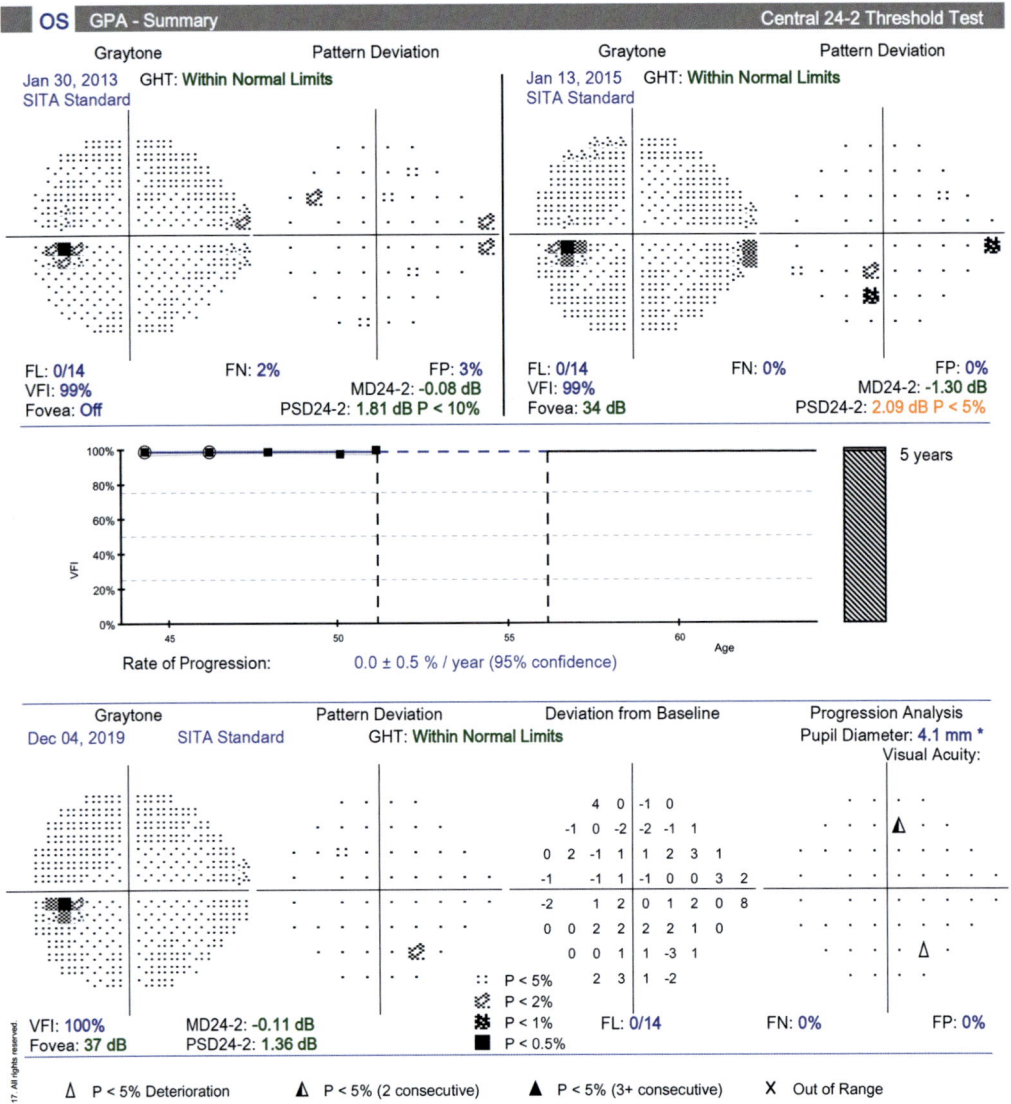

Both eyes have stable GPA for 6 years.

Rate of progression for OD: 0.0 ± 0.7%/year; for OS: 0.0 ± 0.5%/year (95% confidence).

OU: VFI bar: future extrapolation shows no progression for next 5 years on GPA.

5.11 Case 2

A patient of POAG in both eyes.
 OS GPA between 46 and 49 years. (2016–2019).

5.11.1 OS ONH Color Photo

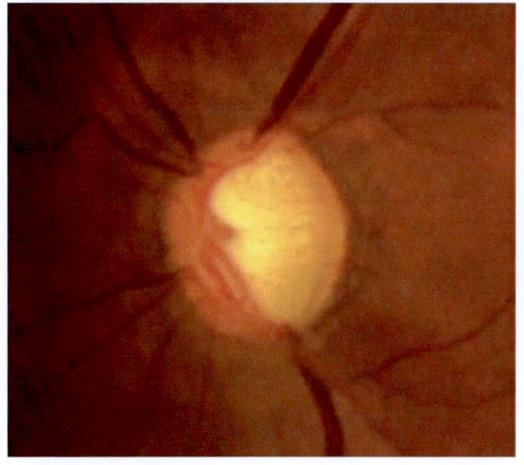

5.11.2 OS ONH Red-Free Photo

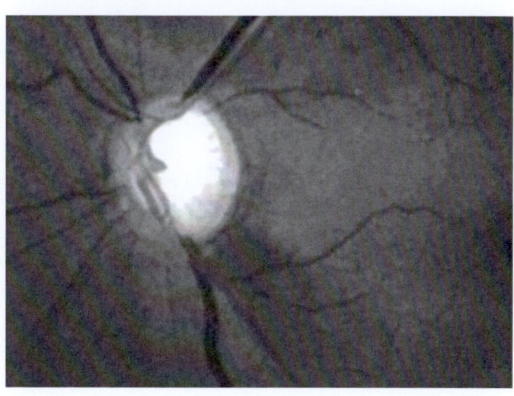

5.11.3 OS OCT

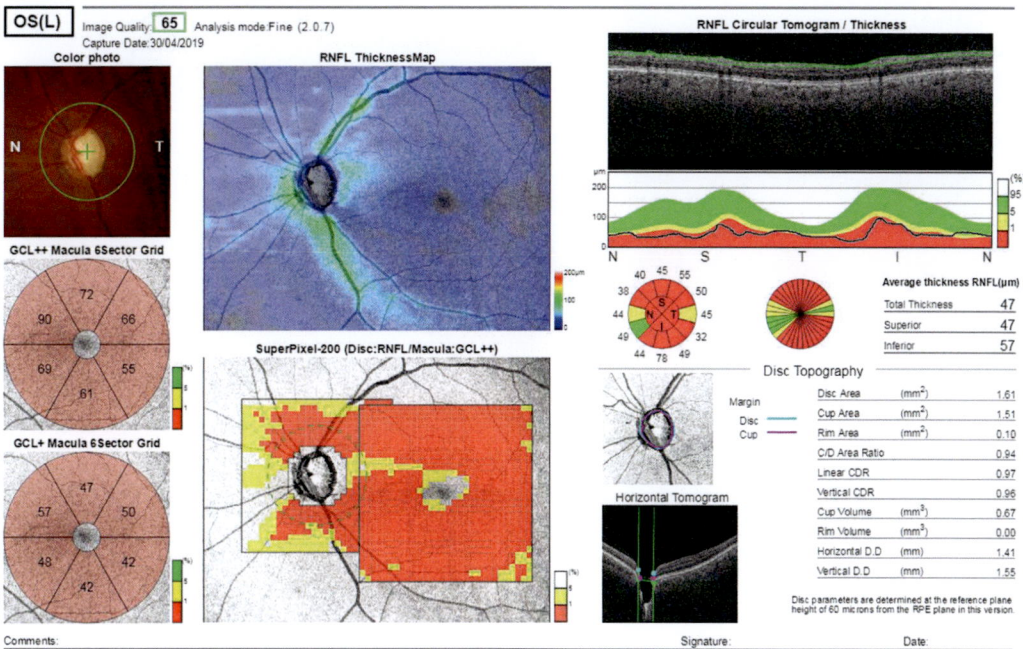

OS ONH color and red-free photos show RNFL thinning in superotemporal and inferotemporal quadrant. OS OCT shows small disc, high C/D with extensive RNFL, and RGC thinning.

5.11.4 OS GPA

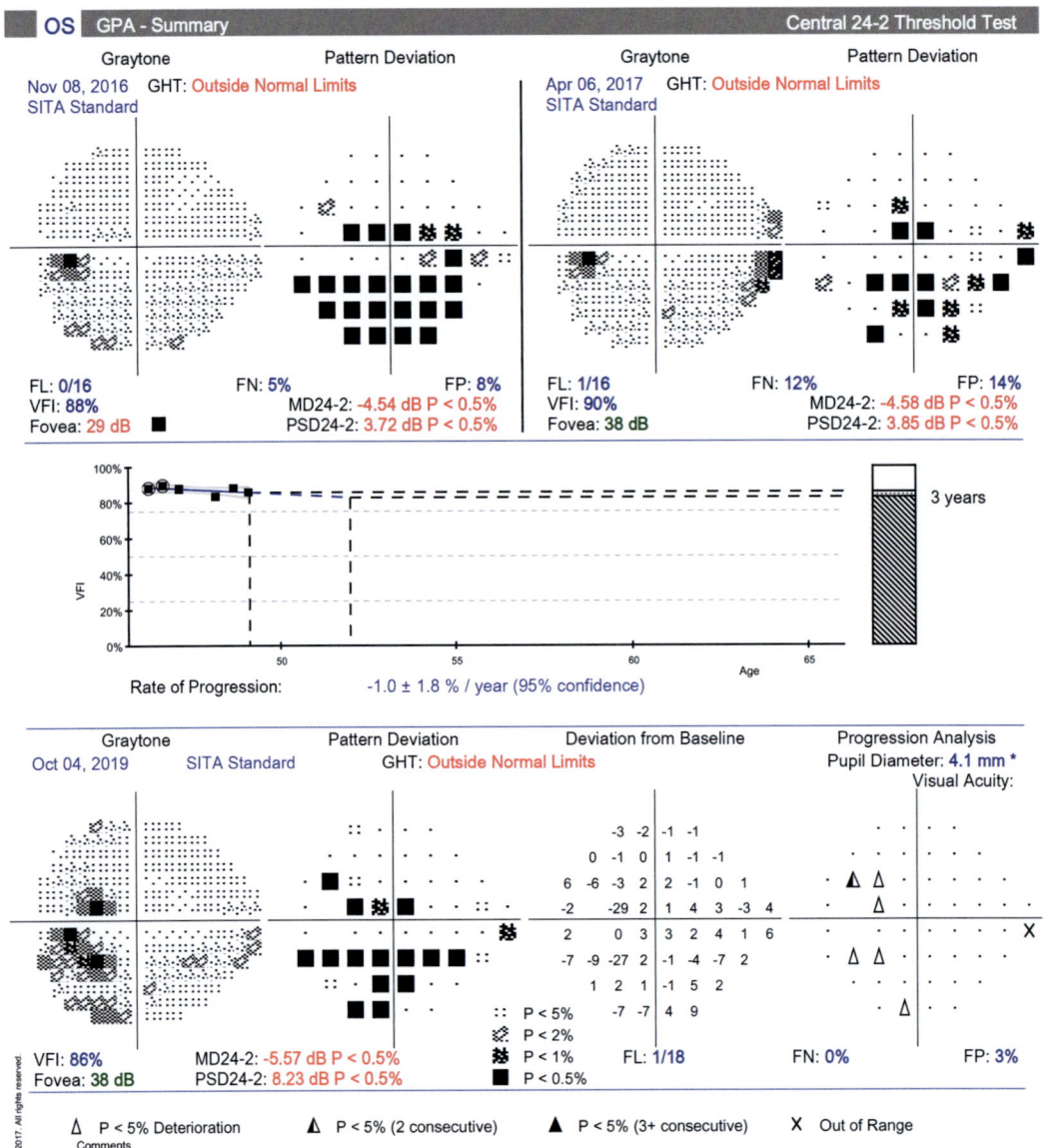

Rate of progression: −1.0 ± 1.8%/year (95% confidence).

In the left eye, structural loss is much more than functional loss. Also functional loss shows very slow progression on GPA.

5.12 Case 3

A patient who was initially diagnosed as OHT, progressed to POAG.

OD GPA between 2014 and 2020 (49–55 years).

5.12.1 OD ONH Colour Photo

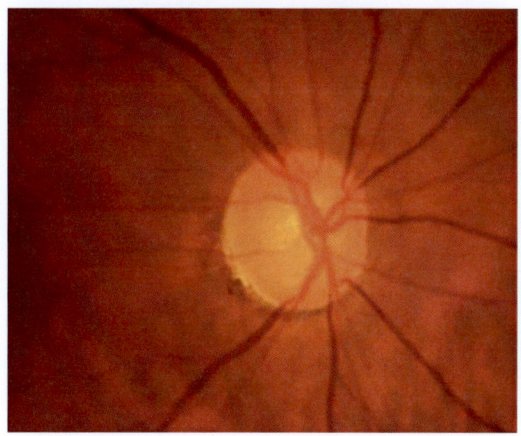

5.12.2 OD ONH Red-Free Photo

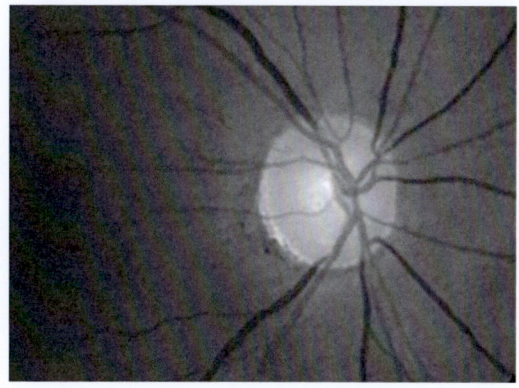

5.12.3 OD GPA

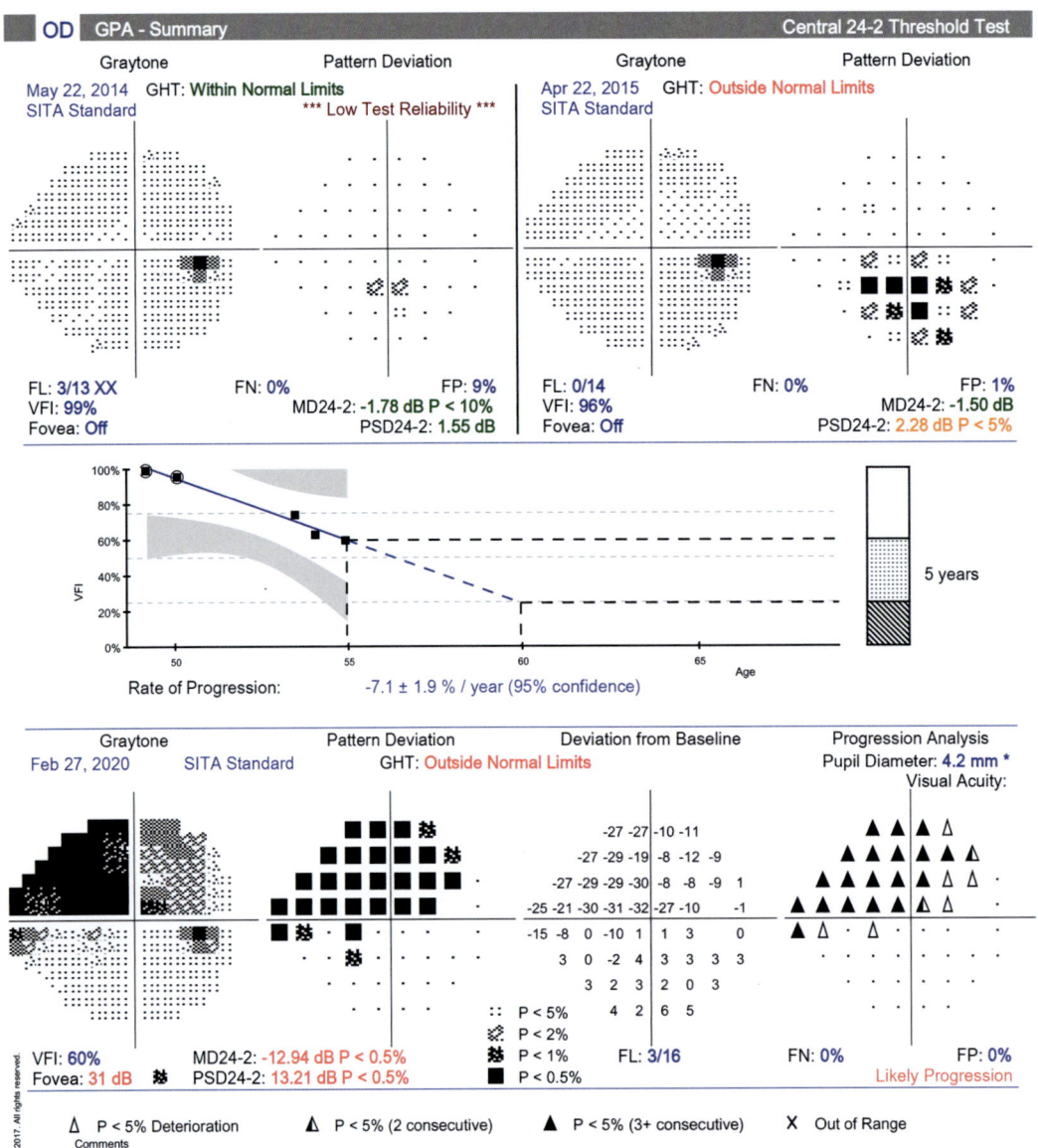

A patient of low compliance, who did not report for eye examination for 4 years. Patient has low compliance for prescribed antiglaucoma medications also.

OD ONH photo shows thinning of NRR, especially in inferotemporal quadrant.

OD GPA shows significant rate of progression −7.1 ± 1.9%/year (95% confidence).

Progression analysis shows multiple test points, which show progression on three consecutive tests (closed triangles). GPA alert is likely progression. There is development of dense superior arcuate defect.

There may be a need to establish a new baseline once the IOP is controlled. As patient has low compliance for antiglaucoma medical management, there may be need to change the management strategy to other management options or surgical intervention.

5.13 Case 4

A patient of Juvenile glaucoma in both eyes.

OS GPA between 26 and 31 years (2014–2019).

5.13.1 OS ONH Color Photo

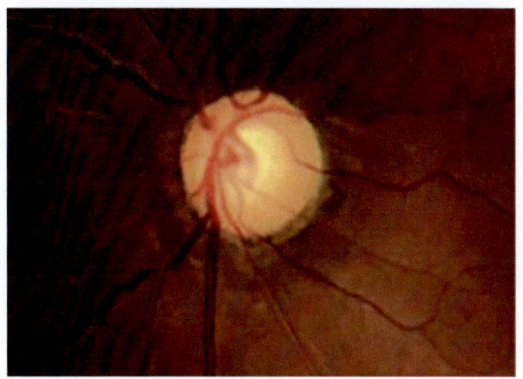

5.13.2 OS ONH Red-Free Photo

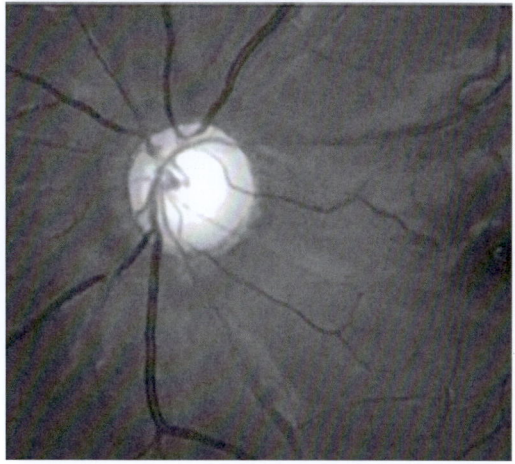

5.13.3 OS GPA

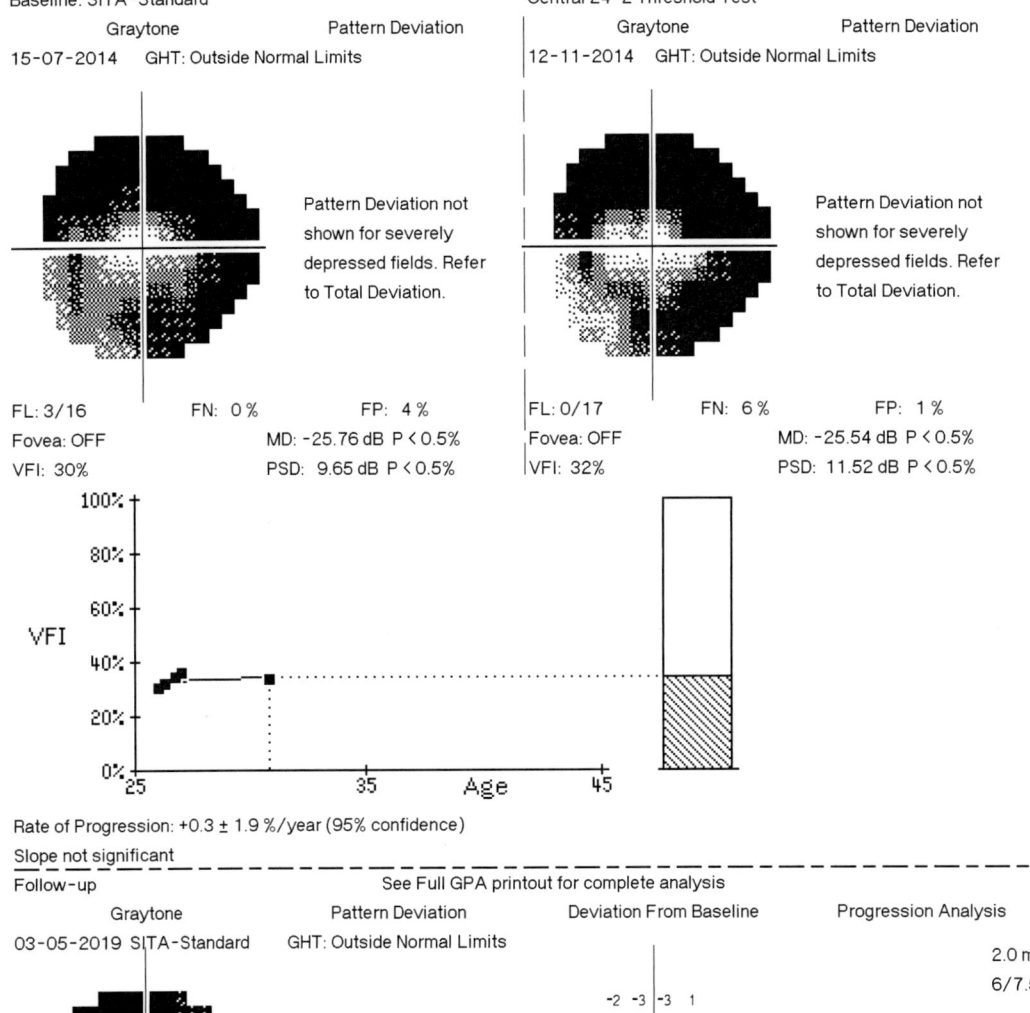

On July 15, 2014 patient presented with very high IOP of 42 mm Hg in the left eye. After initial control of IOP, surgery in the form of trabeculectomy with Ologen implant was advised and was performed on August 1, 2014. Subsequent perimetry shows stable fields. Patient went out of country after 1 year and reported after almost 4 years. As the fields are severely depressed, pattern deviation is not given. Rate of progression is +0.3–1.9%, where the slope is not significant. (+) sign may indicate stability or that there may be improvement.

5.14 Case 5

A patient with advanced glaucoma in the right eye.

OD GPA between 73 and 80 years (2013–2020).

5.14.1 OD ONH Colour Photo

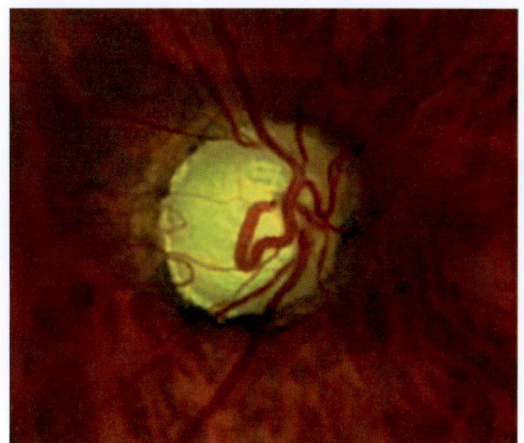

5.14.2 OD ONH Red-Free Photo

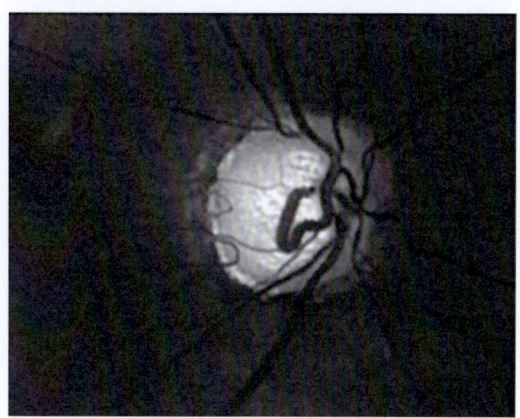

5.14.3 OD GPA

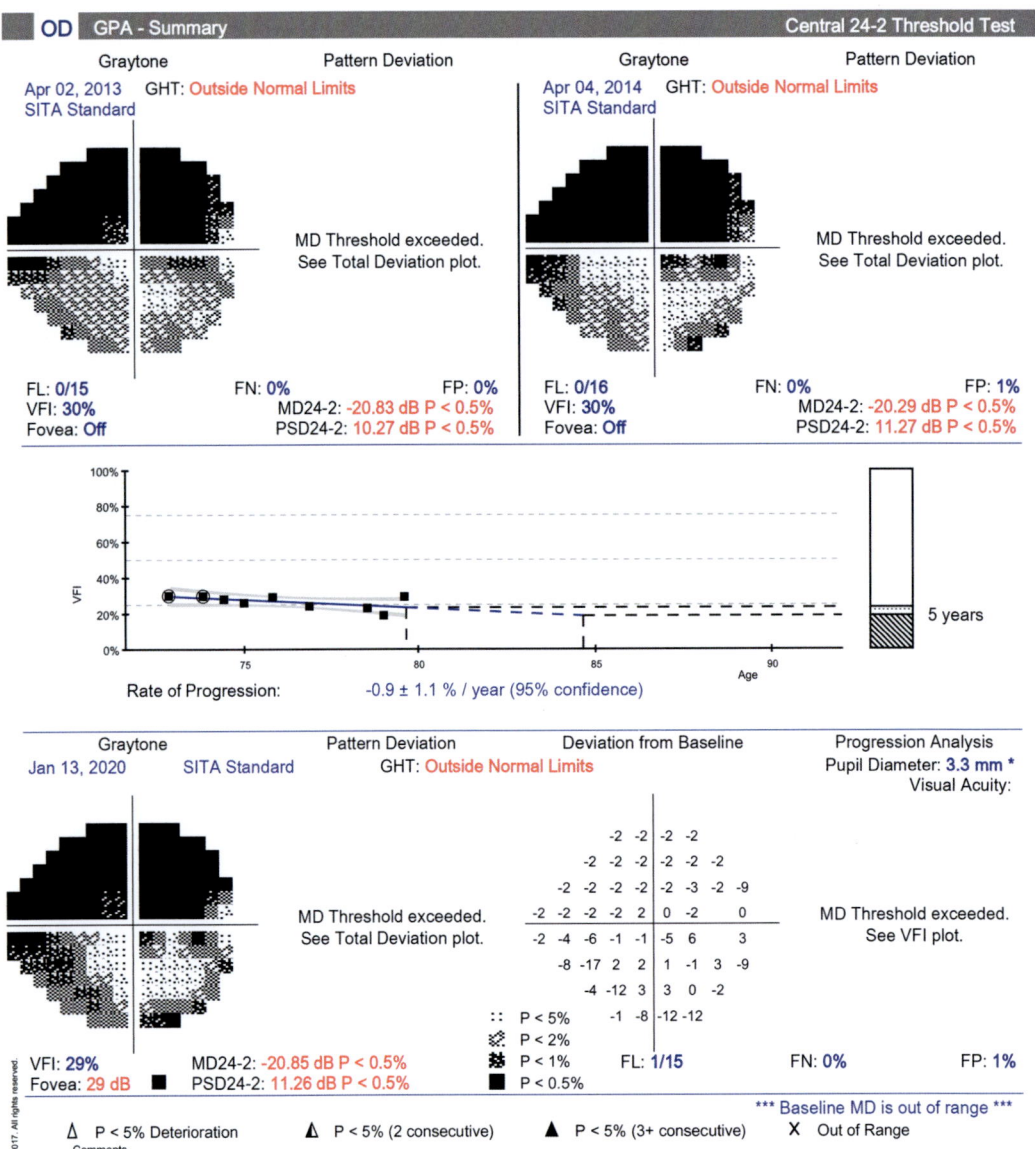

5.14.3.1 Advanced Glaucoma

Baseline MD is out of range. Pattern deviation is not shown. Change in decibel values given in "Deviation from baseline" needs to be monitored. Also progression analysis is not possible for severely depressed fields. VFI progression plot shows "borderline progression."

Rate of progression −0.9 ± 1.1%/year (95% confidence).

Projection for next 5 years shows slow progression on GPA.

In patients with advanced field loss and severely depressed fields, it is necessary to compare serial 10–2 tests with overview. GPA is not available for 10–2.

5 Evaluating Progression on Perimetry

OD 10-2 overview

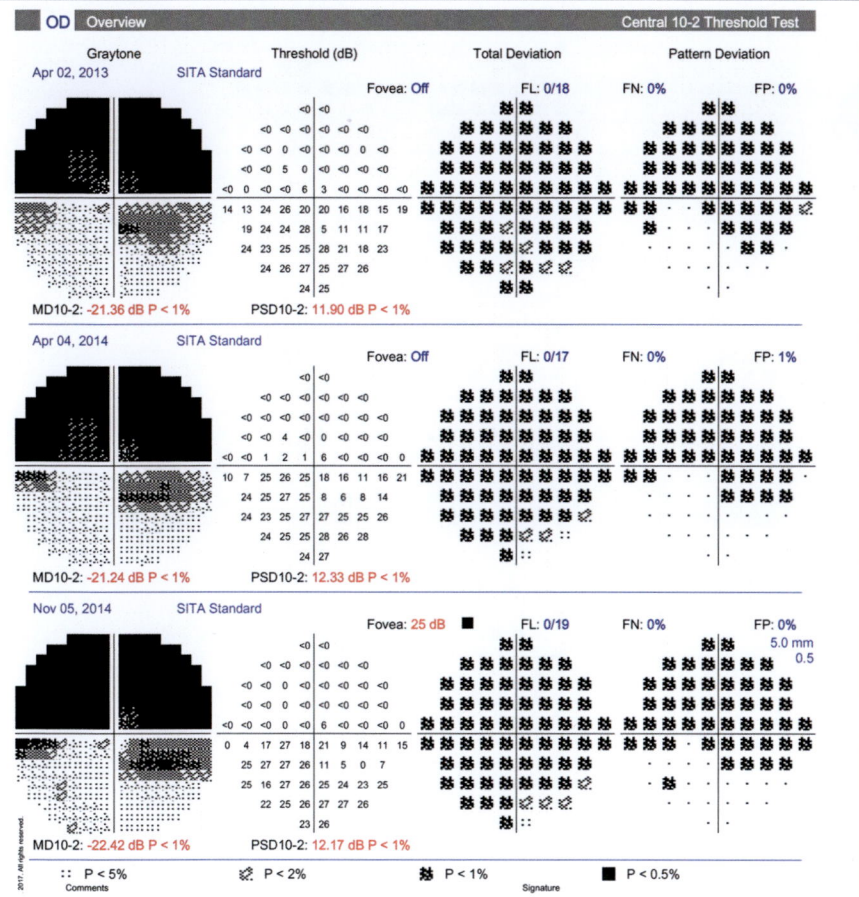

OD 10-2 shows threat to fixation in superior 2 quadrants

OD 10-2 overview

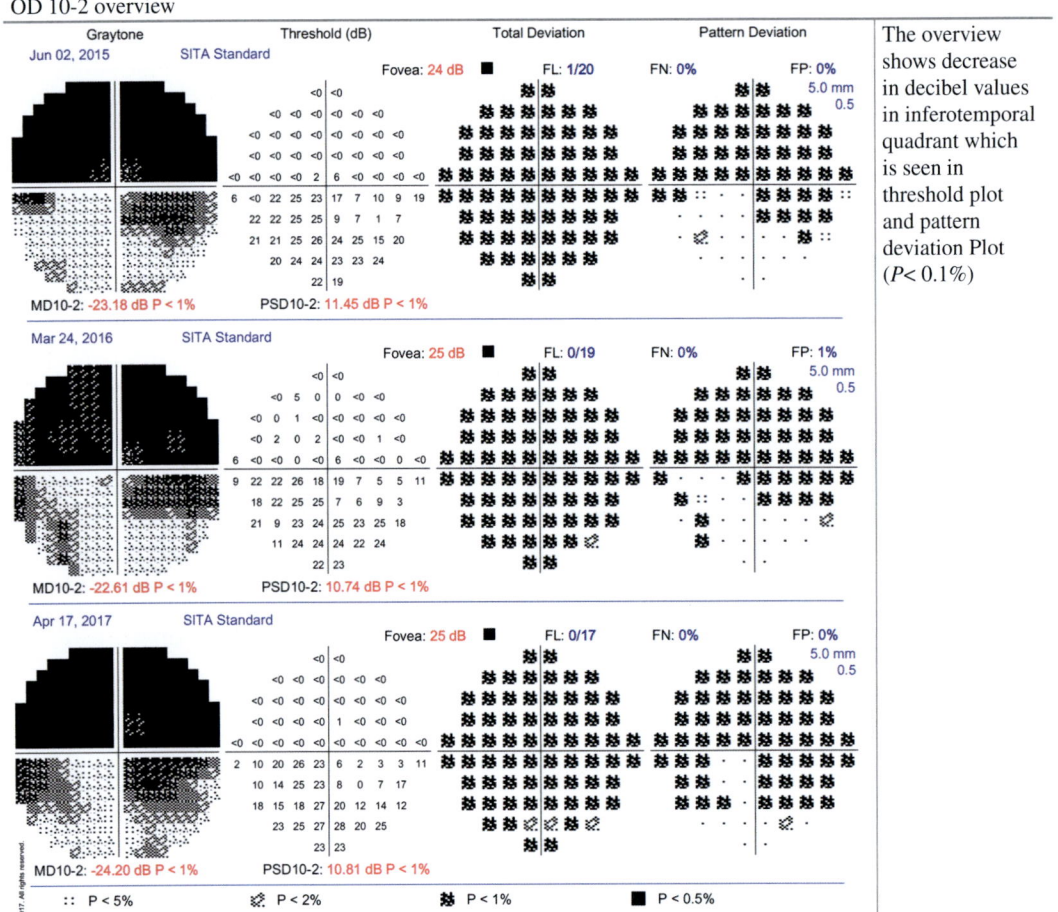

The overview shows decrease in decibel values in inferotemporal quadrant which is seen in threshold plot and pattern deviation Plot ($P < 0.1\%$)

OD 10-2 overview

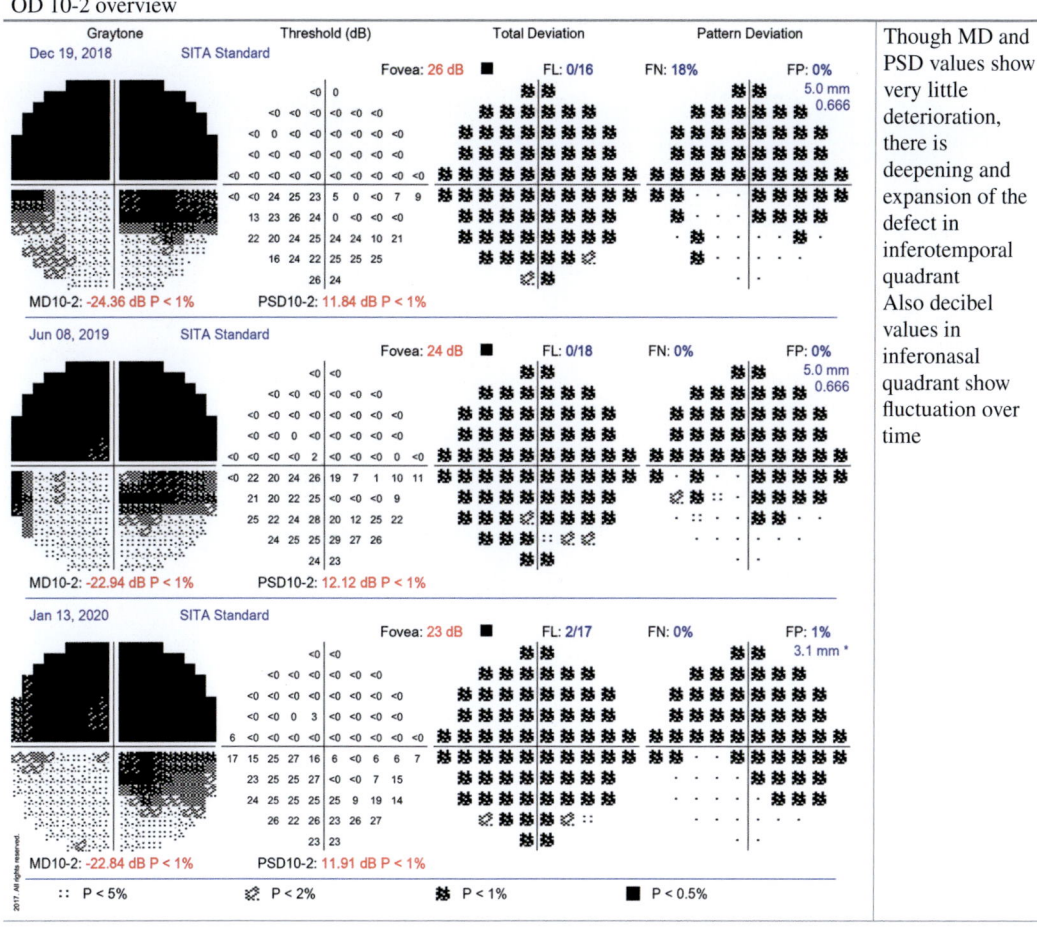

Though MD and PSD values show very little deterioration, there is deepening and expansion of the defect in inferotemporal quadrant
Also decibel values in inferonasal quadrant show fluctuation over time

5.15 Case 6

46 years old patient, diagnosed as right eye acute angle closure glaucoma with IOP of 48 mm Hg.
OD GPA between 46 and 48 years (2017–2019).

5.15.1 OD ONH Colour Photo

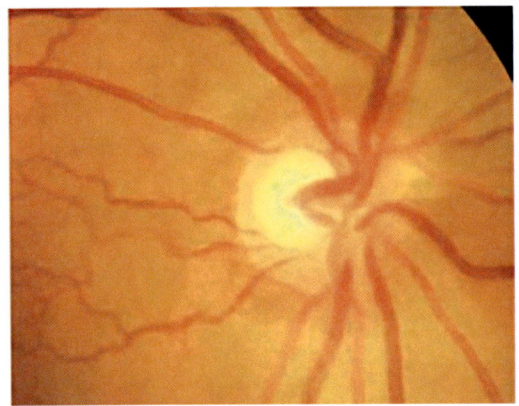

5.15.2 OD ONH Red-Free Photo

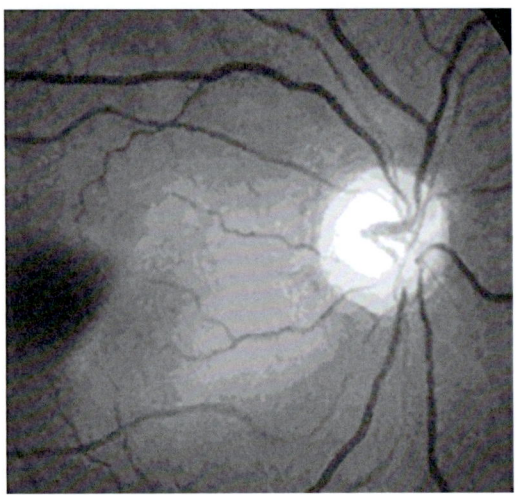

5.15.3 OD GPA 1

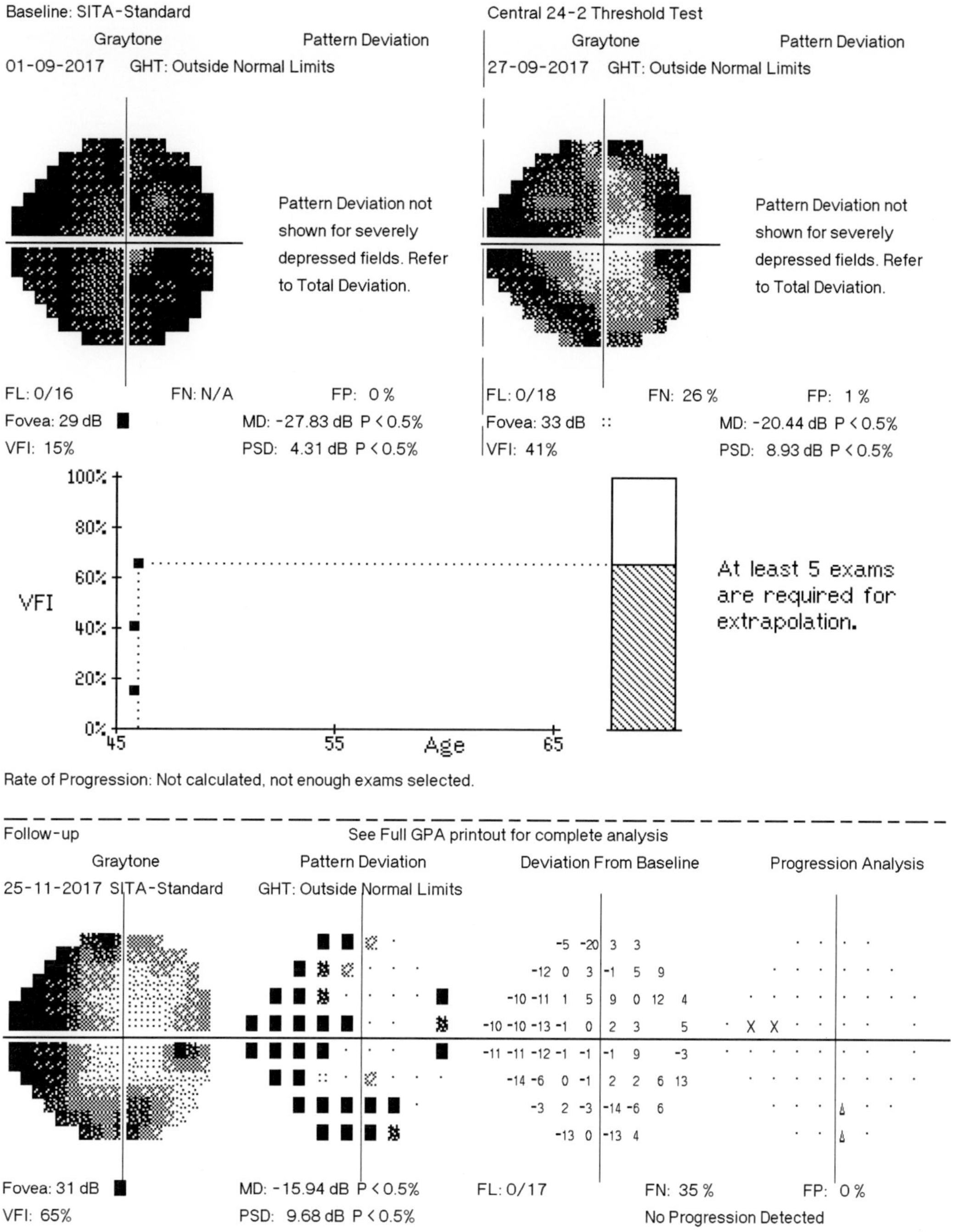

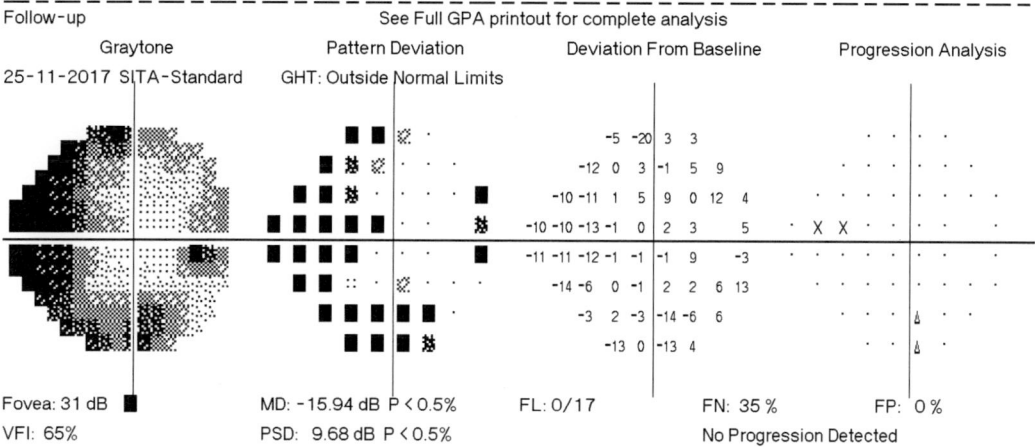

Rate of Progression: Not calculated, not enough exams selected.

Right eye angle remained closed in 3 quadrants even after Nd YAG peripheral iridectomy. There is improvement in field of vision after control of IOP with medications. Field of vision improved further after trabeculectomy.

Baseline MD is out of range due to severely depressed field, note that false negatives are more in each field.

5.15.4 OD GPA 2

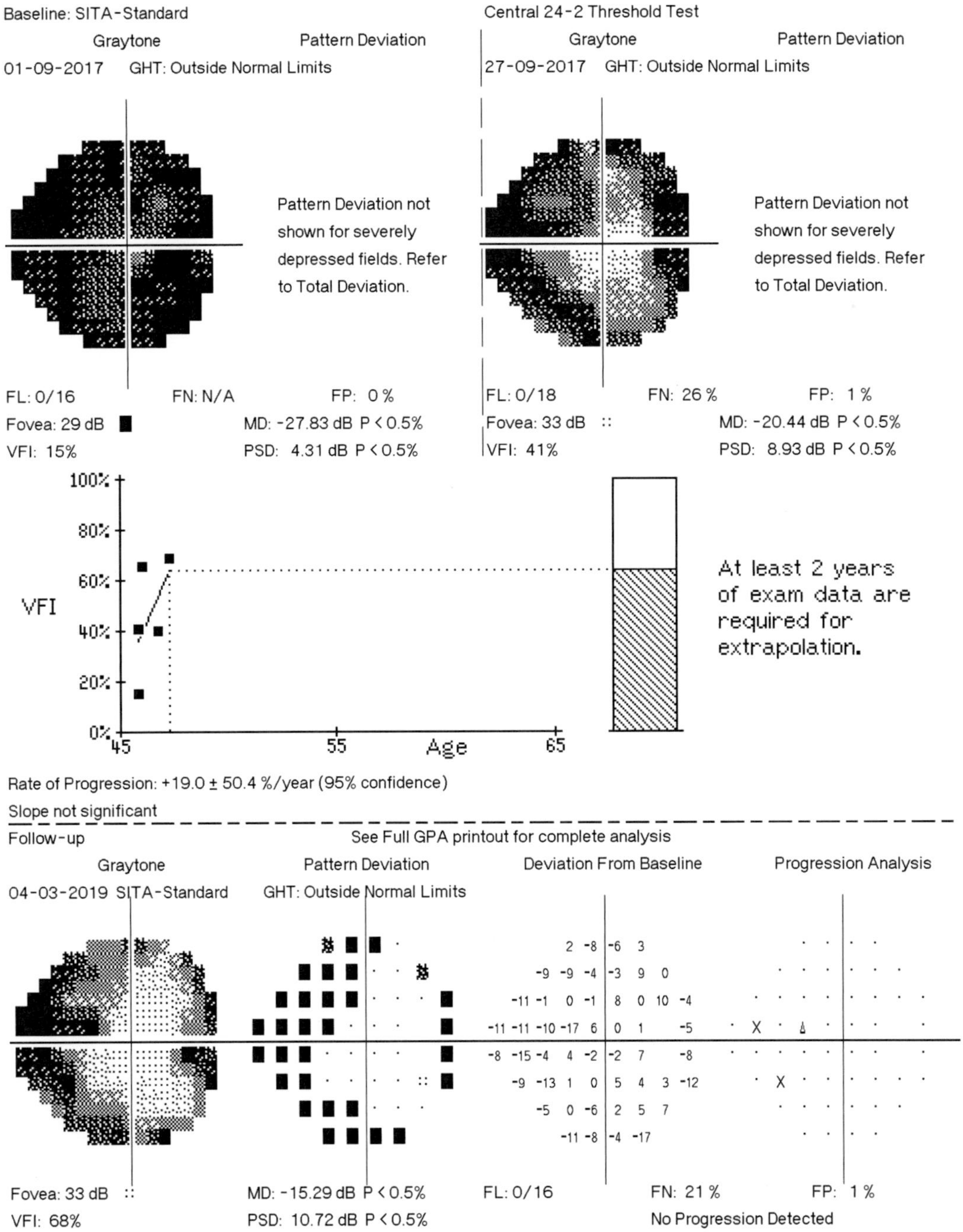

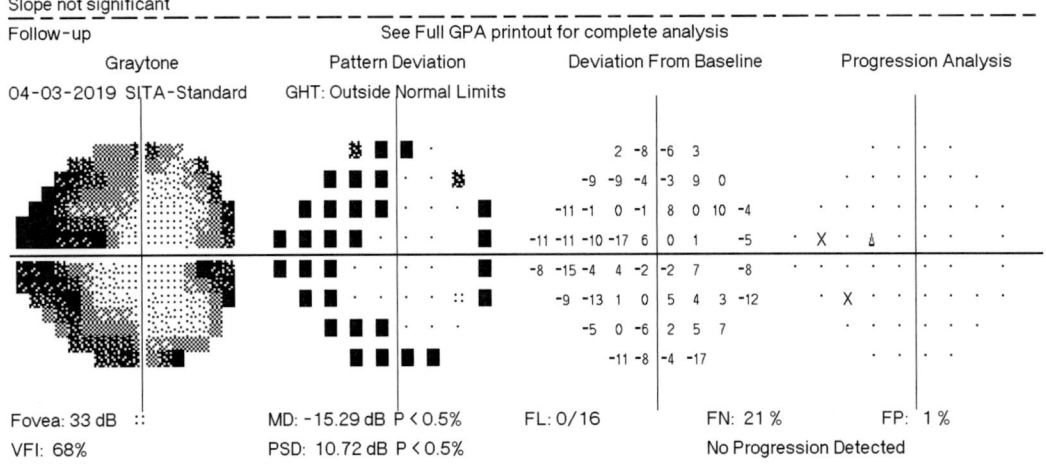

Rate of progression +19.0 ±50.4% per year, (+) sign shows improvement from the first field. Fourth visual field was unreliable.

There is a need to establish a new baseline for this patient, after control of IOP following surgical intervention, to find out progression or worsening in future.

5.16 Case 7

A patient with moderate myopia and family history of advanced glaucoma.

OD GPA between 28 and 31 years (2016–2019).

5.16.1 OD GPA 1

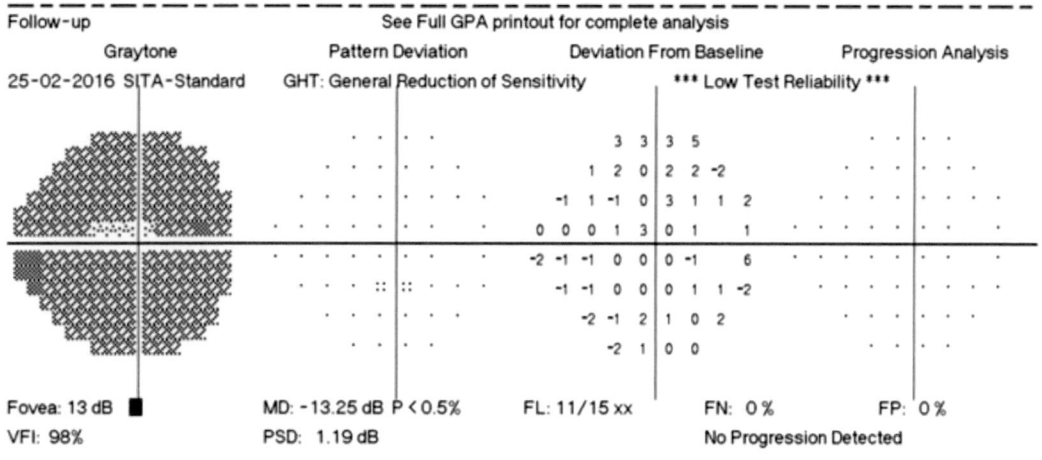

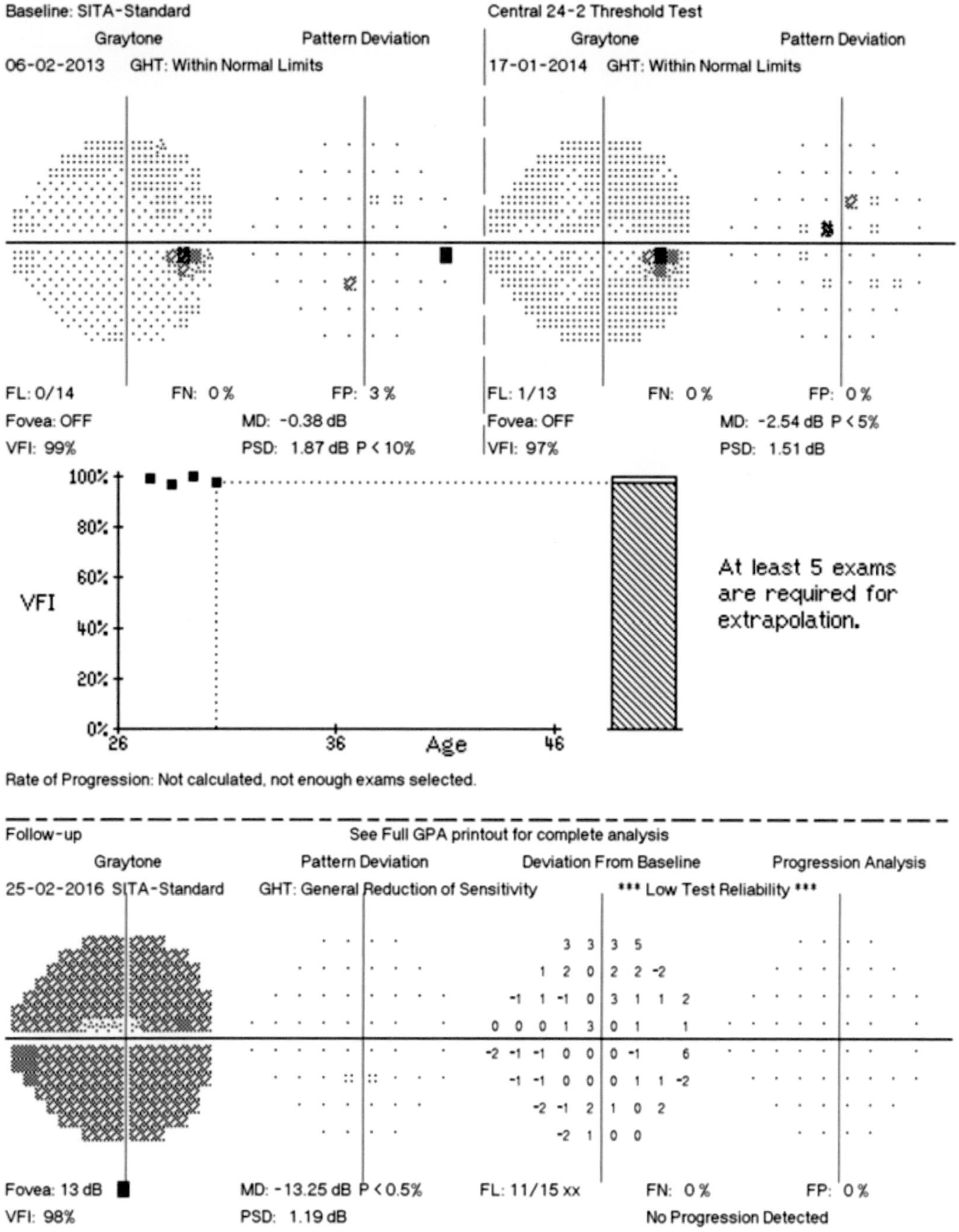

Refractive error was not corrected in visual field test (done on February 25, 2016) inadvertently. "Low test reliability" message is displayed, as there are high fixation losses. (Fovea: 13 db).

Patient's MD shows low value (−13.25 dB), but it does not reflect in VFI progression plot.
GPA alert shows no progression detected.

5.16.2 OD GPA 2

Test was repeated after 2 days with proper correction.

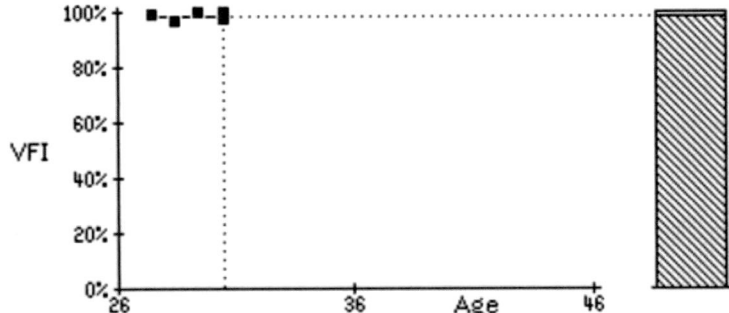

After correction of refractive error, MD is −2.17 dB. There is not much difference in PSD values. Also note improvement in foveal threshold from 13 to 34 dB.

5.17 Case 8

A 62 years patient with diagnosis of secondary glaucoma in the right eye. High IOP (35–38 mmHg) was noted 2 weeks post cataract surgery. IOP became stable after initial aggressive medical management. Now IOP is stable with one antiglaucoma eyedrop daily.

OD GPA between 62 and 66 years (2015–2019).

5.17.1 OD ONH Color Photo

5.17.2 OD ONH Red-Free Photo

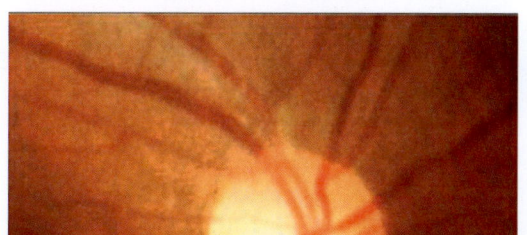

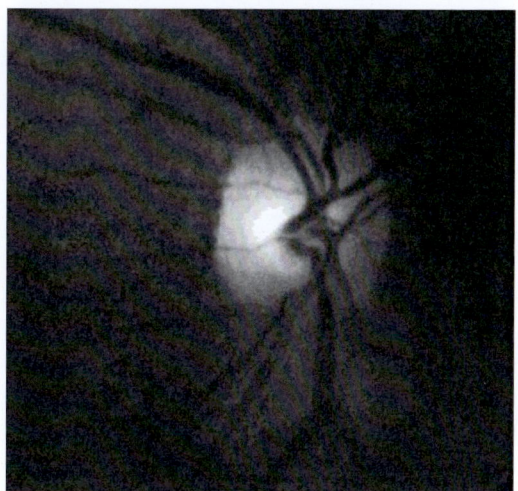

5.17.3 OD GPA

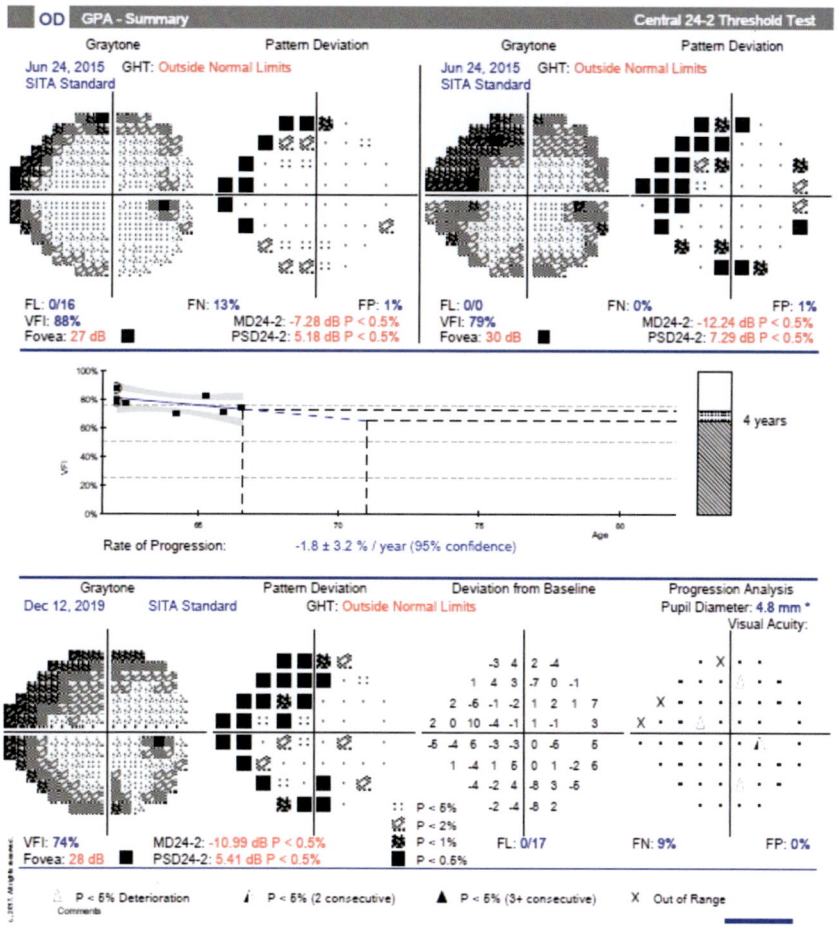

OD ONH color and red-free photos do not show features of glaucomatous optic neuropathy, still visual field shows changes. This may be due to short duration of raised IOP.

First VF was done after control of IOP, which shows borderline false negatives. Test was repeated on the same day and after a week after explaining properly. There is generalized loss of decibel values (MD −7.28 dB in first field). This may be due to resolving corneal edema initially, but later on also confounded by early posterior capsular opacification which may need YAG laser capsulotomy in future.

After four and half years, rate of progression is −1.8 ± 3.2%/year (95% confidence).

VFI bar shows future progression if the same rate continues.

Progression bands: (Ref: Fig. 5.3) The gray bands in GPA indicate the statistical significance of the regression analysis. The upper/top band represents 97.5% significance for the upper edge and 90% significance for the lower edge.

The edges of the lower/bottom band represent 10% significance upper edge and 2.5% significance lower edge.

5.18 Case 9

34 years male patient, with diagnosis of steroid-induced glaucoma in both eyes (IOP noted 35 mm Hg 5 years back). Patient was using topical steroids for allergic conjunctivitis for 4 to 5 years, before developing high IOP. There is evidence of minimal posterior subcapsular cataractous changes in both eyes.

GPA between 34 and 41 years (2013–2020).

5.18.1 OD ONH Color Photo

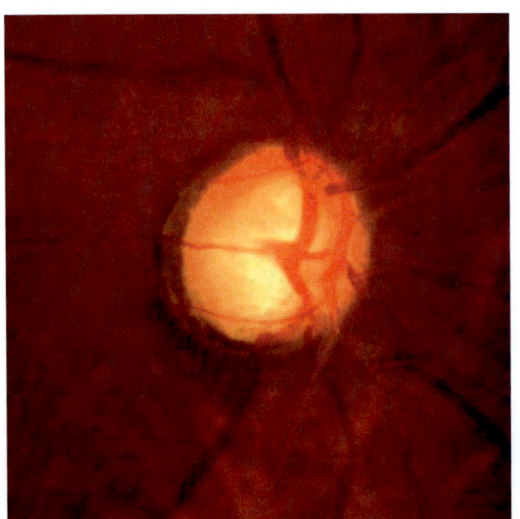

5.18.2 OD ONH Red-Free Photo

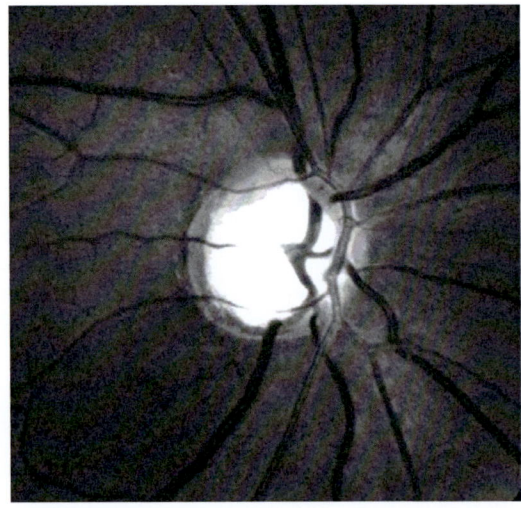

5.18.3 OU Combined Visual Field and ONH OCT Analysis Report

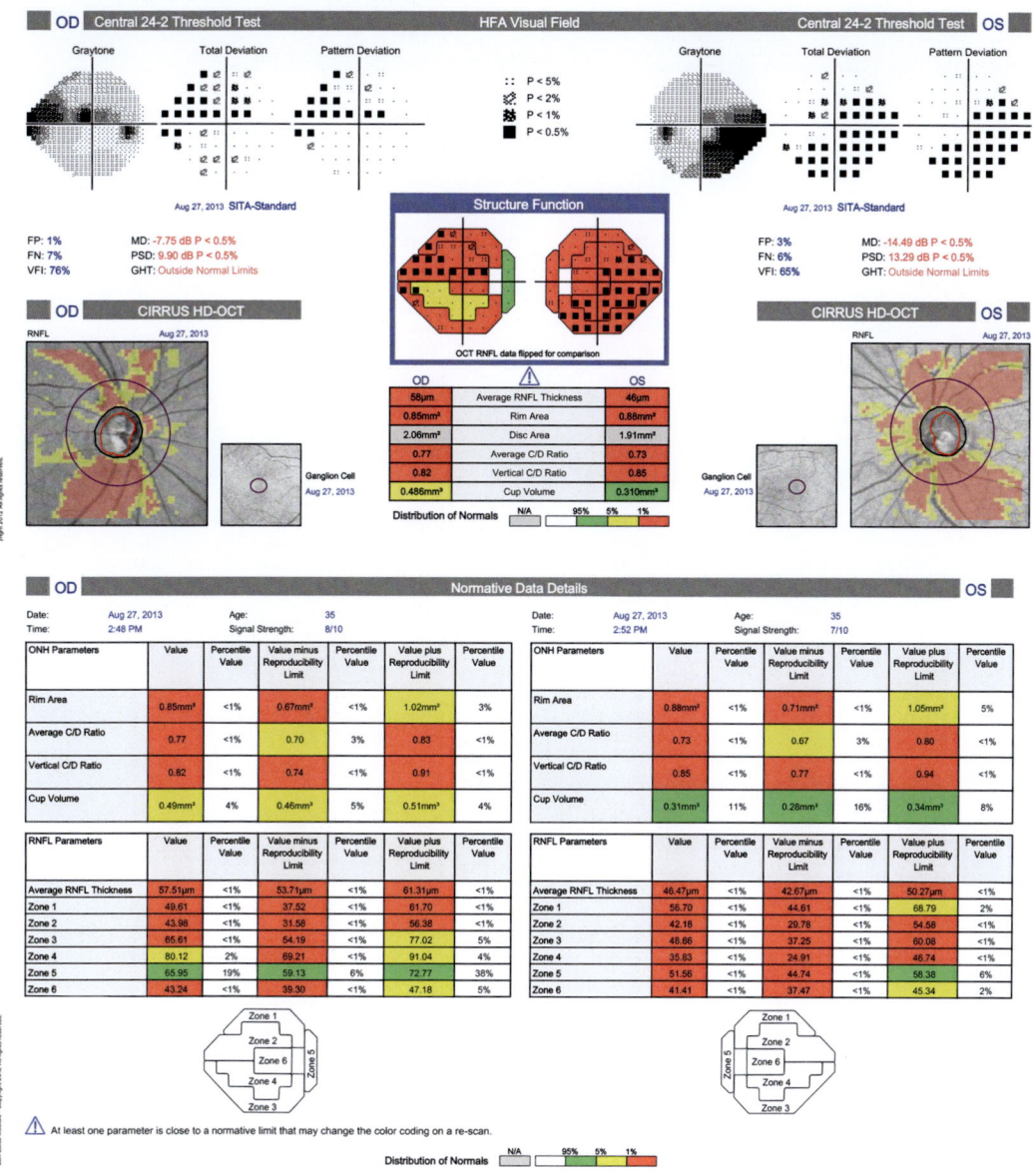

OD ONH photo shows signs of glaucomatous optic neuropathy along with RNFL thinning on OCT. On structure function correlation, structural loss is more than functional loss in both the eyes.

In this example, we will study the right eye in detail.

5.18.4 GPA

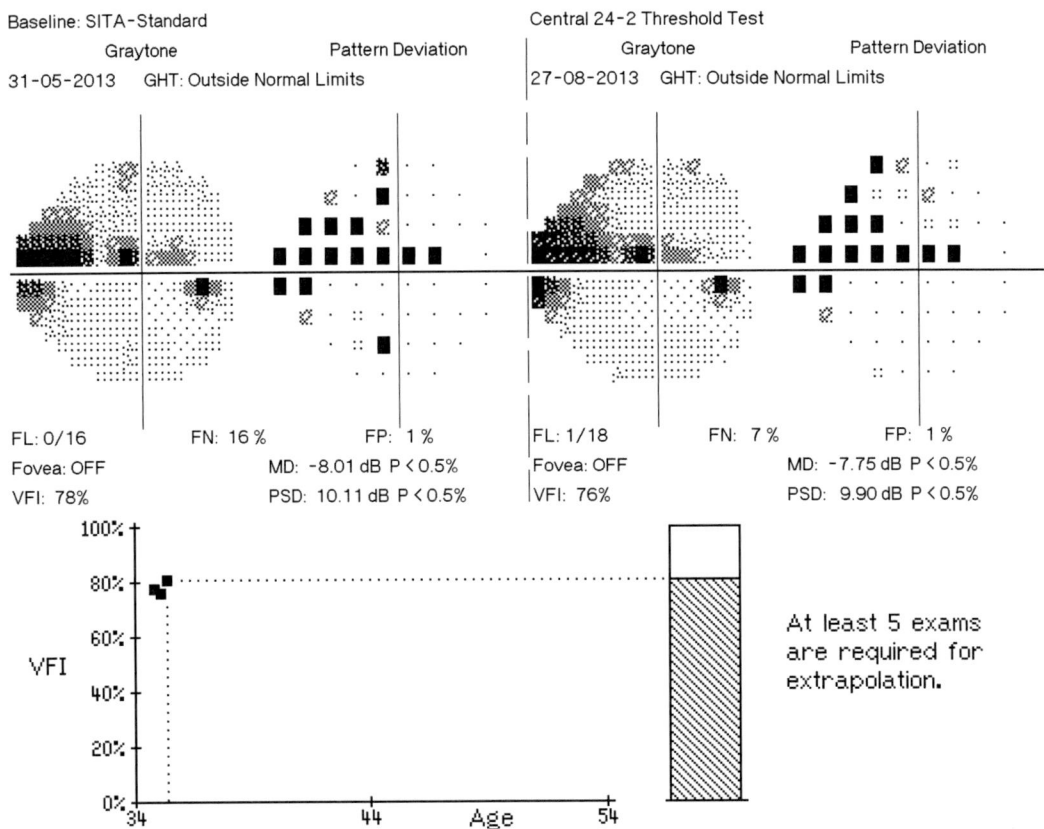

GPA of perimetry tests done on May 2013, August 2013, and December 2013.

Progression analysis shows few examined points out of range. GPA alert shows no progression.

Paracentral defect can be attributed to posterior subcapsular cataractous (PSC) changes.

FI plot graphs of tests from 2013 December to 2015 February

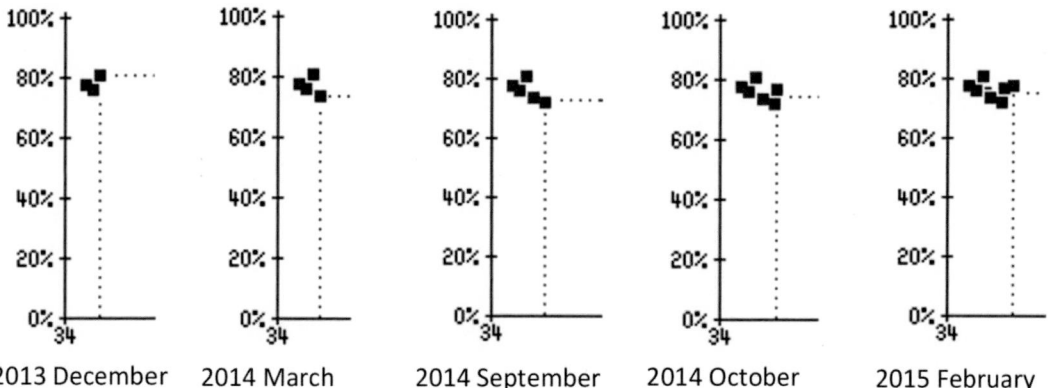

Consecutive GPAs from 2013 December to 2015 February show minimal fluctuation in VFI. Future progression is not shown in these GPAs as 2 years data are required for extrapolation

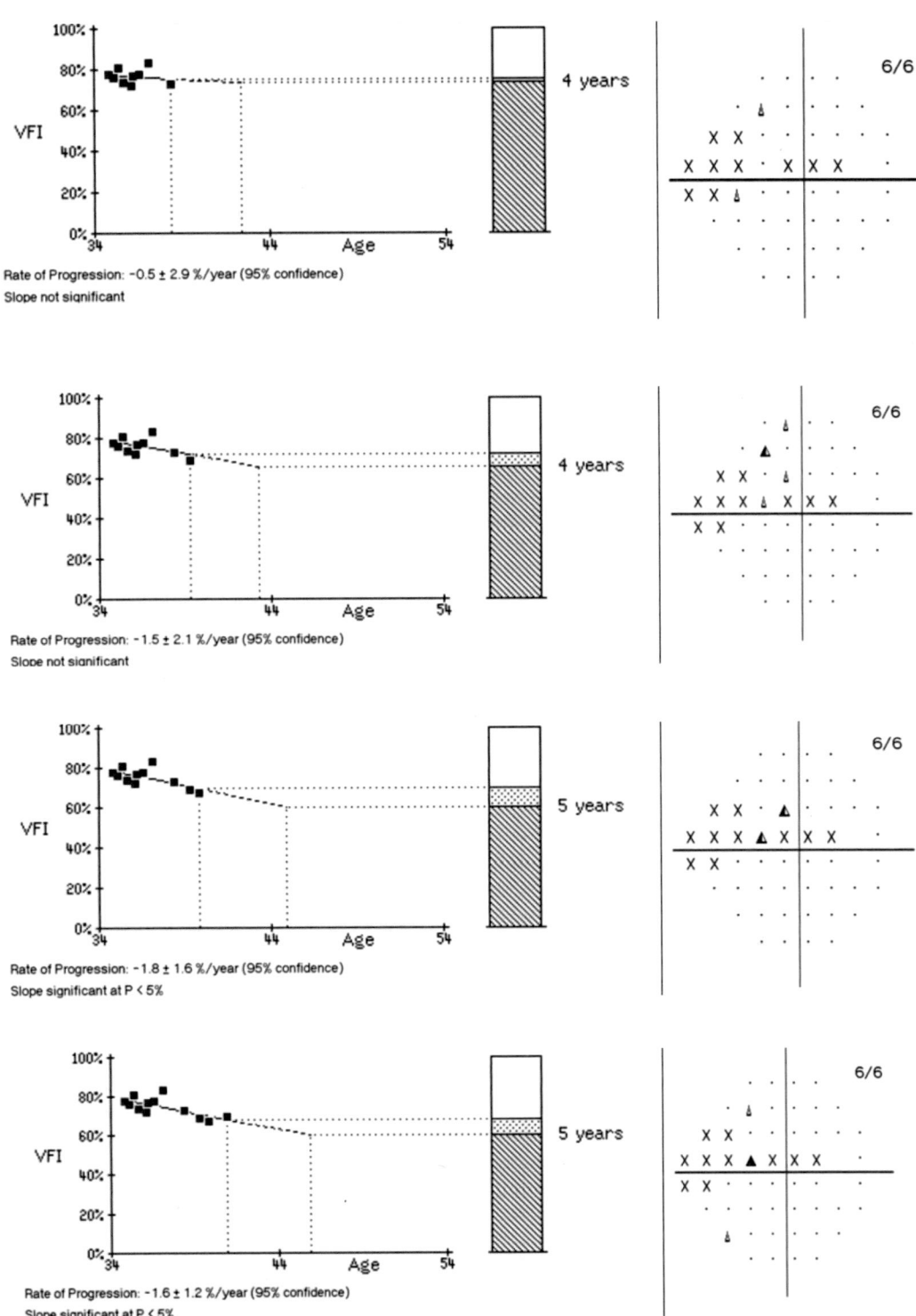

GPAs from December 2016 to June 2019. The patient has a defect near fixation which can be due to PSC cataract. The values near fixation are out of range. There is a development of open triangle next to it on November 2017, which shows deterioration on consecutive tests (half closed on June 2018 and closed triangle on June 2019). Ref: Table 5.2

5 Evaluating Progression on Perimetry

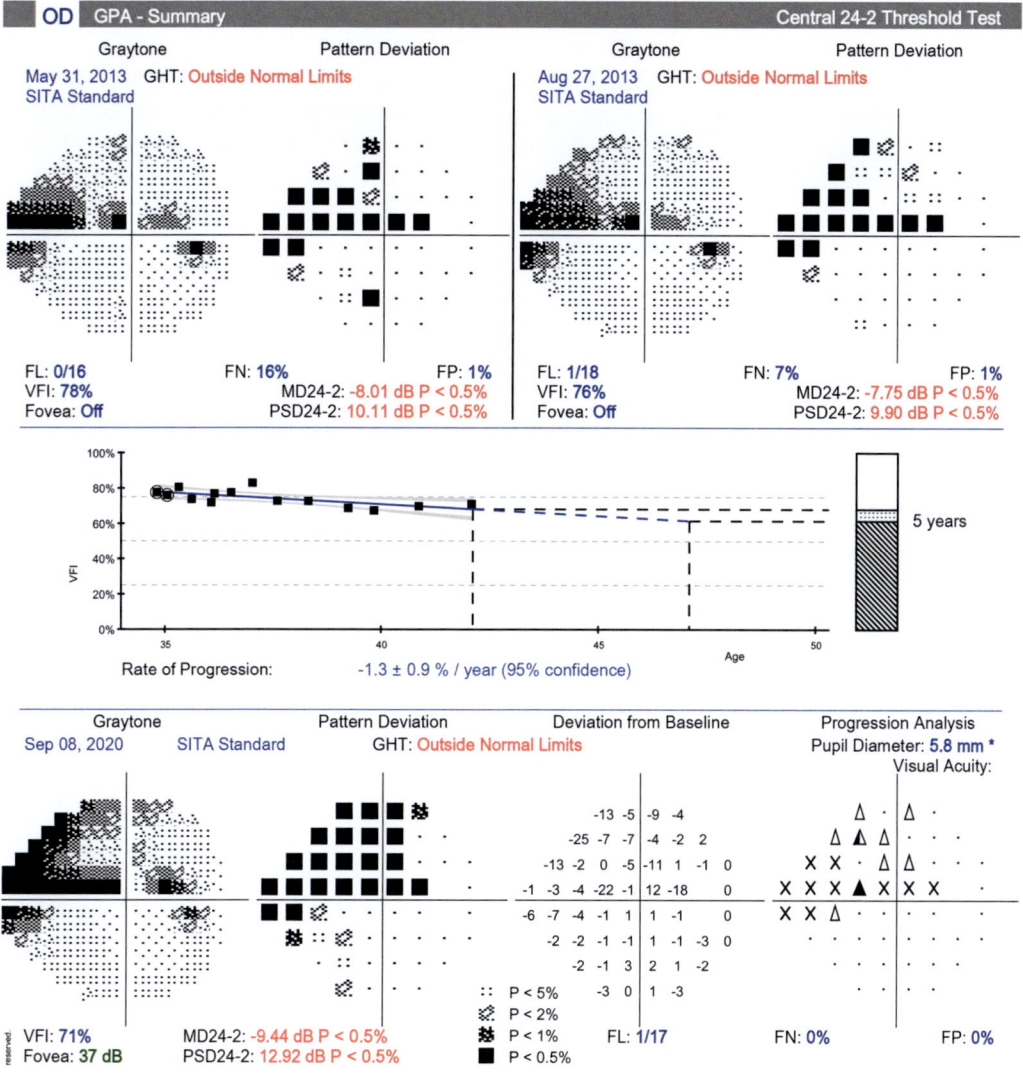

GPA. Recent GPA of the right eye

Date	VFI in %	MD dB	PSD dB	ROP[a] % per year (95% confidence)	GPA alert
2013 May	78	−8.01	10.11	Not calculated	Not available
2013 August	76	−7.75	9.90	Not calculated	Not available
2013 December	81	−6.61	8.83	Not calculated	No progression detected
2014 March	74	−7.97	11.02	Not calculated	No progression detected
2014 September	72	−10.64	12.62	−4.7 ± 9.0	No progression detected
2014 October	77	−7.91	9.78	−2.7 ± 6.7	No progression detected
2015 February	78	−7.71	10.37	−1.2 ± 4.9	No progression detected
2016 December	73	−9.32	11.26	−0.5 ± 3.2	No progression detected
2017 November	69	−11.49	12.78	−1.5 ± 2.1	No progression detected
2018 June	67	−11.94	12.35	−1.8 ± 1.6	No progression detected
2019 June	70	−10.07	12.39	−1.6 ± 1.2	No progression detected
2020 September	71	−9.44	12.92	−1.3 ± 0.9	Not given

[a]ROP: Rate of progression

Rate of progression is calculated after first five tests, over 17 months, (−4.7 ± 9.0% per year). It appears that the progression is rapid. But in follow-up of 7 years, VFI is reduced by 7% from baseline, MD change is −1.43 dB and PSD change is 2.81 dB. Rate of progression is −1.3 ± 0.9% per year over 7 years (above Table).

The patient has a defect near fixation which can be due to PSC cataract. There is a corresponding open triangle which shows progression November 2017 (above figure "GPAs from December 2016 to June 2019") onwards. After counselling, no surgical intervention was contemplated; as visual acuity as well as IOP remains in lower range (10–12 mm Hg) with single IOP lowering molecule.

This example shows the more visual field examinations you have over time, the better assessment of progression and prediction of future progression can be achieved.

5.19 Case 10

A patient with OD advanced glaucoma with preservation of central island of visual field.

GPA between 59 and 60 years (2013–2014).

5.19.1 OD ONH Color Photo

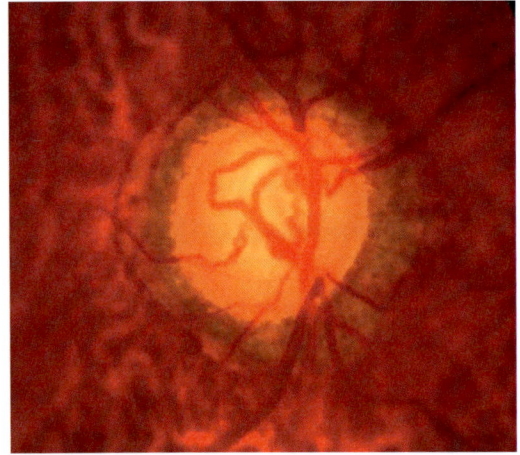

5.19.2 OD ONH Red-Free Photo

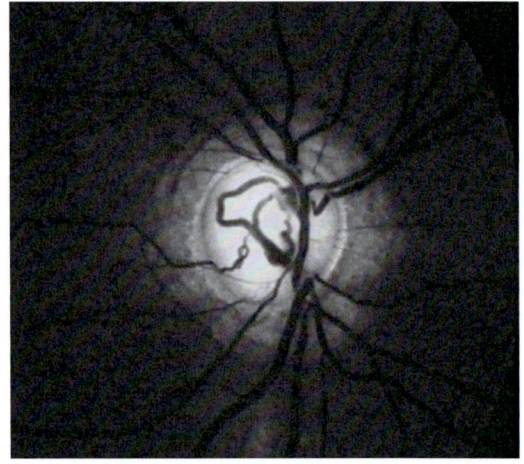

5.19.3 OD GPA

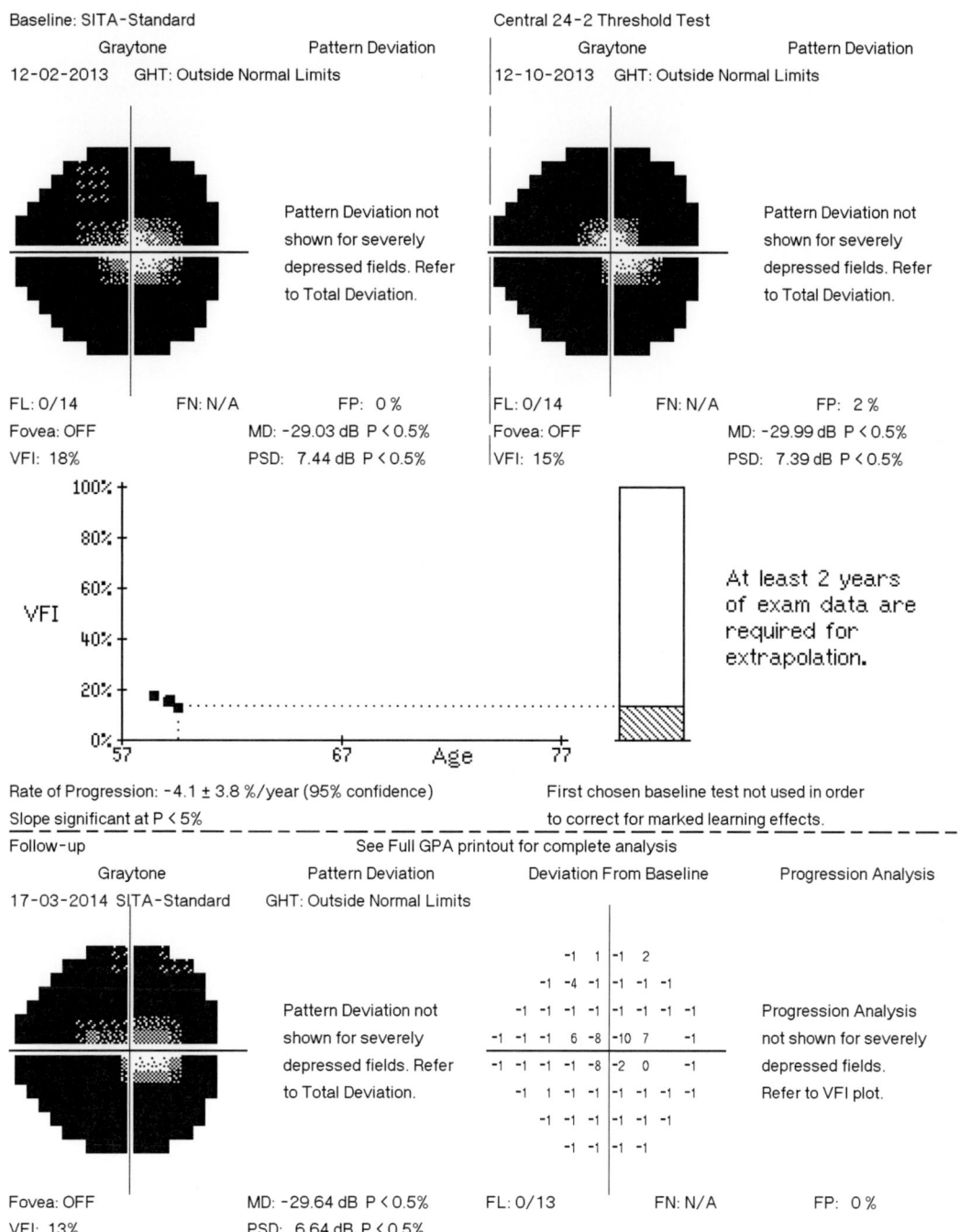

Rate of progression: −4.1 ± 3.8%/year. Slope significant at $P < 5\%$.

Pattern deviation and progression analysis are not shown as the fields are severely depressed. In "deviation from baseline plot," negative decibel values are given which show progression at each point.

5.19.4 OD: 10-2 Overview

OD 10-2 Overview of same patient between 2013 and 2015.

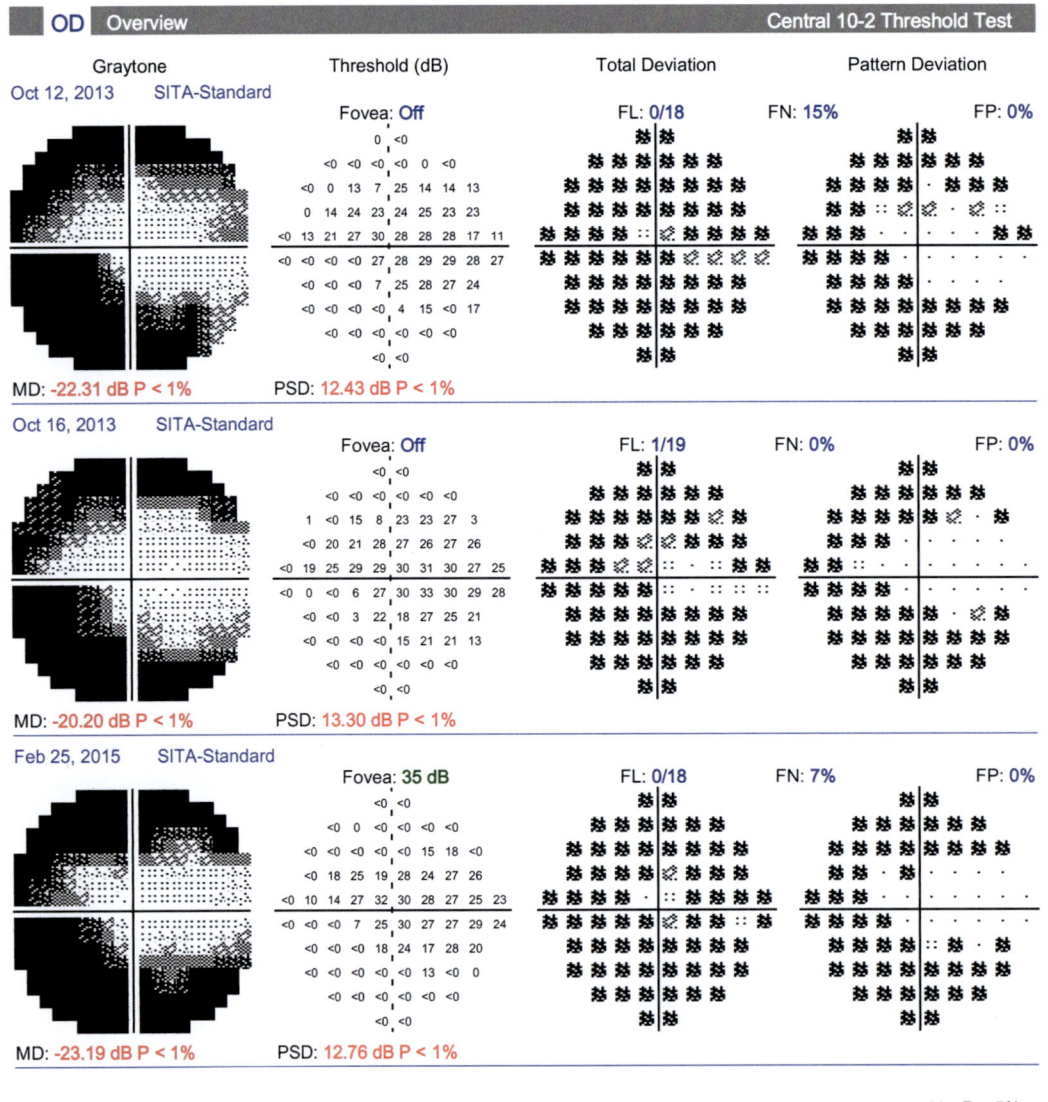

10-2 Overview along with probability symbols.

In advanced glaucoma, it becomes necessary to evaluate serial 10-2 visual fields. There is no GPA for 10-2 analysis. The overview also provides MD and PSD values for comparison. There is a need to check for individual decibel values along with probability symbol, to check if the central remaining field is stable or progressing.

References

1. Heijl A, Patella VM, Bengtsson B. The field analyzer primer: effective perimetry. 4th ed. Carl Zeiss Meditec; 2012.
2. Tanna AP, Desai RU. Evaluation of visual field progression in glaucoma. Curr Ophthalmol Rep. 2014;2:75–9. https://doi.org/10.1007/s40135-014-0038-4.
3. Nevalainen J, Paetzold J, Papageorgiou E, et al. Specification of progression in glaucomatous visual field loss, applying locally condensed stimulus arrangements. Graefes Arch Clin Exp Ophthalmol. 2009;247(12):1659–69. https://doi.org/10.1007/s00417-009-1134-2.
4. Hodapp E, Parrish RK II, Anderson DR. Clinical decisions in glaucoma. St. Louis: The CV Mosby Co; 1993. p. 52–61.
5. Anderson DR, Chauhan B, Johnson C, et al. Criteria for progression of glaucoma in clinical management and in outcome studies. Am J Ophthalmol. 2000;130(6):827–9.
6. Zeiss Mastering GPA Instruction Manual [Internet]. 2021 [cited 28 June 2021]. Available from: https://manuals.plus/zeiss/zeiss-mastering-gpa-manual-pdf.
7. Weinreb RN. Progression of glaucoma: the 8th consensus report of the world glaucoma association. Amsterdam: Kugler Publications; 2011.
8. Bengtsson B. Prediction of glaucomatous visual field loss by extrapolation of linear trends. Arch Ophthalmol. 2009;127(12):1610–5.
9. Heijl A. Reduction of intraocular pressure and glaucoma progression. Arch Ophthalmol. 2002;120(10):1268–79.
10. Weinreb RN. Diagnosis of primary open angle glaucoma: the 10th consensus report of the world glaucoma association. Amsterdam: Kugler Publications; 2017.
11. Bengtsson B, Heijl A. A visual field index for calculation of glaucoma rate of progression. Am J Ophthalmol. 2008;145:343–53. https://doi.org/10.1016/j.ajo.2007.09.038.
12. Bengtsson B, Lindgren A, Heijl A, Lindgren G, Asman P, Patella M. Perimetric probability maps to separate change caused by glaucoma from that caused by cataract. Acta Ophthalmol Scand. 1997;75:184–8.

Interpretation of Octopus Visual Fields

6

N. R. Rangaraj and P. Sathyan

6.1 Introduction to Octopus Perimeter

The basic concept to the first prototype of the automated static perimetry was developed by Fankhauser et al. in Berne, Switzerland in 1972 [1]. The initial development work was started in 1957 on an automated kinetic perimetry, and this was abandoned in favor of an automated computer-assisted static perimetry which was introduced as the Octopus 201 in 1975. The mathematical and statistical approaches for the optimal test points in the program and the approach to determine the differential sensitivity or the strategy were refined to give a reliable and reproducible central visual field report that was due to the extensive work by Fankhauser and Bebie.

There was continuous development in the programs from the initial P32 (30-2) to the G program introduced by Flammer in 1985 [2]. The strategy introduced in the first machines was the full threshold testing, subsequently the Dynamic (Weber) [3] and TOP (Gonzalez de la Rosa) strategies [4] were added to the versatile

N. R. Rangaraj (✉)
Premier Eye Care and Surgical Center, Chennai, India

P. Sathyan
Sathyan Eye Care Hospital and Coimbatore Glaucoma Foundation, Coimbatore, India

perimeter. The newer strategies were able to match the full threshold with an economy of time and test points. The modern Octopus 900 incorporates the static and kinetic perimetry [5] in one machine with the cupola similar to the original Goldmann manual perimeter. The Octopus 600, the smaller sibling is a standalone static only automated perimeter used in compact clinics and spaces for central visual field testing featuring the same programs and strategies.

6.2 Interpretation of a Visual Field Test Report

The visual field test report is structured to give the best representation of the raw values measured during the visual field examination of the patient. The EyeSuite software in the Octopus perimeter generates the "7 in 1" and the "9 in 1" printout of single measured fields. The representations in an Octopus printout are of three types; 1. The values or measured values from the visual field test; 2. Comparisons or values indexed to normal age match data; and 3. Corrected comparisons or values derived after correcting for diffuse defects, which highlight focal defects.

The other representations in the printout are derived from the above representations providing unique graphic statistical significance at each tested point. The cumulative defect curve or the

© The Author(s), under exclusive license to Springer Nature Singapore Pte Ltd. 2021
S. Patyal, M. Gandhi (eds.), *Resolving Dilemmas in Perimetry*,
https://doi.org/10.1007/978-981-16-2601-2_6

Bebie curve ranks the best to the worst sensitivity values from the left to right. The probability plots are representation from the numeric value of the comparisons and corrected comparisons. The global indices reduce all numeric values in the tested locations to a single numeric value.

6.2.1 Values: Sensitivity Threshold Display

The perimeter measures the differential light sensitivity values as dB (decibels) and presents the raw data of the visual field test as the values table. These values are represented as the two-dimensional gray scale values (Fig. 6.1) and as numerical values (Fig. 6.2). The gray scales as they are so called is a historical legacy term when there was only a monochrome printer. The gray scale representations are now displayed in color. The color/monochrome representation gives a good idea of the hill of vision. Each color or the shade of gray in the gray scale table represents a range of 5 dB. The color gray scale graph gives a better visual impression of the dynamic range of sensitivities along with the topography in the pattern of visual field loss. The gray scale can be used to counsel the patient on the loss of visual fields.

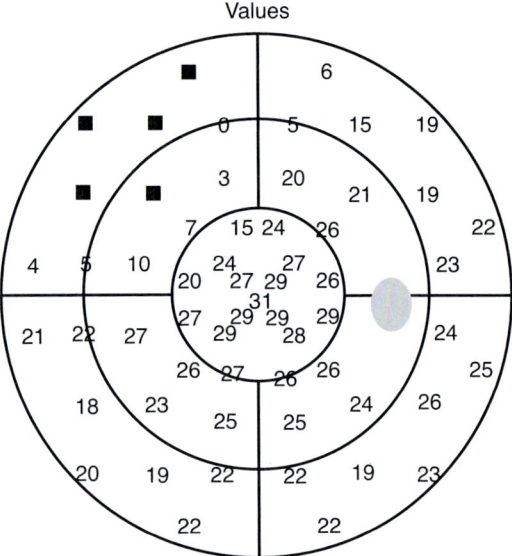

Fig. 6.2 Numeric values

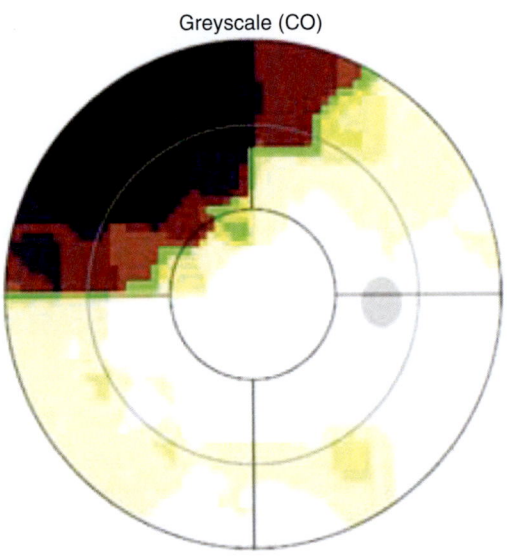

Fig. 6.1 Gray scale

6.2.2 Comparisons: With Normal Age Match

The comparisons table represents the deviation from the age match taking account of the location of the tested point. The sensitivity of the peripheral test point location is less than the central points. A meaningful representation normalizes each of the test point to age and location to reduce the clutter. This table represents the index of deviation from the normal. The representations are in the form of "+" which are normal values with numerical values denoting deviations of more than 4 dB from normal values (Fig. 6.3). The comparisons gray scale plots the graph from the comparisons table highlighting the topography of the pattern of defect. Octopus allows the selection of the gray scale graph from either the raw values (Fig. 6.4) or the age and location matched values (Fig. 6.5) which highlights the topography of defect with no clutter at intervals of approximately 10 dB intervals.

6 Interpretation of Octopus Visual Fields

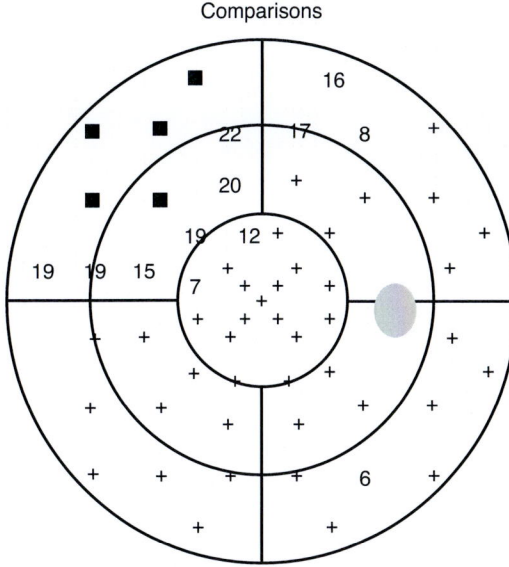

Fig. 6.3 Comparisons

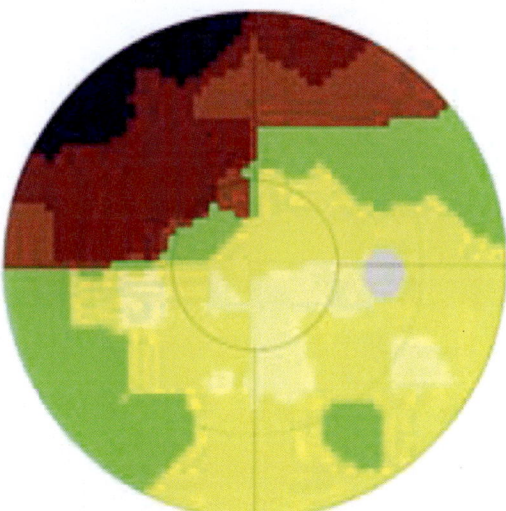

Fig. 6.4 Gray scales from raw values

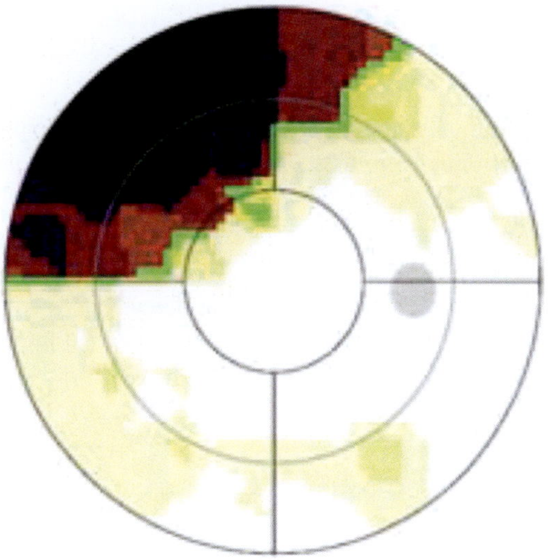

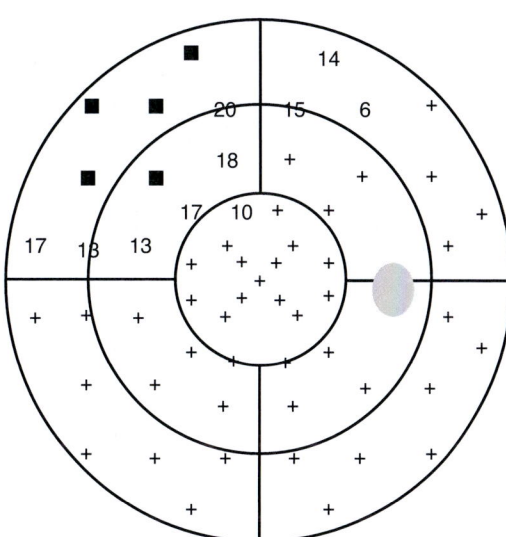

Fig. 6.5 Gray scales from age indexed values

Fig. 6.6 Corrected comparisons

6.2.3 Corrected Comparisons: Eliminate the Effect of Diffuse Defect

Corrected comparisons are numerical tables derived after subtracting the effect of diffuse defects from the comparisons values which are already corrected for age-match normative values (Fig. 6.6). The representations are marked "+" when within bandwidth of 4 dB and numerical values when deviated at each test locations. The value to be subtracted from the comparisons is derived from the cumulative defect curve (Fig. 6.7). Comparisons unmask focal defects when hidden in a diffuse defect.

6.2.4 Cumulative Defect Curve: The Bebie Curve

The graphic representation is based on comparisons value (Fig. 6.8). The sensitivity values from the age-corrected comparisons table are ranked left to right, from the smallest to the worst values, respectively. The defect curve does not indicate the topography of the defect. The defect curve also gives the normative bandwidth of upper and lower normal limits (extent of 90% normal) (Fig. 6.9) [6].

The defect curve shows a uniform parallel downward shift in diffuse defect (Fig. 6.10). Focal defects show a drop in the right-hand side of the curve (Fig. 6.11). A combination of diffuse and local defect is also well displayed (Fig. 6.12).

6.2.5 Probabilities Plots

The probabilities plot represents the probability that the tested location is within normal limits or not for a given age with normal visual field sensitivity. These plots are derived from the comparisons and corrected comparisons tables with a statistical symbolic representation. The two plots reflect the deviation with a probabil-

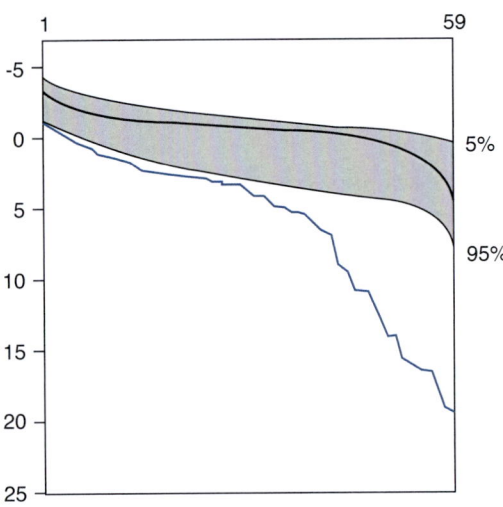

Fig. 6.7 Cumulative defect curve

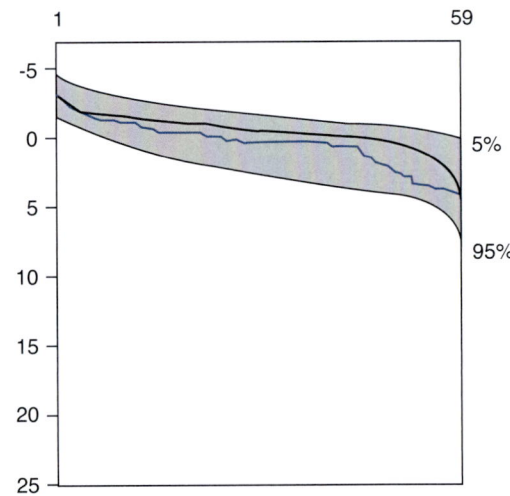

Fig. 6.9 Normal bandwidth of values

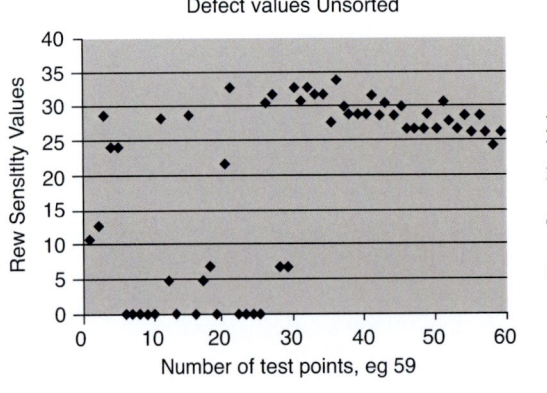

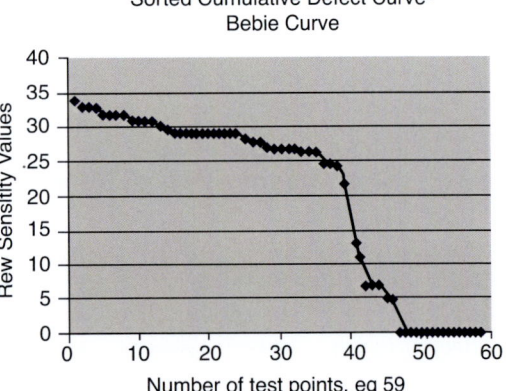

Fig. 6.8 Test points when sorted from high values on the left to low values on the right

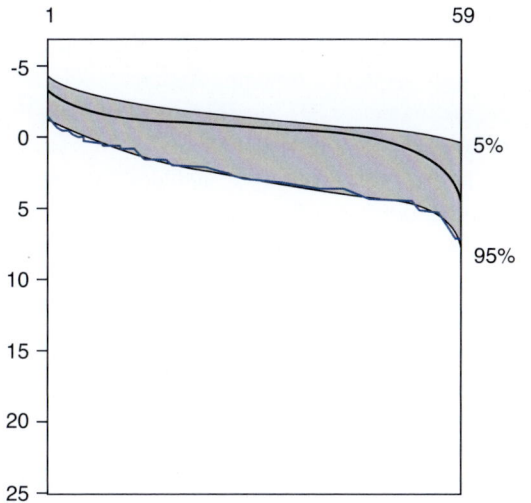

Fig. 6.10 Uniform down shift

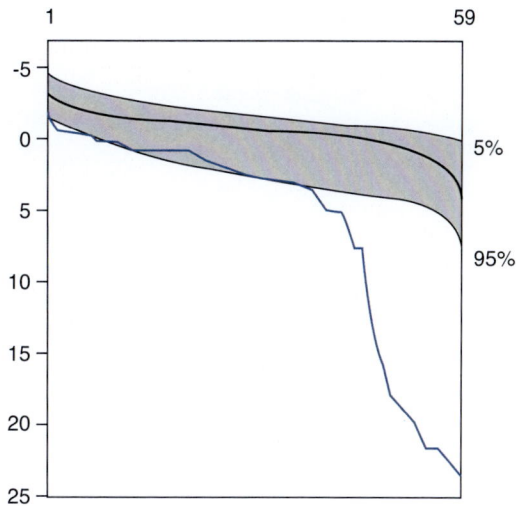

Fig. 6.12 Defect curve displays the diffuse and focal defect

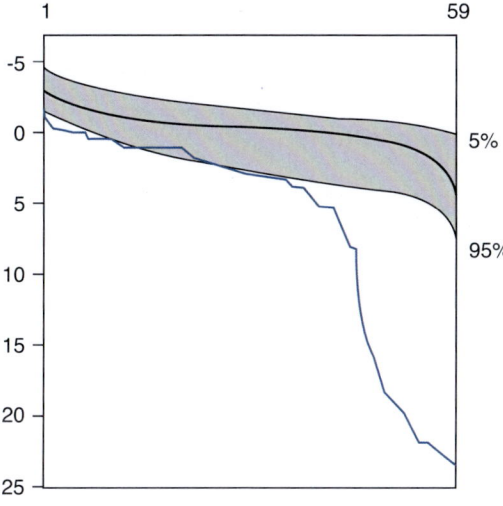

Fig. 6.11 Focal defect on the left

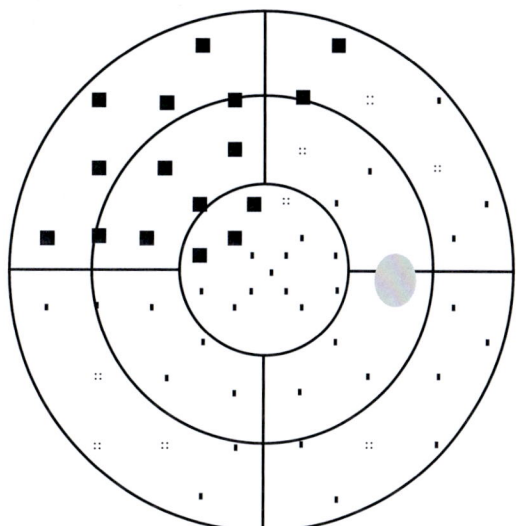

Fig. 6.13 Comparisons plot

ity of $P > 5\%$, $P < 5\%$, $P < 2\%$, $P < 1\%$, and $P < 0.5\%$ of being normal in the normal visual fields. (Figs. 6.13 and 6.14).

6.2.6 Visual Field Global Indices

The indices are global summary of the entire visual field. They serve three purposes: (1) summary of the status of visual field, (2) assess and classify the severity of the loss in visual function, and (3) the numerical values help track change over time. (Table 6.1). The color printout of the result flags the high values in red, along with the "p" value significance. Hence one need not remember the abnormal values.

6.2.7 Patient and Examination Data

The patient data contains information of the patient; these include name, gender, date of birth,

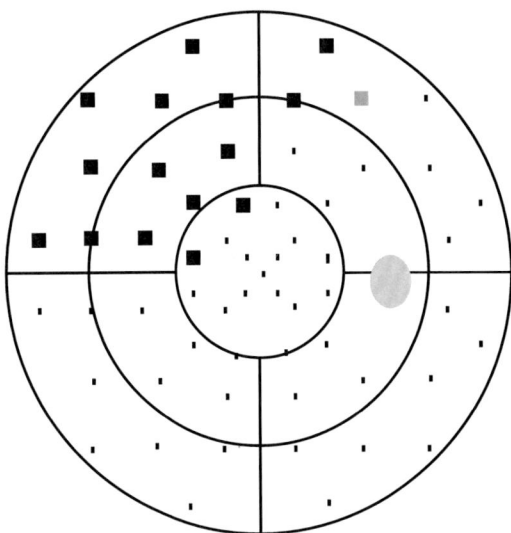

Fig. 6.14 Corrected comparisons plot

Table 6.1 Global indices—octopus perimeters [7]

Mean defect—MD	Arithmetic mean of the sensitivity values in the comparisons representations. MD is independent of age. Normal MD value is zero. 90% of normal visual fields are in the range of −2 to +2. MD indicates global damage
Square root of loss variance—sLV	Provides a measure of variability across the visual fields. sLV is large in local defects and small in diffuse defects
Diffuse defect—DD	DD is calculated from the 20th to 27th percentile which determines the shift from average normal defect curve representative of that location on the graph (Fig. 6.11)
Local defect—LD	LD identifies the presence of local progression. Quantifies the dB derived from the defect curve (Figs. 6.12 and 6.16)
Mean sensitivity—MS	Average of all the measured values of sensitivity in dB and has low clinical value

and ID number. These data need to be entered correctly only once now in the EyeSuite software since subsequent follow-ups are a mere selection of the name or ID number and starting the required follow-up examination.

The examination data includes the demographic data, reliability parameters, program, strategy, type of perimetry, stimulus size, and pupil size. The demographic data and eye are in bold letters so as to not mismatch the examination and the patient being examined. Understanding the reliability indices enhances the value of the examination. Perimetry is a subjective test hence reliability and reproducibility of the visual fields provide data for better follow-up over time. (Fig. 6.15).

False-positive (FP) answers are common in trigger happy patients. Response is recorded even when there is no stimulus presented. The false-positive rate is calculated as the ratio of false-positive answers to the total number of positive catch trials presented.

False-negative (FN) detects fatigue, loss of attention, and fixation losses while testing the visual fields. FN occurs in areas close to scotomas when no responses to brighter stimulus at the same test location where a positive response to a dimmer stimulus was affirmative previously. The FN rate is calculated as the ratio of the false-negative answers to the total number of negative catch trials presented.

6.2.8 Symbols and Representations

The symbols and representations are summarized at the bottom of the printout. The note above the shaded portion of the visual field printout gives the details of the stimulus used, size, brightness,

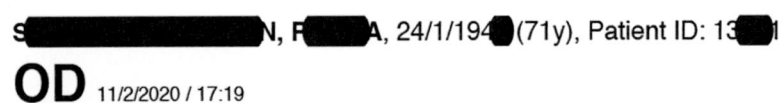

Fig. 6.15 Patient and test data

OD 11/2/2020 / 17:19

Examination parameters: G, TOP, SAP, White/White, III
Refraction, lens (S/C/A), pupil: -2.0/-0.75/85, +1.0/-/-, 4.1 mm

False Positives/Negatives: 0% (0/3), 0% (0/3)
Duration, questions/repetitions: 01:57, 69/2
Fixation control: Med

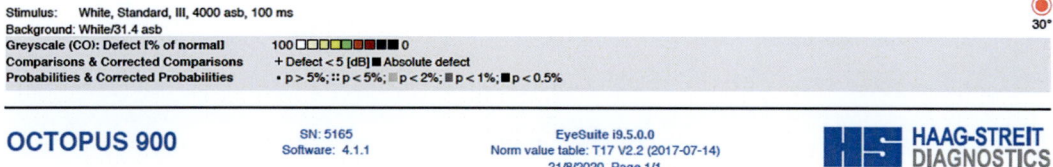

Fig. 6.16 Testing data and representations in colors and symbols

and time duration of the stimulus. The background brightness is set to white at 31.4 asb. The background light would change to yellow in SWAP perimetry (Fig. 6.16). The shaded portion gives the numerical values of the symbolic statistical representations, including the color scale. The red dot at the bottom right of the page indicates the visual field is a 30° visual field.

6.3 Interpretation and Reporting of the 7 in 1 Single Field

Reporting a visual field as in Fig. 6.17. Below is sample of the complete reporting of the 7 in 1 visual field illustrating the wealth of data presented by the printout. Visual fields need not be reported elaborately. The positive highlights would be sufficient.

Step 1: Patient and examination data: The printout is a visual field (VF) of a 71-year-old. Right eye VF was performed with the G program and TOP strategy, white on white, default size III stimulus and adequate pupil size of 4.1 mm. (Pupil size measurement is automatic in Octopus). The FP and FN are not flagged, the duration was 1 min 57 s, and 59 test points was presented with 69 questions with 2 repetitions of stimulus presentations.

Step 2: Values table: The measured data has few central dB values within the high 20s with the periphery showing lower values (low 20s or high teens). The superior temporal quadrant above the horizontal meridian shows test locations of very low values in the peripheral 30° to 20° and with five absolute defects (black square, sensitivity 0 dB). Most values within the central 10° are high 20s. The value of MS (mean sensitivity) is 19.2 dB, which shows a rather low overall height in the hill of vision with a steep cliff in the superior temporal quadrant. These are measured values that are not adjusted for age and diffuse defects.

Step 3: Gray scale (CO): The gray scale highlights the dark and darker area in the superior temporal quadrant respecting the horizontal meridian. The darker area is also impinging in the superior nasal quadrant too. The two inferior quadrants show light areas. The topography of the defect points to an arcuate type of VF defect present in glaucoma. (The gray scale when derived from raw values would be full of clutter as in Fig. 6.4).

Step 4: Comparisons (CO): The central 10° shows "+" symbols with two numerical values. Majority of the test locations in the superior temporal and nasal quadrants show numerical values (indicating the amount of deviation from normal age match) and black squares indicating absolute defects (0 dB). There is large difference in dB values across the test locations at the nasal horizontal raphe. The superior hemi field test locations of the VF has significant depressed sensitivity values.

Step 5: Defect/Bebie curve and global indices: The dB values of almost two-thirds of the test locations lie horizontally within the lower normal of the age match. The dB values of the rest of the one-third test locations are in the steep arm dipping down the graph. This example shows the diffuse defect (DD). The shift of the horizontal arm is not yet affected despite being in the lower normal, with value of 1.8 dB with $p > 10\%$. The MD value of 6.2 dB in red ($p < 5\%$) is affected since almost two-thirds of the sensitivity values are in the low normal. The rest of the one-third test locations lie in the steep arm of the graph that shows numerical values of

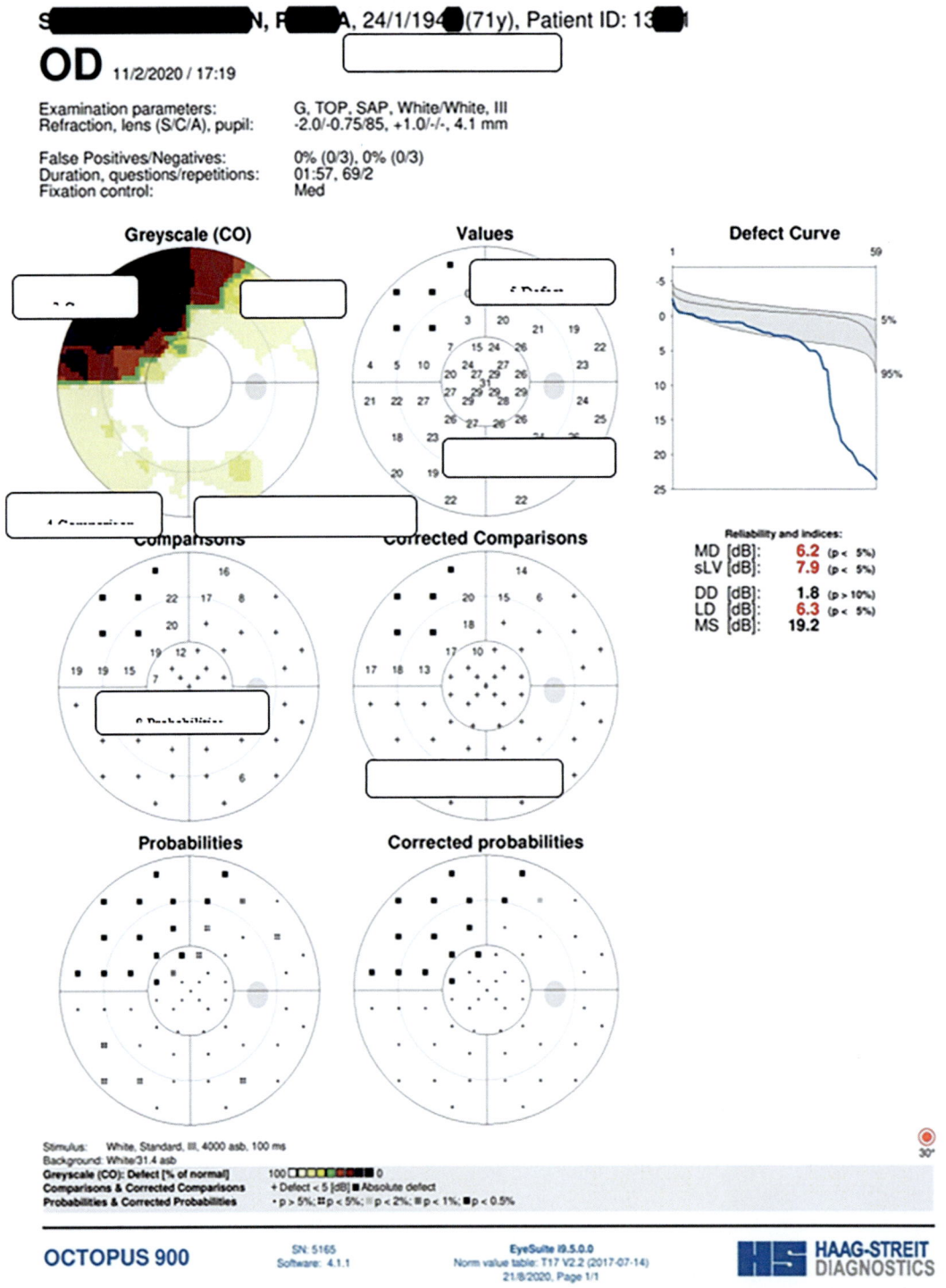

Fig. 6.17 The suggested interpretation sequence in a 7 in one printout

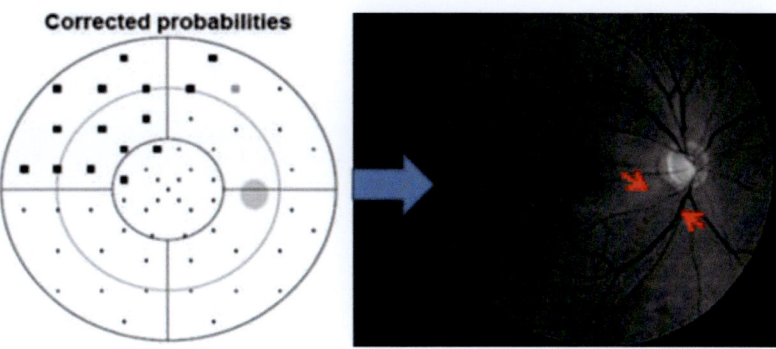

Fig. 6.18 Correlating superior visual function loss in visual field and inferior temporal RNFL structural loss in a red-free fundus picture

considerable deviation along with black squares which represent 0 dB. These one-third of tested locations are indicative of a deep local or focal defect with severe loss of sensitivity. This is the sLV (square root of loss variance) which is 7.9 dB in red with $p < 5\%$. The LD (local defect) is the average of sensitivity from the fourteenth to the fifty-ninth ranks in this test. LD is 6.3 dB with $p < 5\%$, being sensitive to any increase in focal defect.

Step 6: The probability plot for both comparisons and corrected comparisons displays the symbolic statistical deviation from normal age match, and these plots at a glance show the superior arcuate defect with the symbolic representation indicating the statistical significance at each of the test locations.

Impression: Superior arcuate defect with a low hill of vision right eye. Visual field represents the visual function which should be correlated with structural defect (Fig. 6.18).

6.3.1 Summary

1. Patient data and examination data—Details of the patients and examination done.
2. The value table or representation—Presents all the measured values. All other representations in the printout are derived from this table.
3. The gray scale—Gives an idea of the topography of defect.
4. Comparison table—Presents the tested values at each location corrected with normative age data.
5. Defect curve and global indices—Summarize the visual fields into a line graph and a few numbers.
6. Corrected comparisons—Diffuse defect is subtracted to reveal the true extent of visual field defects.
7. The probability plots—Both comparison and corrected comparison provide the statistical significance at all tested locations.

References

1. Fankhauser F, Koch P, Roulier A. On automation of perimetry. Graefes Arch Clin Exp Ophthalmol. 1972;126–50.
2. Flammer J, Jenni A, Bebie H. The OCTOPUS G1 program. Glaucoma. 1987;9:67–72.
3. Weber J, Klimaschka T. Test time and efficiency of the dynamic strategy in glaucoma perimetry. German J Ophthalmol. 1995;4:24–31.
4. González de la Rosa M, Rodríguez J, Rodríguez M. Flicker-TOP perimetry in Normals and Patients with ocular hypertension and early Glaucoma; Perimetry Update 1998/1999. p. 59–66.
5. Schiefer U. Realization of semi-automated kinetic perimetry (SKP) with the Interzeag 101 Instrument. In: International Perimetric Society (IPS) Meeting. 2002.
6. Bebie H, Flammer J, Bebie T. The cumulative defect curve: separation of local and diffuse components of visual field damage. Graefes Arch Clin Exp Ophthalmol. 1989;227:9–12.
7. Visual field Digest 6th Edition 2016, Haag-Streit AG, Koniz Switzerland (ISBN 978-3-033-06001-2).

Progression Monitoring with an Octopus Perimeter

N. R. Rangaraj and P. Sathyan

7.1 Introduction to Visual Field Progression on Octopus Perimeter

Visual fields can be analyzed for point-wise trends over time with global indices MD (mean defect), sLV (square root of loss variance), DD (diffuse defect), and LD (local defect). Cluster trend analyze the subtle changes in the nerve fiber bundle regions that are divided into five clusters in each hemisphere. The polar trend gives a perspective to the structural damage by interpolating the visual field trends as a structural representation. The EyeSuite software is enabled for local area network viewing stations to assess all the parameters and representations of the visual fields over time with selection and deselection of clinically assessed inconsistently performed tests. The EyeSuite software selects the last six visual fields to evaluate the current trends, with a manual selection option.

7.2 The EyeSuite Progression Analysis of Octopus Perimeter

The EyeSuite progression analysis is presented in three logical representations: 1. global trend analysis (GTA) (Fig. 7.1), 2. cluster and corrected cluster trend analysis (CTA and CCTA) (Fig. 7.2), and 3. polar trend analysis (PTA) (Fig. 7.3) [1]. Patterned visual field analysis in Octopus provides location, orientation, and depth of the visual field loss. The cluster trend, for example, highlights the clusters worsening near the fovea that calls for more aggressive intervention. The values from comparisons and corrected comparisons table are the basis of the CTA and CCTA that display the sector of nerve fiber bundle affected by progression or worsening over time. The polar trend derives the values from the comparisons to provide a structural orientation (Fig. 7.3) to the worsening.

7.2.1 Global Trend Analysis (GTA)

In Octopus perimetry EyeSuite follow-up software has four indices which track the differential light sensitivity of the tested visual fields over time (Fig. 7.4). These indices summarize the visual field changes into a single number.

MD (mean defect): The overall average sensitivity of all the tested locations in the visual field is summarized in the MD. Worsening of visual

N. R. Rangaraj (✉)
Premier Eye Care and Surgical Center, Chennai, India

P. Sathyan
Sathyan Eye Care Hospital and Coimbatore Glaucoma Foundation, Coimbatore, India

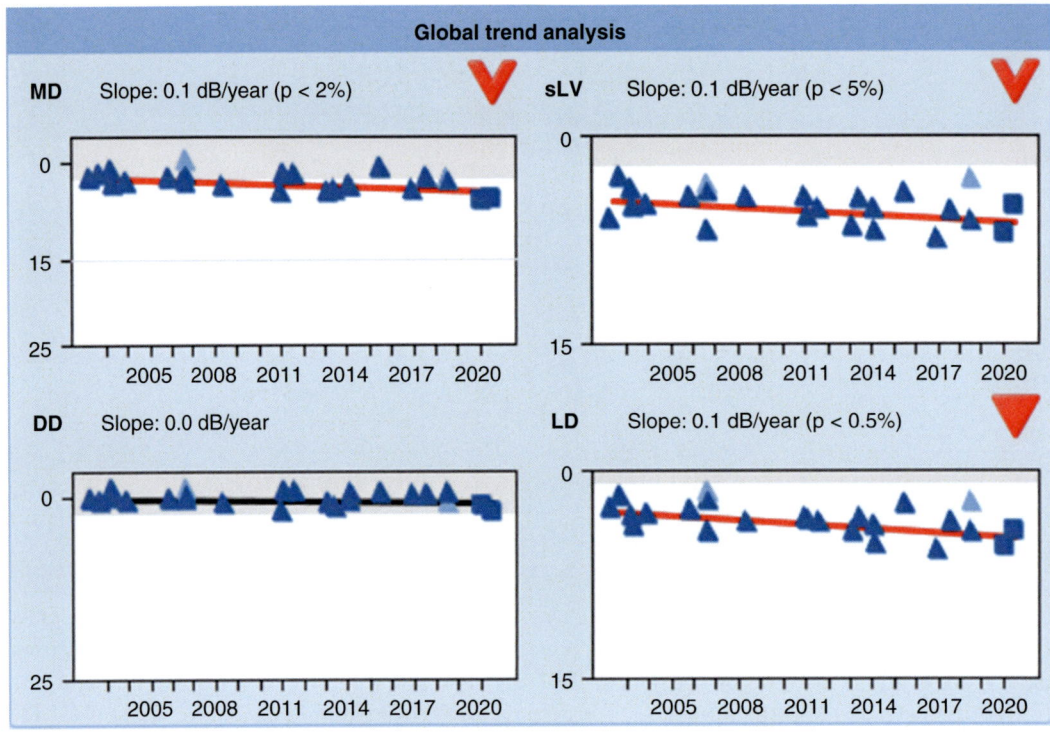

Fig. 7.1 Global trend analysis of visual field indices

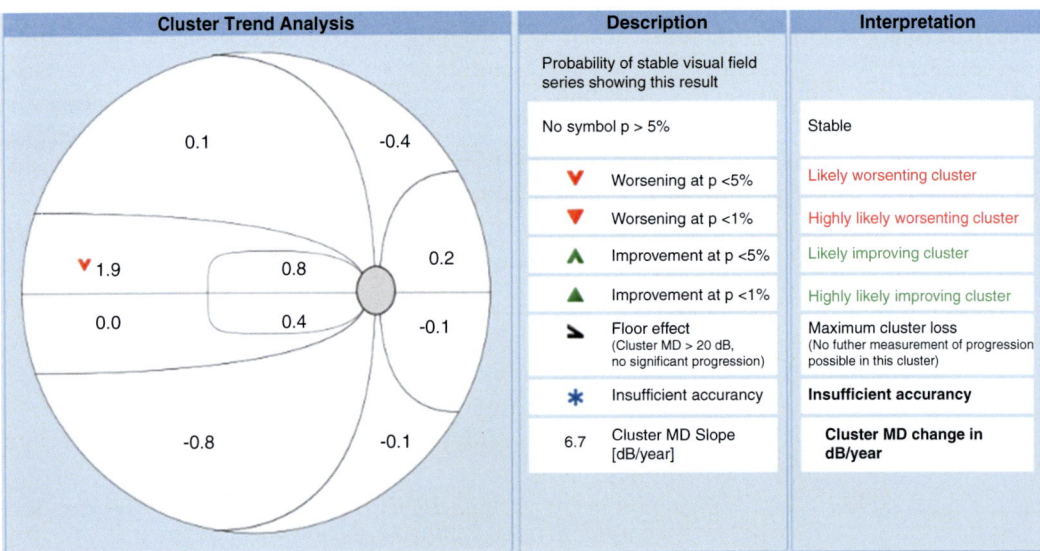

Fig. 7.2 Cluster and corrected cluster trend analysis with symbolic statistical representation

fields over time changes the MD value even though it may be small. MD is good index to track overall visual fields changes.

DD (diffuse defect): Allows the assessment of the overall diffuse change due to media opacity or diffuse neuronal loss over time.

LD (local defect): This index identifies the local changes in the visual fields. The LD is calculated from the defect curve. LD typically tracks the changes in early and moderate visual field damages in glaucoma especially when adjacent sectors worsen. DD and LD trend analysis can

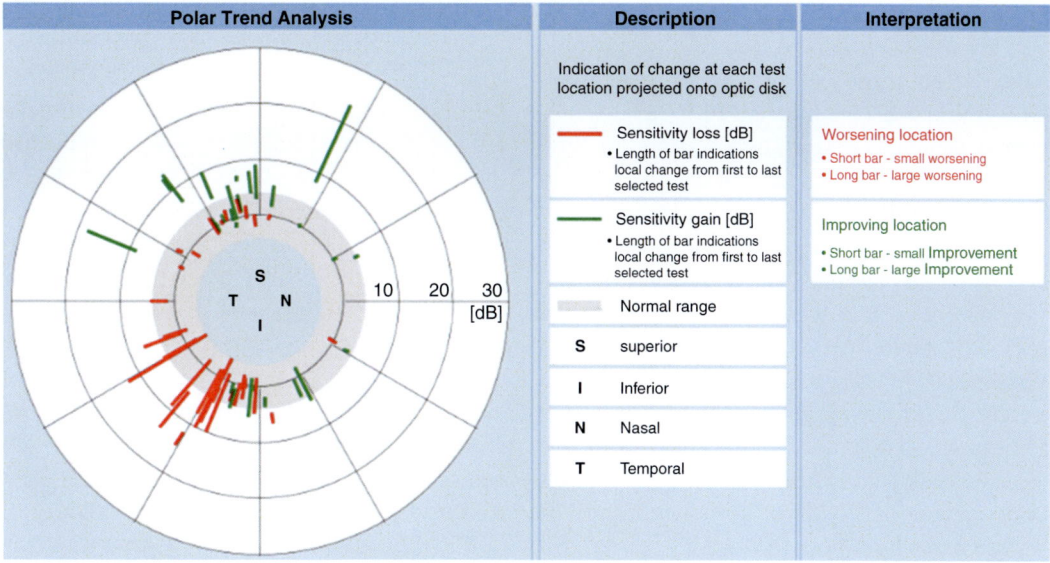

Fig. 7.3 Polar trend analysis shows progressing worsening in the inferior temporal areas

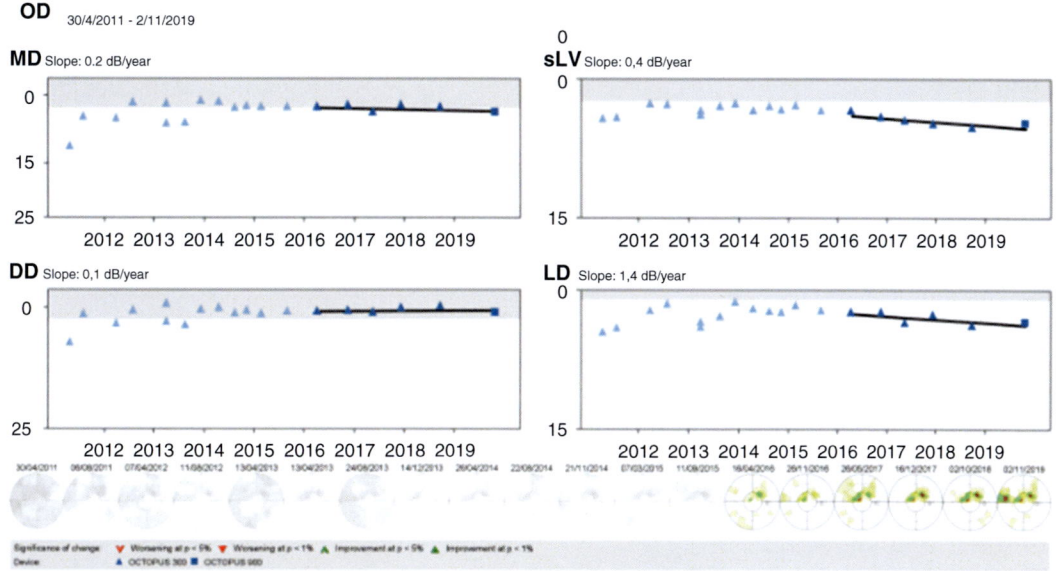

Fig. 7.4 Global trends with timeline and gray scale representation in a single view

distinguish between diffuse and local sectorial changes.

sLV (square root of loss variance): This index is a measure of inhomogeneity in a visual field. The sLV trend provides information on the depth of the focal defects when progressing from early to moderate visual field defects.

The trend analysis printout gives symbolic statistical representations which facilitate interpretation. While viewing online the mouse over gives the "P" values too.

Closed inverted ▼ Worsening at $P < 1\%$.
Open inverted ▽ Worsening at $P < 5\%$.
Floor effect ◣ When there is more than 20 dB sensitivity loss, determination of progression or stability is not possible due to advance disease.

The following Table 7.1 gives an overview of the significance of the global trend analysis.

Global trends printout case example Fig. 7.5.

This serial visual field data of a 69-year-old lady on follow-up with the global trends MD, DD, sLV, and LD are not flagged for any significant worsening. These are typical trends in long-term follow-up. She underwent cataract surgery in 2015 with MD values improving. She then discontinued her topical medications between 2016 and 2017 and presented with significant worsening of MD. The topical medications were restarted, and the last six VF show no significant worsening of MD, sLV, and LD. The global trends printout presents the series of global Indices in comparisons gray scale with the selected tests highlighted with the normal reference values and symbols for significance of change in the last row.

Table 7.1 Typical behavior of global trend analysis from early to moderate loss

	MD	sLV	DD	LD
Stable				
Diffuse progression	▼		▼	
Local progression	▼	▼		▼
Diffuse and local progression	▼	▼	▼	▼

Assessment of progressions with trend analysis requires a minimum of three reliable follow-up fields. The number of visual fields in the first 2 years of diagnosis would be three visual fields test per year. The visual field strategy should be short and smart, e.g., TOP or Dynamic. The G program test locations are along the nerve fiber bundles. The global indices are used for follow-up and reflect the change when there is worsening. The short strategies make it patient friendly to perform visual fields tests reliably for good data that is used for assessment of progression over the lifetime of the patient.

When assessing global trends, the history, media changes, and unreliable visual fields are to be considered before assuming progression.

The effect of selecting last 10 tests (Fig. 7.6) in the same example shows MD, sLV, and LD flag worsening at 1% significance, when in reality the visual fields have stabilized in the last six selections over 3 years since she was restarted with the topical medication (Fig. 7.5).

In summary, the global trends indices provide a sensitive indicator of diffuse, focal, and sectorial worsening that calls to the attention of the

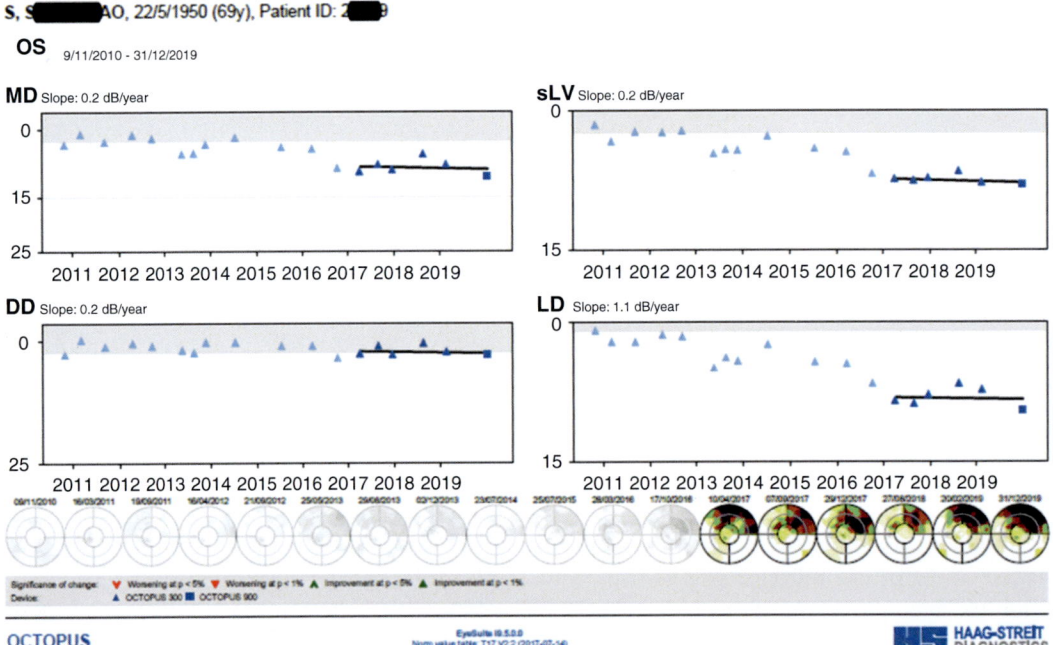

Fig. 7.5 Typical default selection of last six visual field tests with no deterioration in sensitivities

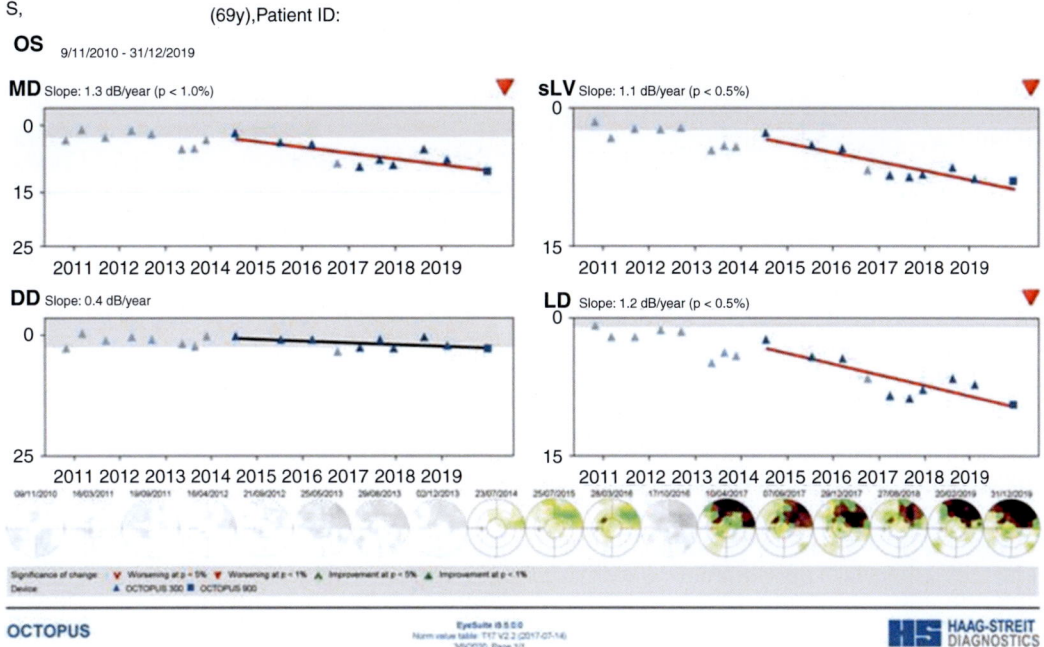

Fig. 7.6 The inverted red triangle shows worsening at $P < 1\%$ when the last 10 visits were selected

clinician, to consider appropriate therapeutic intervention. To flag a worsening, a short strategy with test locations reflecting the nerve fiber bundles is done at ideal intervals that best highlight the change early. Good communication with the patient helps in achieving this ideal follow-up.

7.2.2 Cluster Progression of Visual Field Defects in Glaucoma

Retinal nerve fiber bundles in the retina when damaged affect clusters of adjacent areas that cause typical glaucomatous visual field defects. Small localized defects do not influence the MD values, yet the local MD value of the cluster would be below the normal values and amenable for tracking early worsening. There are ten clusters that are followed up, five in each hemisphere (Fig. 7.7). The papillomacular, nasal step, and arcuate fibers are well represented to highlight change and monitor progression clinically. The main function of the cluster and corrected cluster analysis is to highlight sectorial worsening. Early glaucomatous changes are mostly local, and the

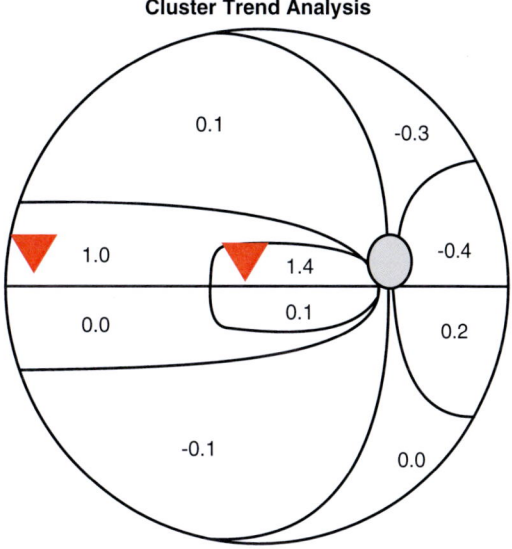

Fig. 7.7 Cluster trend analysis highlighting the sectorwise worsening

averaging method used to derive the global MD could mask these changes. Hence sector/cluster analysis being a local averaging is an early indicator of change. Clusters of test location in a sector indicate change better than single test point event analysis. The number displayed in each sector is worsening from the expected sector/local MD average. The cluster trend analysis also corrects for diffuse defect and displays the corrected cluster trend analysis [2].

7.2.3 Polar Trend Analysis

Polar trend analysis is a unique Octopus EyeSuite representation of the visual function that provides a structural orientation to the visual field progression. The structural changes are detected at the optic disc, and visual field damage is at the represented retinal location. Early glaucomatous changes are subtle and require a structural and functional correlation if possible. The polar trend orients the clinician to the worsening in the visual field to the structural damage in the optic disc. The length of the red bar indicates the dB loss per year. The graph has a gray ring that indicates the normal expected sensitivity of the test locations represented at the fiber angle. A cluster of red bars indicate corresponding worsening for the affected test locations in the sector along with the loss in dB per year. The polar trend analysis looks at the point-wise trend analysis to determine the trend line. The trend line is the best fit from the date first selected to the last selected date of the visual field. This line is then marked on the polar grid to the corresponding test location from where the nerve fibers arrive. Worsening in dB per year is indicated with the length of the red line. (Fig. 7.8) [3].

7.2.3.1 Case Example [4]
Case example of an early to moderate primary open angle glaucoma that show cases the representations that display progression in Octopus perimetry EyeSuite software (Fig. 7.9) [4].

This 68-year-old female presented for her regular glaucoma follow-up with discomfort. Her IOP was 22 mmHg in both eyes. Fundus in 2001 showed mild slit like RNFL loss at 7 o'clock

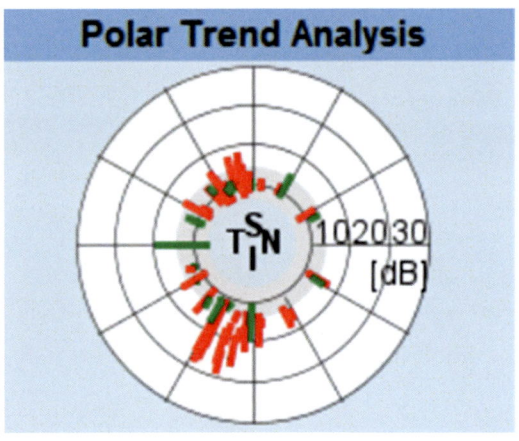

Fig. 7.8 Polar trend analysis

position, with no obvious neuroretinal rim thinning (NRR) or notching. Fundus in 2008 shows RNFL loss at 6–8 o'clock (inferior temporal) positions indicating progression.

7.2.3.2 Interpretation
- Gray scale series shows expansion of superior nasal defect to a superior arcuate defect from 2001 to 2008.
- Significant ($P < 1\%$) but with MD worsening at 0.4 dB/year due to fast progression has affected superior clusters (cluster MD change 1.1–2.1 dB/year).
- Large progression at 6–8 o'clock position in polar trend analysis (length of the red line), giving the structural orientation to the visual function.
- Rim thinning and RNFL loss spreading from 7 o'clock position towards 6 and 8 o'clock position.
- The global trends, cluster analysis, and polar analysis are representations from the same data set, yet gives a unique set of representation to better understand the progression and provide timely therapeutic intervention.

The global indices, cluster trends, and polar trends are only as good as the data that is col-

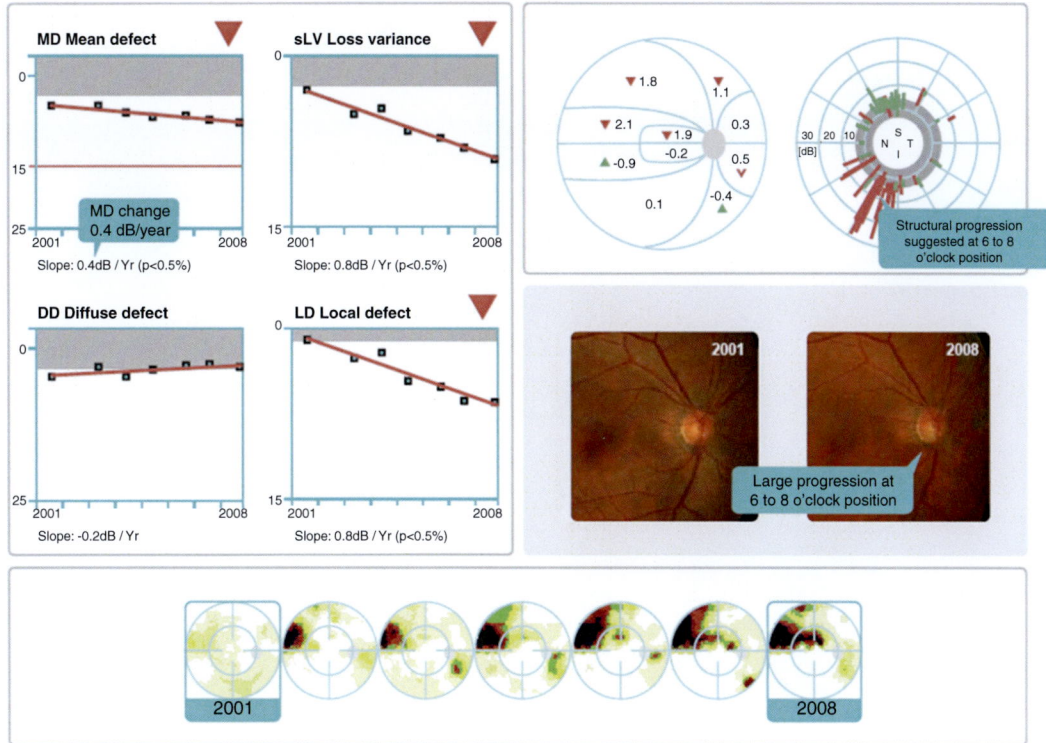

Fig. 7.9 Typical example which highlights the worsening graphically over time

lected. The frequencies of perimetric examination per year along with trustworthy performance of the test play an important role in determining the quality of trend analysis. Three visual field tests in the first year, after taking learning effect into account, set the tone for a good follow-up. Once diagnosis is made, proper selection of perimetry program based on the nerve fiber bundle with a short strategy helps in making the follow-up patient friendly.

References

1. European Glaucoma Society. Terminology and guidelines for glaucoma. 4th ed. Savona: PubliComm; 2014.
2. Naghizadeh F, Holl G. Detection of early glaucomatous progression with octopus cluster trend analysis. J Glaucoma. 2014;23:269–75.
3. Holl G, Naghizadeh F. Evaluation of Octopus Polar Trend Analysis for detection of glaucomatous progression. Eur J Ophthalmol. 2014;24:862–8.
4. Visual field digest 6th edition, A guide to perimetry and Octopus perimeter.

Structure–Function Relation in Humphrey Perimetry

Col Madhu Bhadauria and Jyoti Bhat

Understanding role of structure and function in glaucoma diagnosis has been an enigma right from outset till now due to variable presentation of the same [1]. Automated perimetry has given a very fundamental understanding of sensitivity of visual function at multiple points in the field of vision which can be documented, analysed, reproduced and finally be correlated with corresponding structural change in optic disc as well as in retinal nerve fiber layer (RNFL) [2]. The first fundamental question that needs to be answered is as to why do we need to correlate and understand structure function relationship? We need to do it to understand the presence or absence of glaucoma, severity of glaucoma damage, natural course of disease and the impact that it will make on quality of life of a glaucoma patient. The origin of structure and function change lies in the loss of retinal ganglion cells (RGC) and their axons which are clinically seen as RNFL and neuroretinal rim (NRR) [3]. Hence the degree of neuroretinal rim thinning and RNFL damage with their corresponding visual field (VF) changes are used to grade presence and severity of glaucoma in clinical setting as well as in clinical trials.

It is vital to be able to conceptualize anatomical basis for the origin of visual field changes. Firstly, the layout of RNFL and relation to optic nerve head and then to be precisely able to locate the exact site of RGC loss at different locations leading to changes in RNFL thickness and NRR which cause VF defects at the corresponding sites like macular fibres insert on temporal rim whereas superior and inferior arcuate fibres occupy superior and inferior poles.

Another important component is getting accurate measurements of structural changes like optical coherence tomography (OCT) images, disc photos and visual fields which are subject to many errors due to patient factors like cataract, corneal opacities, refractive errors, pupil size, head position, etc. The challenge arises in patients with same structural changes but with variable field changes. In other scenarios, some patients have only structural changes without any field changes and vice versa. Therefore, the diagnosis and grading of severity should be done after assessing both the parameters. It is possible to have OCT readings of non-neural elements of the optic nerve and some visual function on Humphrey visual fields (HVF) with no visible neuroretinal rim or retinal nerve fibre layer changes in a blind eye. The methods to measure structure could be disc drawing of the optic nerve head (ONH) and RNFL images, OCT and Heidelberg retinal tomography (HRT) [4]. Both these devices provide ONH parameters in mm [2], RNFL thickness in μm and

C. M. Bhadauria (✉)
Regional Institute of Ophthalmology, Sitapur Eye Hospital, Lucknow, India

J. Bhat
Indira Gandhi Netra Chikitsalaya, Sitapur Eye Hospital, Lucknow, India

macular and ganglion cell complex (GCC) in μm with its analysis compared to normative data stored in database of the machines. All these parameters are linear matrix and can report consistent change in RGC density loss in a linear fashion but their values cannot be compared numerically between HRT and OCT and in OCT with different machines working with different algorithms and wavelengths [5].

In standard automated perimetry (SAP), constant stimulus size is III (0.43 degree in diameter) with constant background illumination at all test locations with variable light intensity on test locations, depending upon patient's sensitivity on those locations and is documented in logarithmic units decibels (dB). Decibels are related to luminance of stimulus related to the background illumination. It is the ratio between background illumination and maximum luminance of perimeter. Hence a Humphry perimeter dB values cannot be compared with dB value of other perimeters. The dB values which are charted by perimeter are not linear hence a change of 3 dB in terms of retinal ganglion cell (RGC) loss amounts to reduction or increase in numbers of RGC by 50%. A 2 dB decrease from 38 to 36 means ten times greater change than same dB changes at 28 dB [6].

Quigley has reported that at least 30–40% RGC should be lost before visible changes are apparent on visual fields [7]. Spaeth et al. studied structure function correlation and found many eyes had visual field changes without supporting changes in the optic discs. These discs were studied by masked ophthalmologists who did not expect visual field changes in optic discs as they felt that they were within normal range. They hypothesized that minimal visual field changes occurred when cup disc ratio (CDR) increased from 0.3 to 0.6, and more progressive change was seen when the threshold of CDR was crossed beyond 0.6 [1]. The concept of pre perimetric glaucoma originated after that, when disc and RNFL changes were detected in presence of normal visual fields. This clinical observation was also supported by histopathological studies by scientist who confirmed loss of RGCs [8, 9].

Number of studies revealed latency in the appearance of visual field defects compared to structural changes, hence a concept of functional reserve came into light. Many studies have shown that structure measured in linear units and VF measured in dB have a curvilinear relationship thus in early glaucoma structure loss appears more and in advanced glaucoma VF change appears more [10–12]. This happens because dB measurements are done in log units and are not linear. If both are plotted in a linear fashion, both correlate well linearly with each other as well as with RGC loss. However, on OCT records, RNFL measurement do not fall to zero even in blind eyes with zero readings on visual fields due to residual glial and vascular tissue [13].

Glaucoma continuum by Weinreb clearly shows that structural loss precedes functional loss [14].The current evidence shows that structure and visual function loss is mostly seen simultaneously but functional loss may be visible before structural loss. In Ocular Hypertension Treatment Study (OHTS), end point for the patient to convert from ocular hypertension to glaucoma was appearance of a visual field or optic disc change. In this study, visual field defect as end point was seen first in 35% of patients with structural change as end point detected in 55% [15]. This is contrary to the belief that structural changes are seen much before visual field changes, as in this study 35% of patients developed visual field changes without optic disc changes. Similarly, European Glaucoma Prevention study found this in 60% and Early Manifest Glaucoma Trial found it in 80% of patients [16]. This can be explained by the concept of RGC dysfunction rather that RGC death as structural measurements will remain unaltered in case of dysfunction due to their physical presence there.

The sources of visual field changes span from retina to optic nerve and brain hence are also affected by retinal diseases and neurological diseases apart from the glaucoma-related visual field changes. Hence, it is imperative to understand their relationship with the causative structure and how to differentiate them from glaucomatous visual field defects.

8 Structure–Function Relation in Humphrey Perimetry

The approach for structure function correlation is based on following factors:

1. Is this VF defect based on some anatomical/structural defect? (Figs. 8.1 and 8.2).
2. What is the source of visual field defect? (Figs. 8.3, 8.4, 8.5, 8.6, 8.7, 8.8, 8.9, 8.10, 8.11, 8.12, and 8.13).
3. Is this reliable and due to glaucoma? (Figs. 8.14 and 8.15).
4. If glaucomatous, is it proportional to the structural change? (Figs. 8.16, 8.17, 8.18, 8.19, 8.20, 8.21, 8.22, 8.23, 8.24, 8.25, and 8.26).
5. If not proportionate to one structural change method, is there another modality to correlate better? (Figs. 8.27, 8.28, 8.29, and 8.30).

Answer 1 Anatomical basis (Figs. 8.1 and 8.2).

8.1 Optic Nerve Head and Visual Fields

The visual field, (shown below) on the right side, shows generalized constriction with normal optic disc. A good counselling after ascertaining the cause showed a normal visual field of the left side correlating well with the disc picture.

Answer 2 Source of visual field defect—visual field defect can arise from (a) optic nerve, (b) retina and (c) brain other than glaucoma. Glaucomatous field defect has been answered in answer 4.

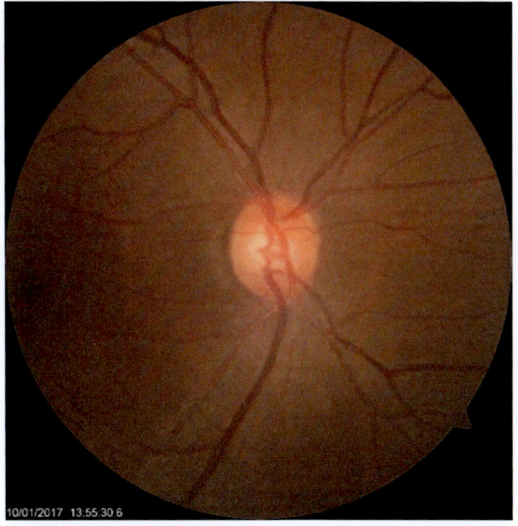

Fig. 8.1 Normal optic disc

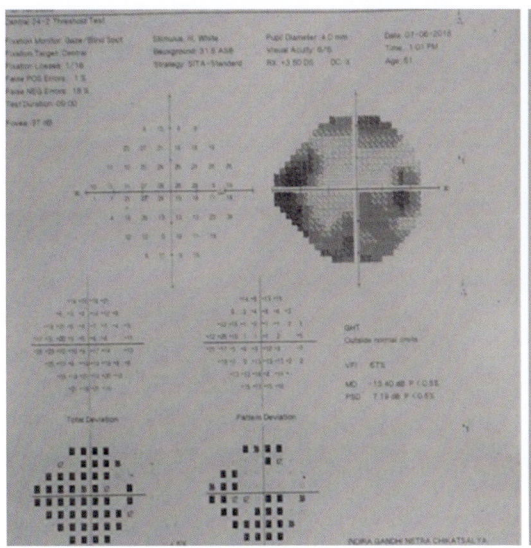 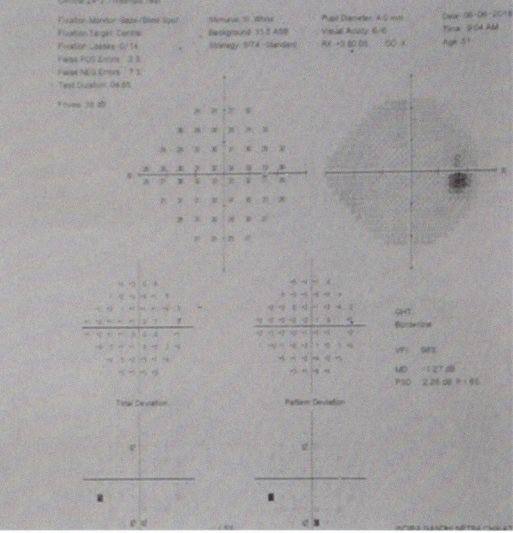

Fig. 8.2 Clover Leaf defect of a malingerer with normal OD Fig. 8.1

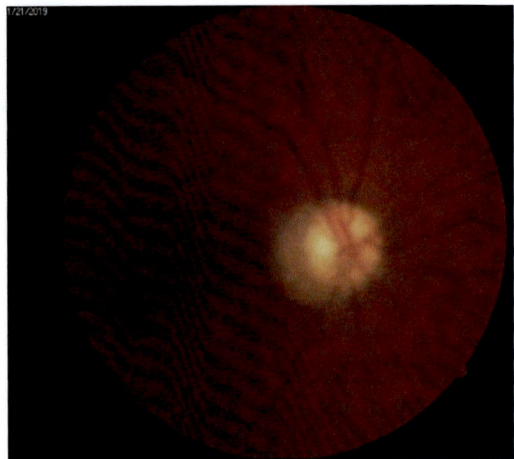

Fig. 8.3 Optic disc OD AION advanced

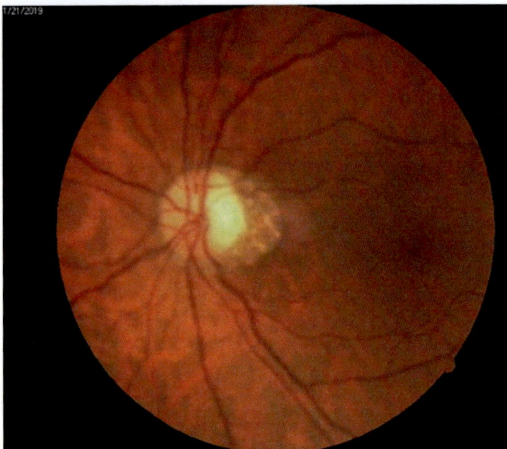

Fig. 8.4 Optic disc OS AION

(a) Optic Nerve Head: Anterior Ischemic Optic Neuropathy (Figs. 8.3, 8.4, 8.5, and 8.6)

55 years male, a known case of diabetes, hypertension and hyperlipidaemia for last 15 years. He came with h/o episode of sudden visual loss in the right eye for the past 7 days and had a similar episode in left eye 6 months ago. He was using one anti glaucoma medication for the last 6 months. On examination OD-BCVA 6/60 with clear cornea, clear posterior capsule, uncomplicated pseudophakia, IOP 17 mmHg with CCT of 532 and diurnal variation showing 2 mmHg change. Optic disc showed pale disc with oedema and HVF showed low test reliability with advanced generalized depression VFI-11% MD −28 dB PSD 6 dB involving all 4 quadrants to variable irregular extent corroborating with pale ischemic disc oedema.

OS-BCVA −6/18 with normal anterior segment except cataract with nuclear sclerosis grade II. IOP was 19 mmHg with CCT 530 and normal diurnal variation of IOP. Disc showed cupping of 0.6 with advanced superior rim loss associated with mild pallor. HVF revealed dense inferior arcuate scotoma with VFI 61% MD −15.3 dB and PSD 11.6 dB consistent with superior rim thinning and pallor. The antiglaucoma drug was discontinued, and IOP was recorded after 6 weeks which did not show any change compared to the first day. Systemic work up revealed long-standing hyperglycaemia with deranged lipid profile. Presence of systemic diseases and a history suggestive of sudden loss of vision with generalized pale disc oedema in OD with generalized visual field loss thus show correlation. Old history of sudden loss of vision with superior rim thinning with equal area of rim pallor OS is also correlating well with field change in form of inferior hemifield loss. This also confirmed diagnosis of anterior ischaemic optic neuropathy which is a glaucoma visual field mimicker as shown from Figs. 8.3, 8.4, 8.5, and 8.6.

(b) Retinal disease—Visual Field Change due to Branch Retinal Vein Occlusion (Figs. 8.7, 8.8, and 8.9)

70 years female, a known hypertensive for past 20 years, reported with sudden blurring of vision in the right eye. She had undergone uneventful cataract surgery 5 and 3 years ago in both eyes. BCVA was RE, 6/24 and LE,

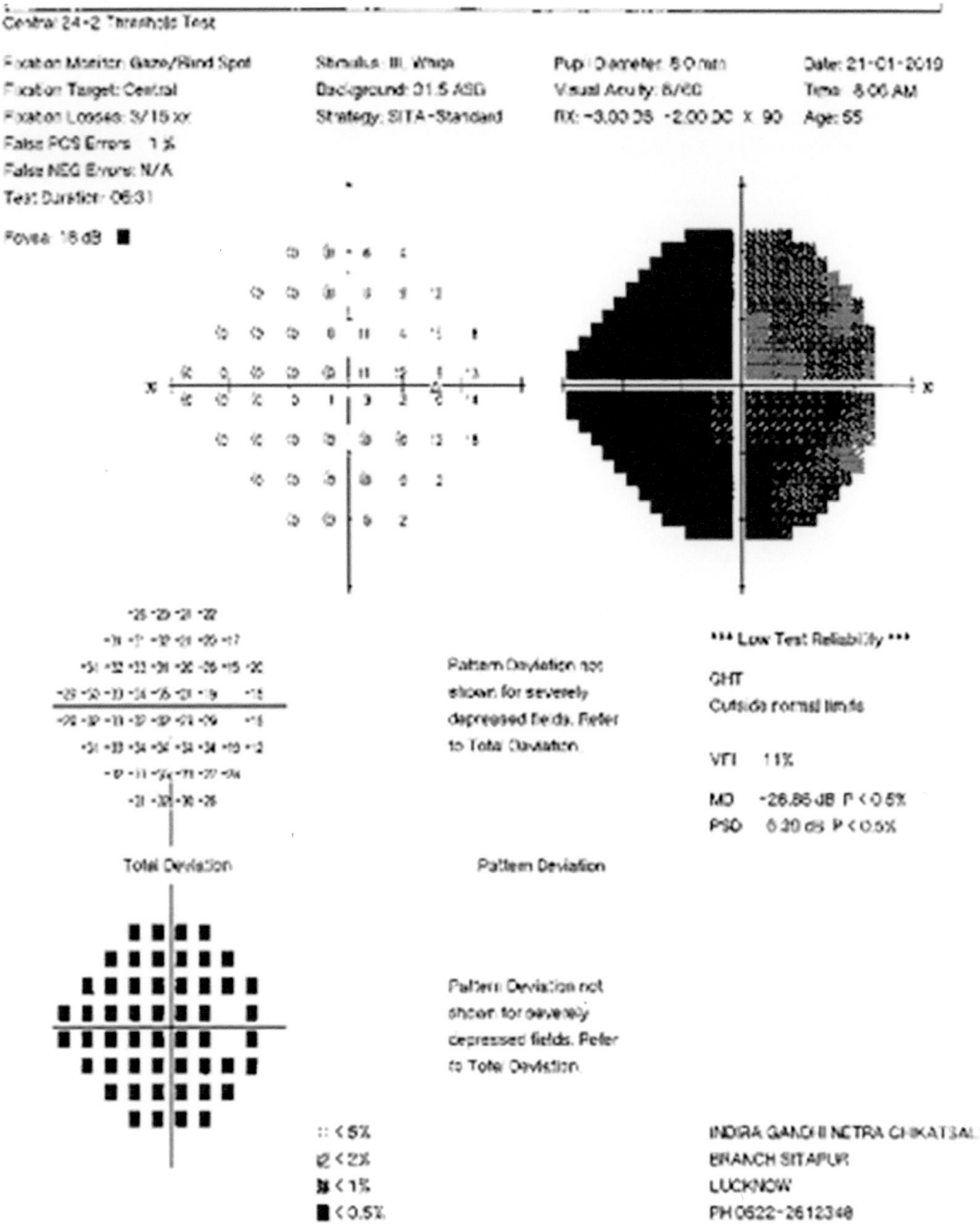

Fig. 8.5 Visual field OD Advanced AION

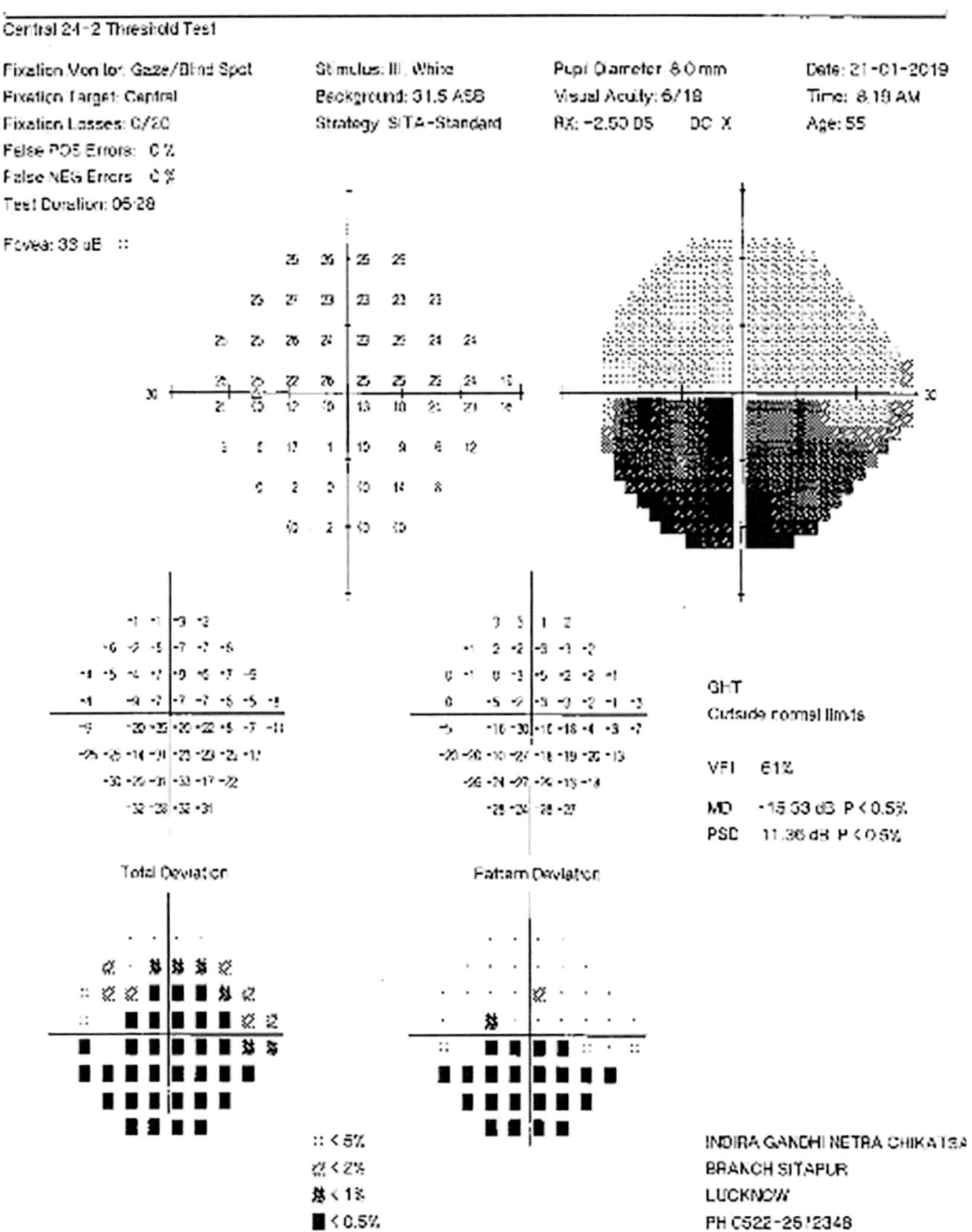

Fig. 8.6 Visual field OS Fresh AION Lower altitudinal defect

6/6. IOP was 13 and 16 mmHg, and she had old visual field printout showing a superior arcuate scotoma and was referred for glaucoma management. A detailed glaucoma work-up was done which was normal and examination of the fundus showed that the optic disc had a large cup due to bipolar rim defect with inferior temporal branch vein occlusion with associated macular changes (Figs. 8.7 and 8.8). Visual field of OS showed

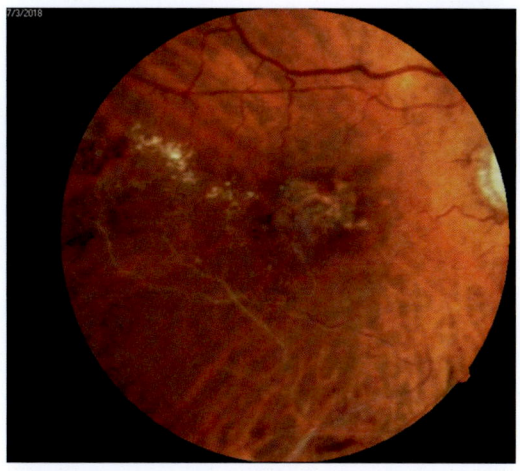

Fig. 8.7 Macular changes BRVO

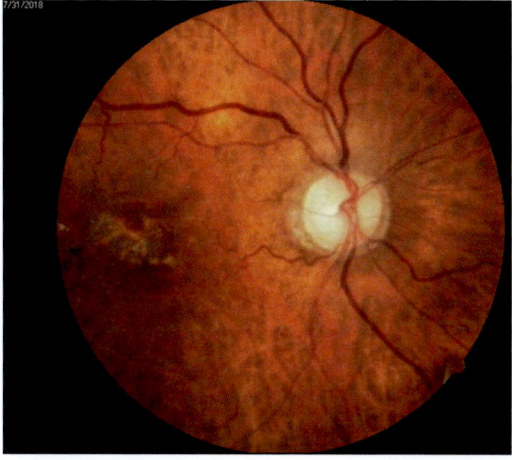

Fig. 8.8 Bipolar rim loss OD with macular changes in same patient Fig. 8.7

upper arcuate scotoma extending into lower hemifield corresponding with bipolar loss (Fig. 8.9). Associated extension of superior arcuate scotoma till fixation is due to macular changes of branch retinal vein occlusion leading to macular oedema and degeneration.

(c) Brain: Intracranial Space Occupying Lesion Mimicking Advanced Glaucoma on Visual Field (Figs. 8.10, 8.11, 8.12, and 8.13)

61 years old female referred as a case of advanced glaucoma for onward treatment. On examination OD-BCVA 6/9 and N/8, normal IOP open angles with shallow cupping of disc with pallor of the temporal rim. Visual field showed temporal hemifield defect along with superior nasal extension across midline. (Figs. 8.10 and 8.12) OS-BCVA 5/60 with shallow cupping 0.9 and profound pallor of the rim. Rim pallor and temporal hemifield loss in OD and partly spared nasal quadrant suggested a neurological cup. (Figs. 8.11 and 8.13). An MRI revealed pituitary adenoma.

Answer 3 Reliability of Visual Fields (Figs. 8.14 and 8.15).

Fixation Losses, false positives and false negatives or fixation losses. High false positives more than 25% seen as white areas and darker areas as false negative (Figs. 8.14 and 8.15).

Answer 4 Glaucomatous and corresponding to structural change.

Glaucomatous changes could be of any severity from (a) mild to moderate and (b) may also be advances in only one in eye hence asymmetric.

(a) Mild to Moderate Glaucoma (Figs. 8.16, 8.17, 8.18, and 8.19).

65 years female with history of diabetes was diagnosed as a case of primary open angle glaucoma OS for the first time. She reported with asymmetric IOP of 18 and 22 mmHg with normal CCT and open angles. OD—disc examination revealed normal size disc with round deep cup and CDR of 0.5. Normal NRR but visible laminar dots (Fig. 8.16). Inferior RNFL showed diffuse thinning. Though visual field does not fit into diagnosis of classical early glaucoma but significant changes seen in superotemporal quadrant with borderline GHT and PSD <2%. (Fig. 8.18)

OS showed CDR 0.8, with inferior notch and splinter disc haemorrhage inferiorly. Classical wedge-shaped RNFL defect is seen below the disc haemorrhage. (Fig. 8.17). VF shows incomplete arcuate scotoma with MD 5.86 and PSD 7.8 $P < 0.5$.

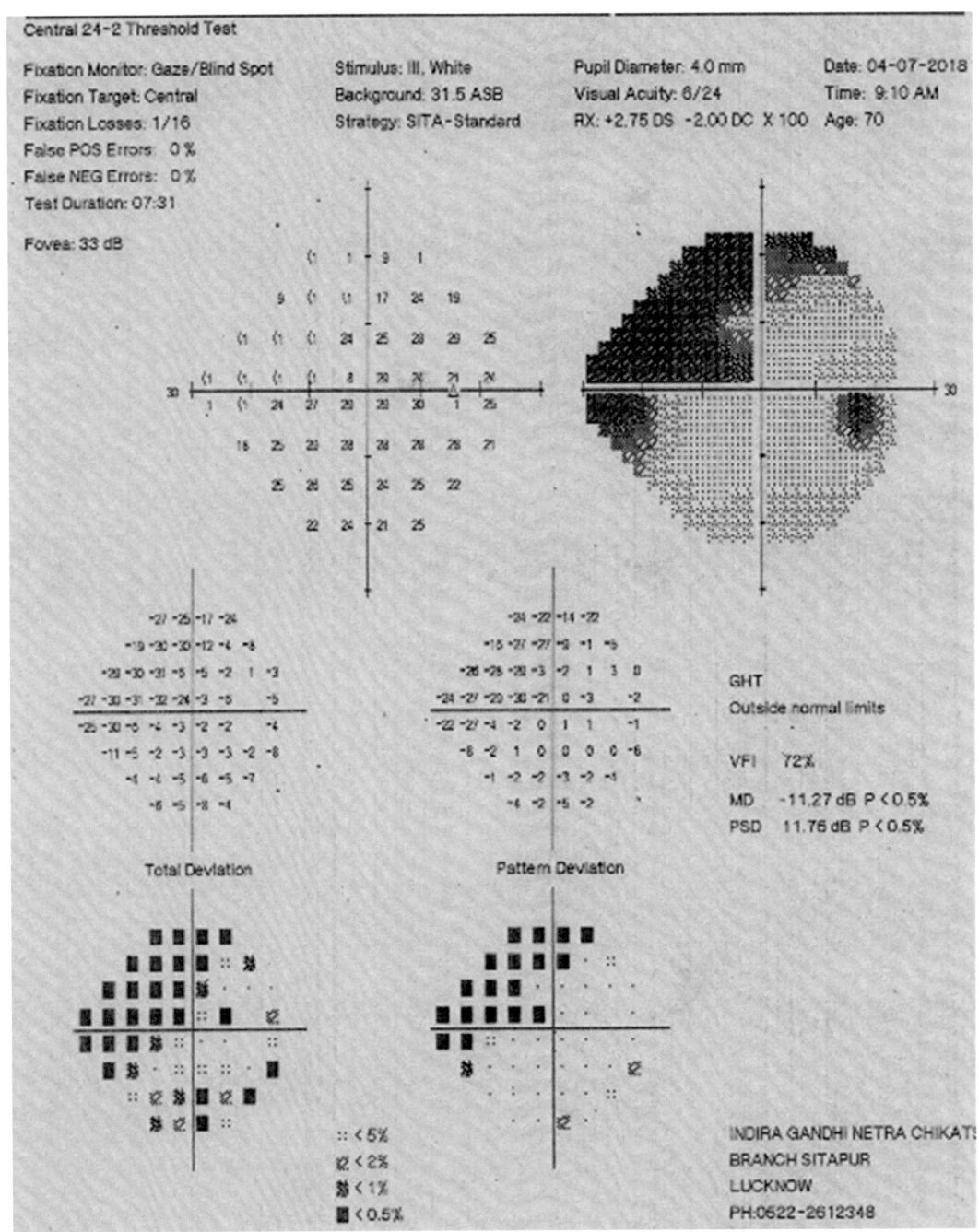

Fig. 8.9 Arcuate scotoma superior with central area involvement and incomplete inferior arcuate scotoma (combined effect of disc and macular changes)

8 Structure–Function Relation in Humphrey Perimetry

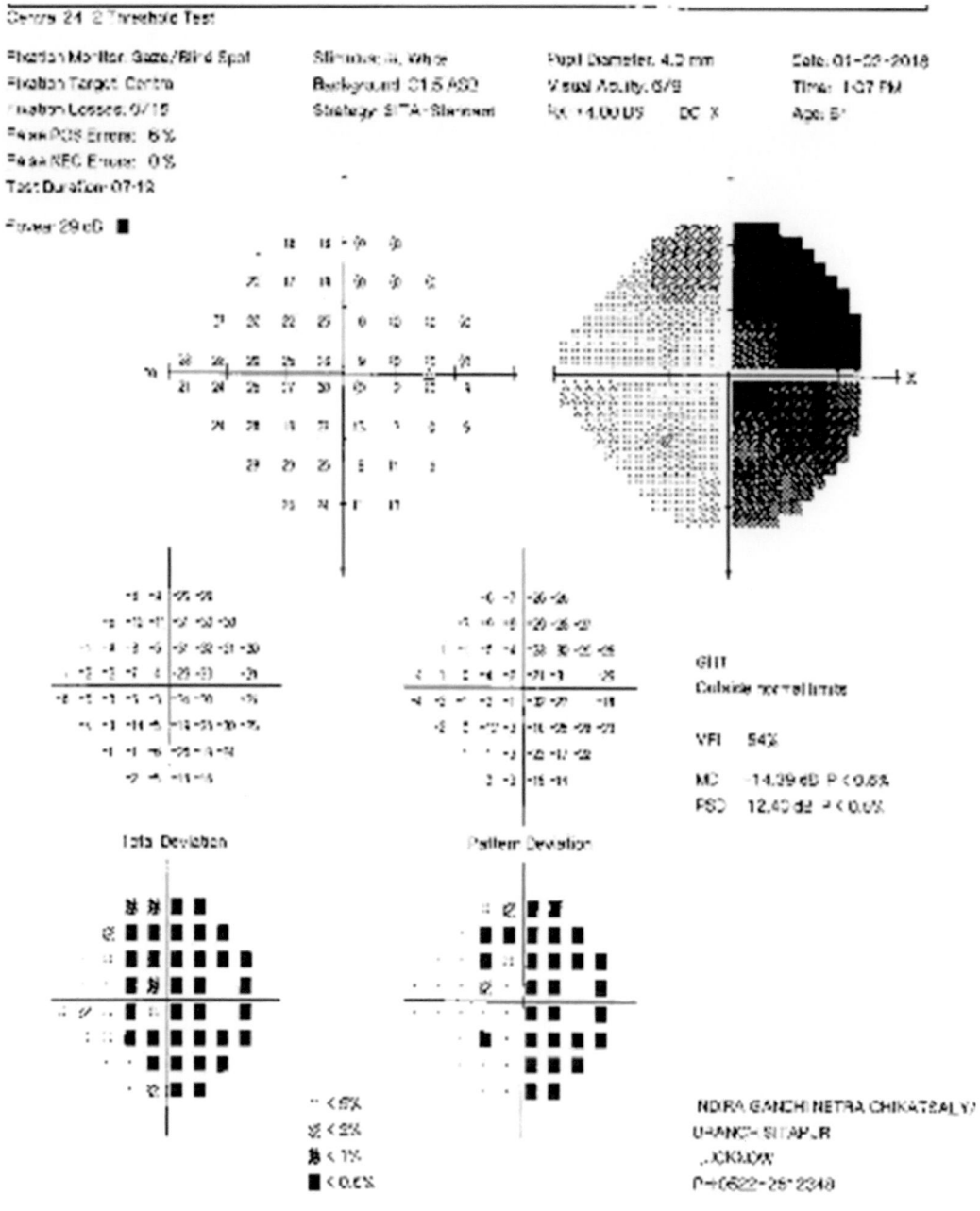

Fig. 8.10 Temporal hemi field defect

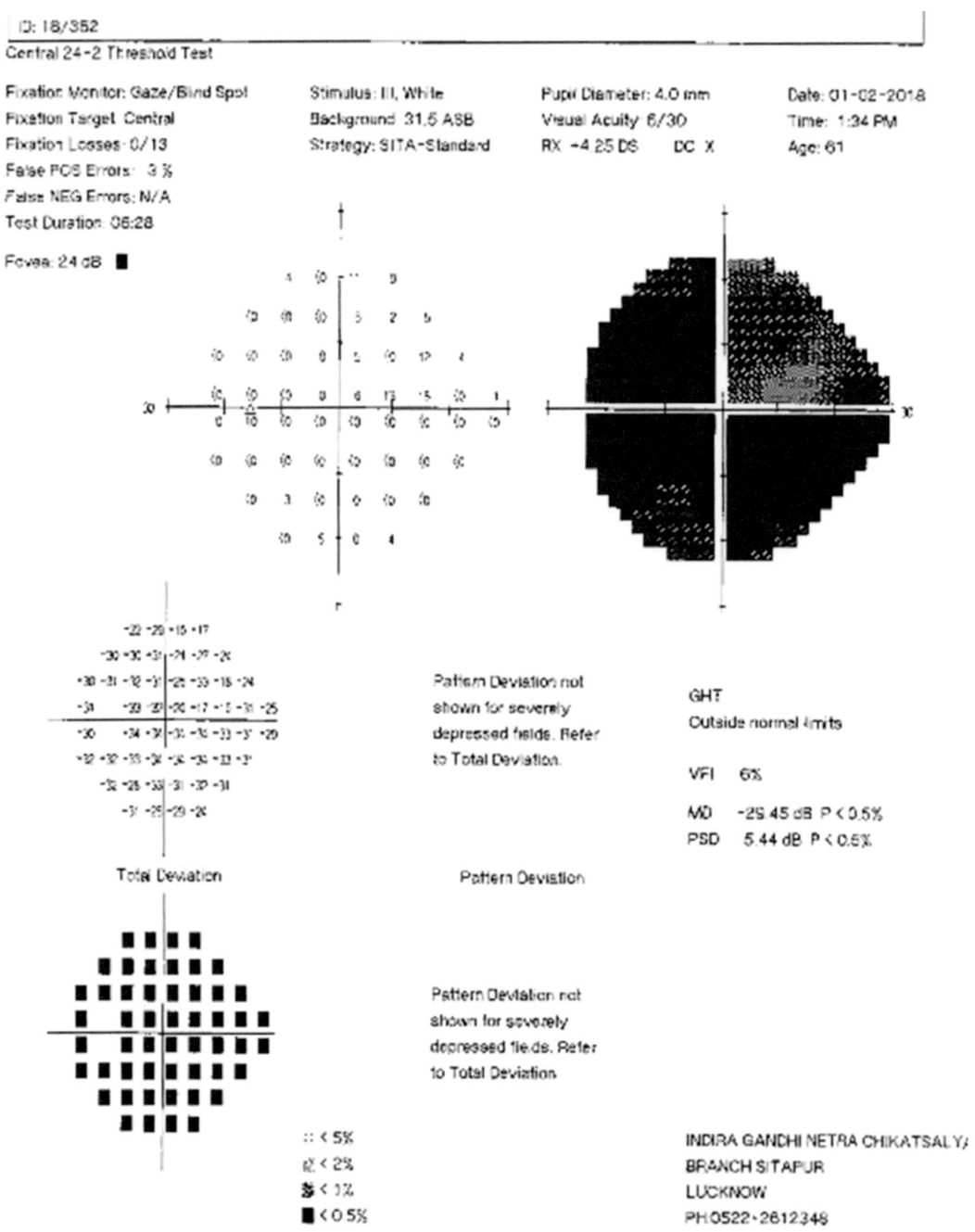

Fig. 8.11 Advanced general field defect

8 Structure–Function Relation in Humphrey Perimetry

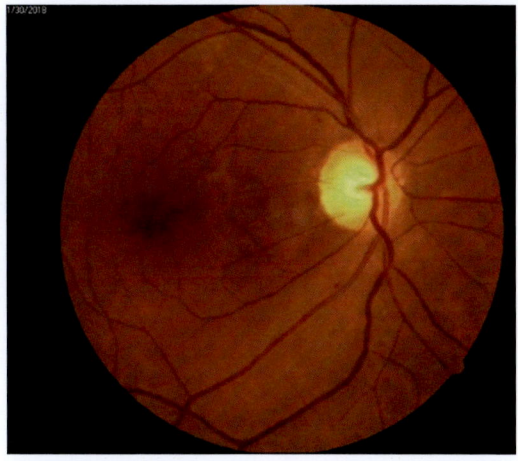

Fig. 8.12 Disc rim pallor

Fig. 8.13 Primary optic atrophy

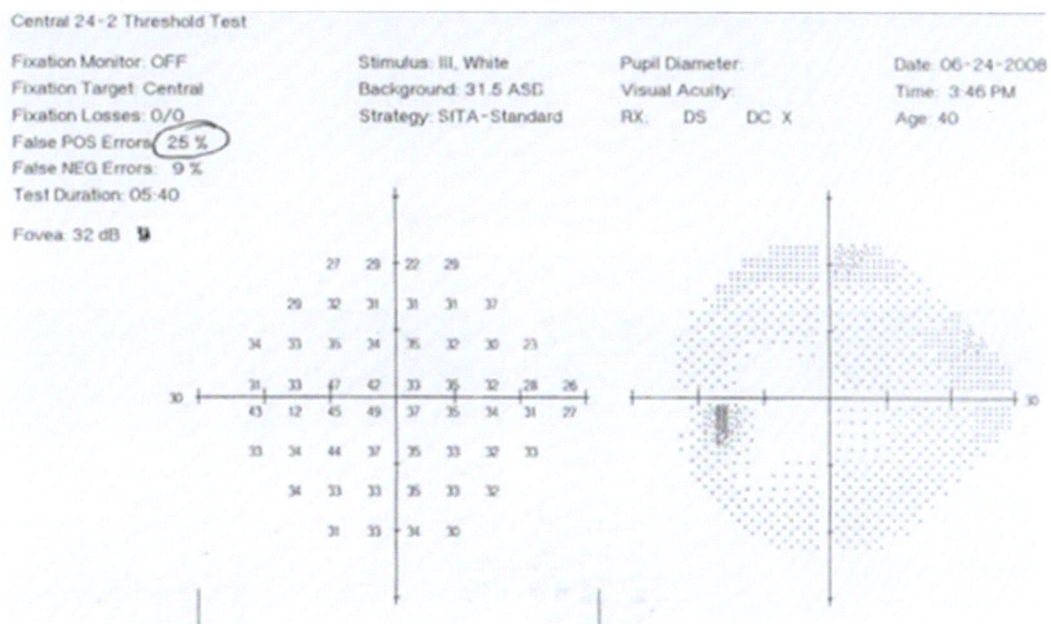

Fig. 8.14 High false positive

Mild to moderate but more moderate glaucoma than mild especially with disc haemorrhage has a positive predictive value for progression. There is good structure function correlation. *Inferior notch with RNFL defect correlates well with incomplete superior arcuate scotoma. (Fig. 8.19)*

(b) Asymmetric POAG: Advanced Glaucoma OD and Ocular Hypertension OS. (Figs. 8.20, 8.21, 8.22, 8.23, 8.24, 8.25, and 8.26)

67-year-old myopic patient was suffering from POAG OD and OHT OS for past 10 years controlled on medical medication. OD shows vertical CDR 0.9 with bipolar rim loss and enhanced myopic crescent as beta zone, and corresponding visual field showing double arcuate scotoma inferior more than superior. She was diagnosed to have advanced glaucoma OD with good structure function correlation. *Bipolar rim loss—superior more than*

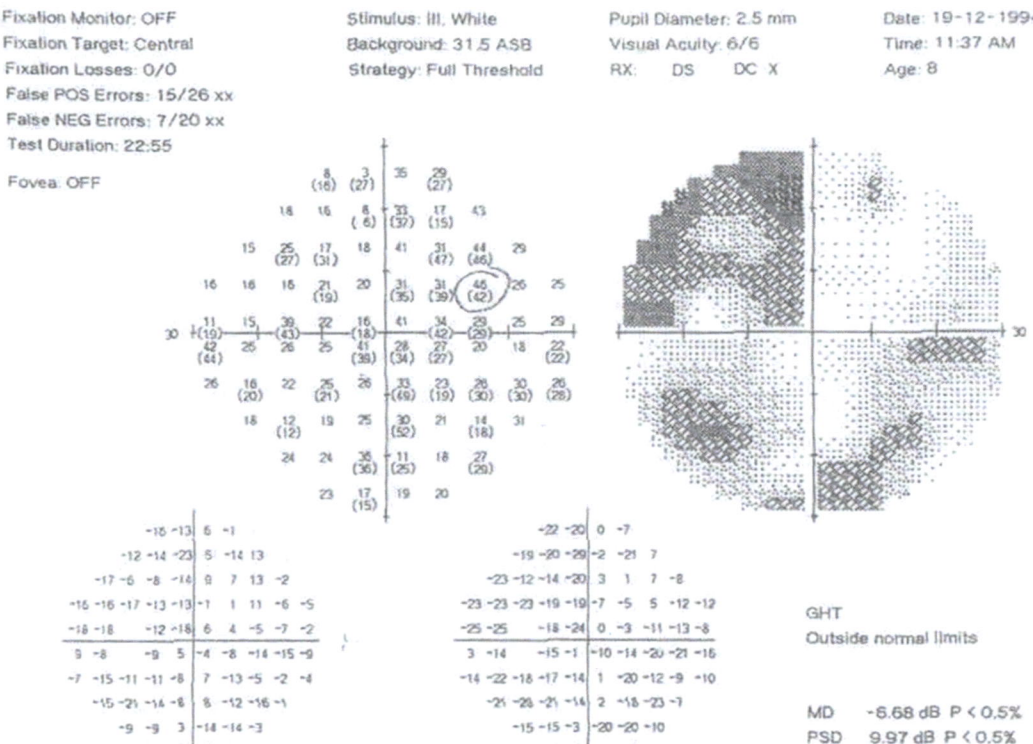

Fig. 8.15 Unreliable fields XX

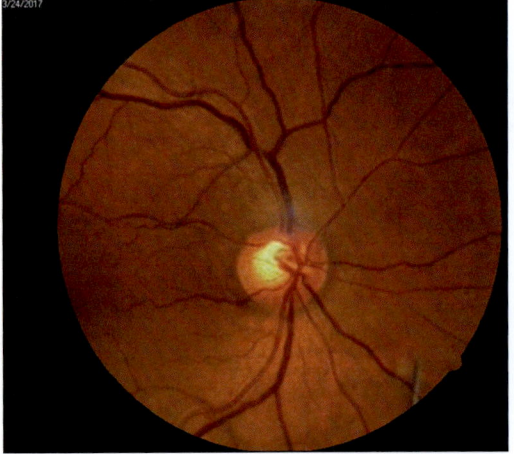

Fig. 8.16 OD Normal optic disc

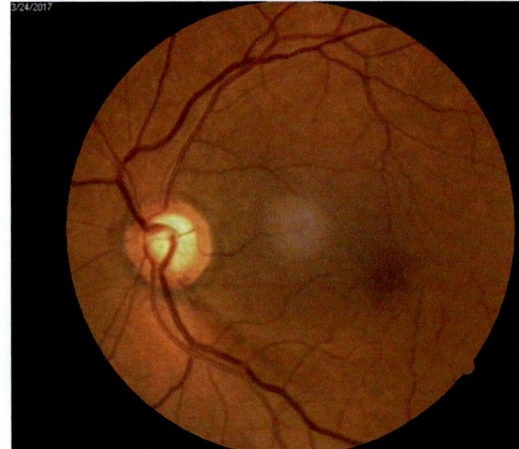

Fig. 8.17 OS inferior notch with RNFL defect

8 Structure–Function Relation in Humphrey Perimetry

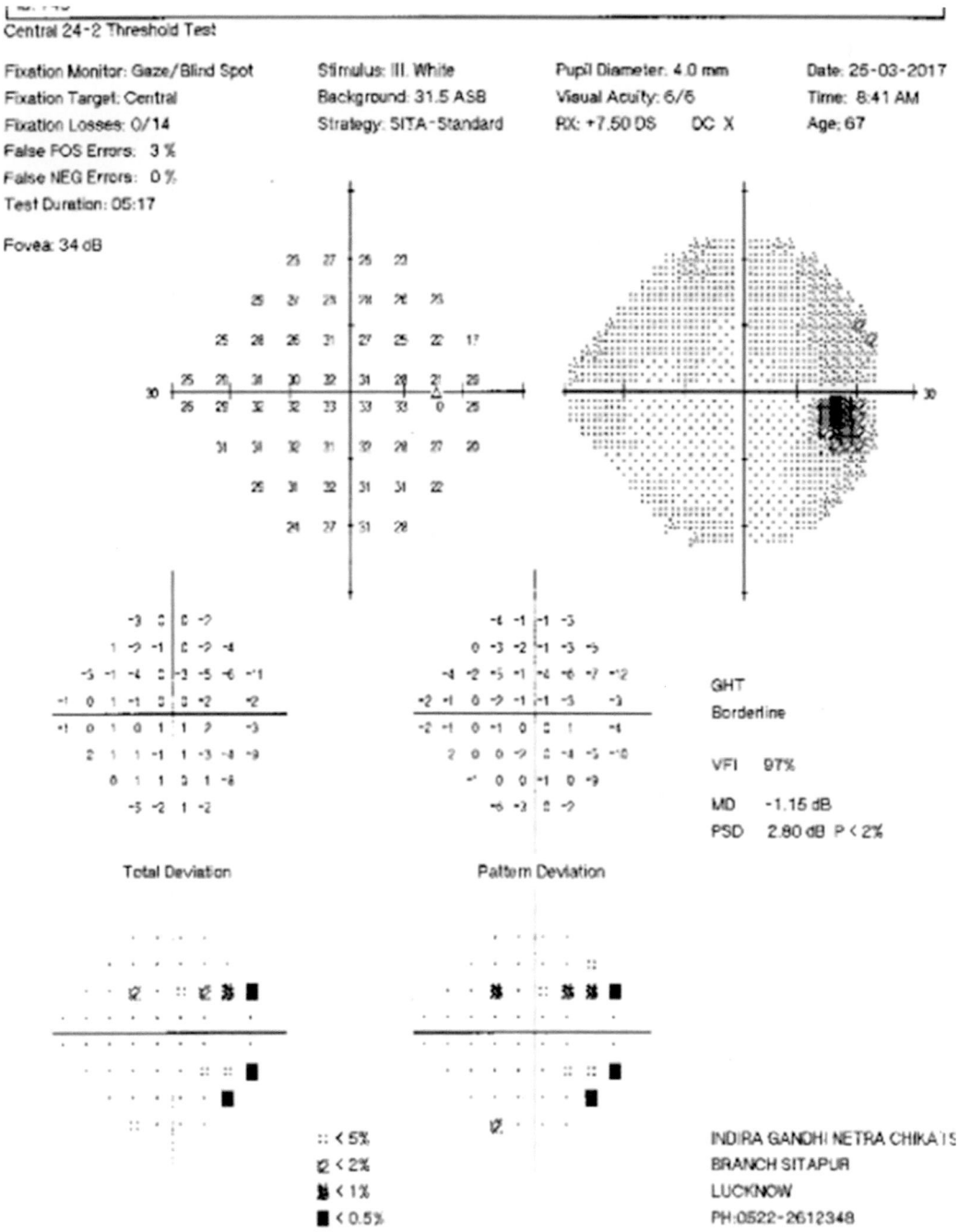

Fig. 8.18 Normal visual field

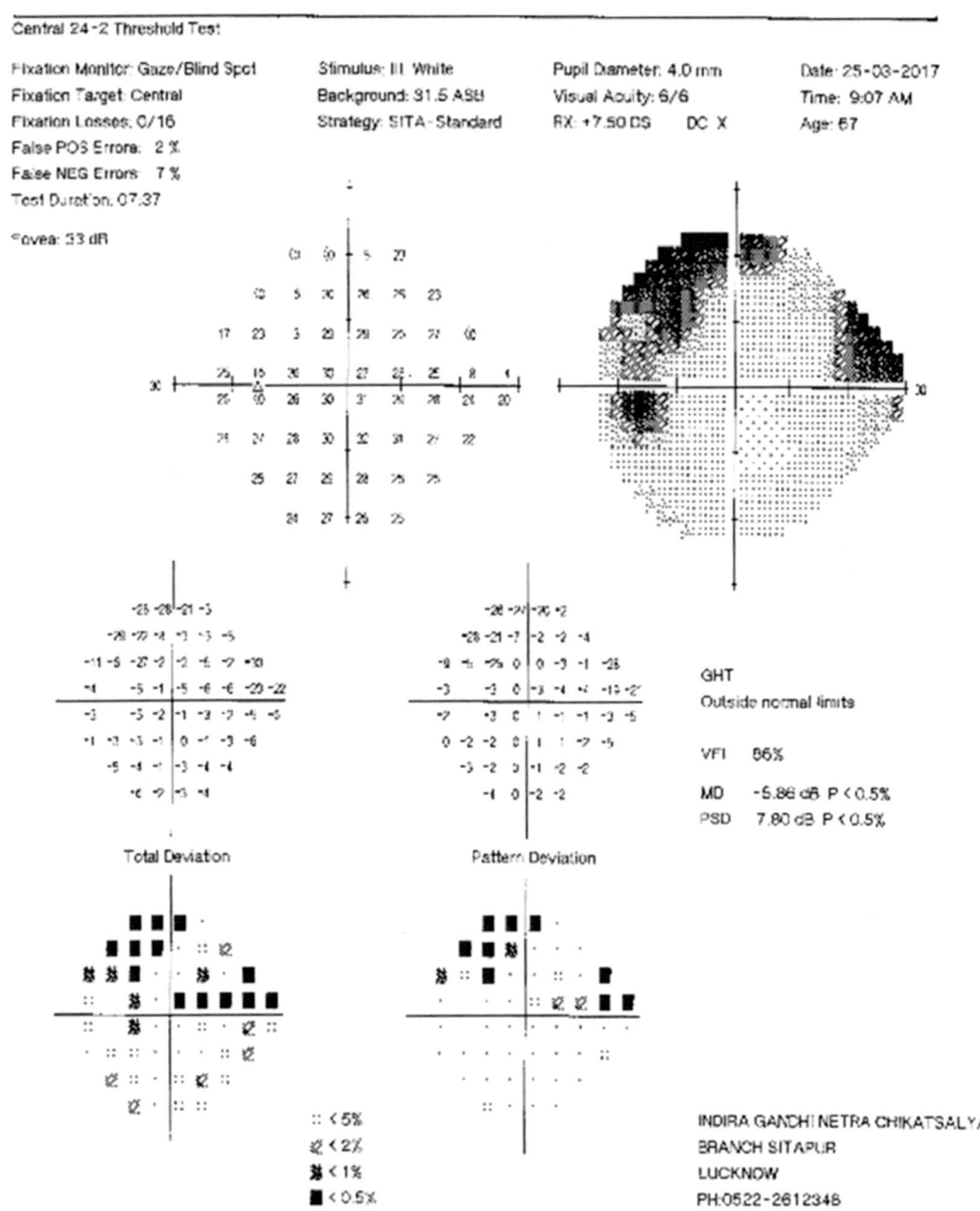

Fig. 8.19 Superior arcuate scotoma

inferior and biarcuate field defects inferior more than superior correlates well as structure function. (Figs. 8.20, 8.21, and 8.24)

OS showed a CDR of 0.3 with normal NRR and RNFL on colour photo as well as red-free photo; however, visual field showed borderline with few depressed points in superonasal area. (Figs. 8.22, 8.23, and 8.25) An OCT was done to confirm the possible changes showed *Normal RNFL with some sectors of macular thinning with field changes of borderline do not*

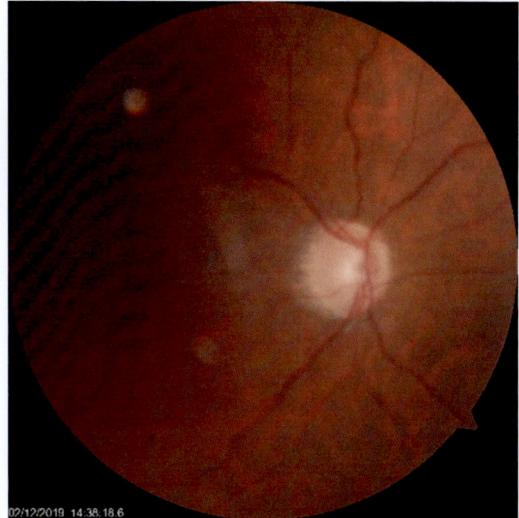

Fig. 8.20 OD CDR 0.9

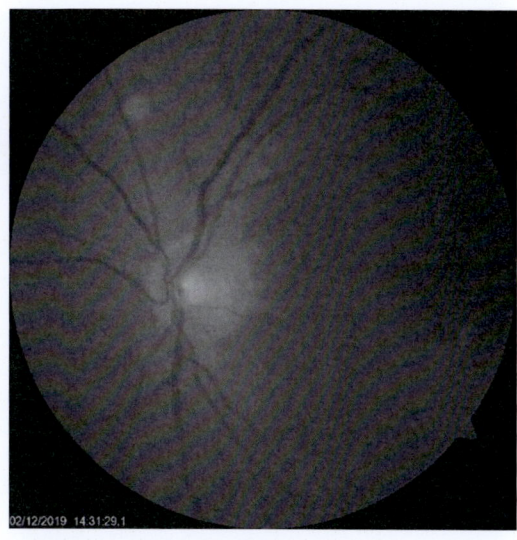

Fig. 8.22 OS CDR 0.3 red-free

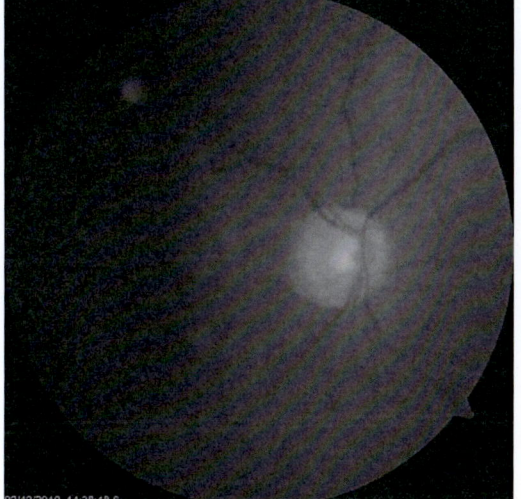

Fig. 8.21 OD Red-free image

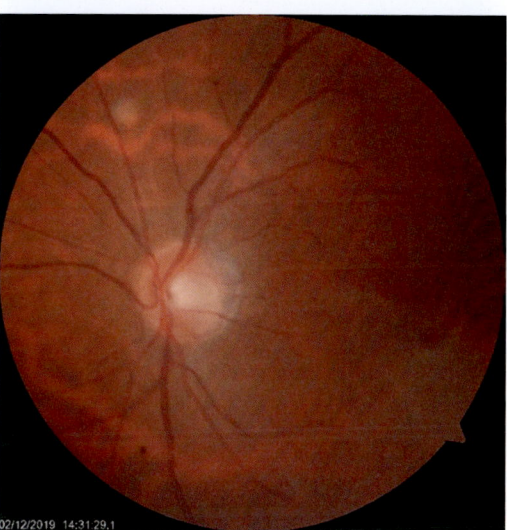

Fig. 8.23 OS CDR 0.3 normal

correlate well. (Fig. 8.26) It is difficult to determine as this is earliest change of glaucoma in presence of normal RNFL or age-related change in macula which were also present in this patient.

Answer 5 When not detected by standard disc photos and visual field, OCT/HRT is next modality to find correlation (Figs. 8.27, 8.28, 8.29, and 8.30).

8.2 Preperimetric Glaucoma

This 30-year-old female with complaints of itching in both eyes had OD-BCVA 6/5 with normal anterior segment. Conjunctiva had mild congestion with few follicles OU. IOP was 16 mmHg and remained so on all visits. Fundus examination showed a CDR of 0.3 with normal NRR and RNFL. OS was same except IOP was 24 mmHg consistently. Fundus examination revealed a CDR

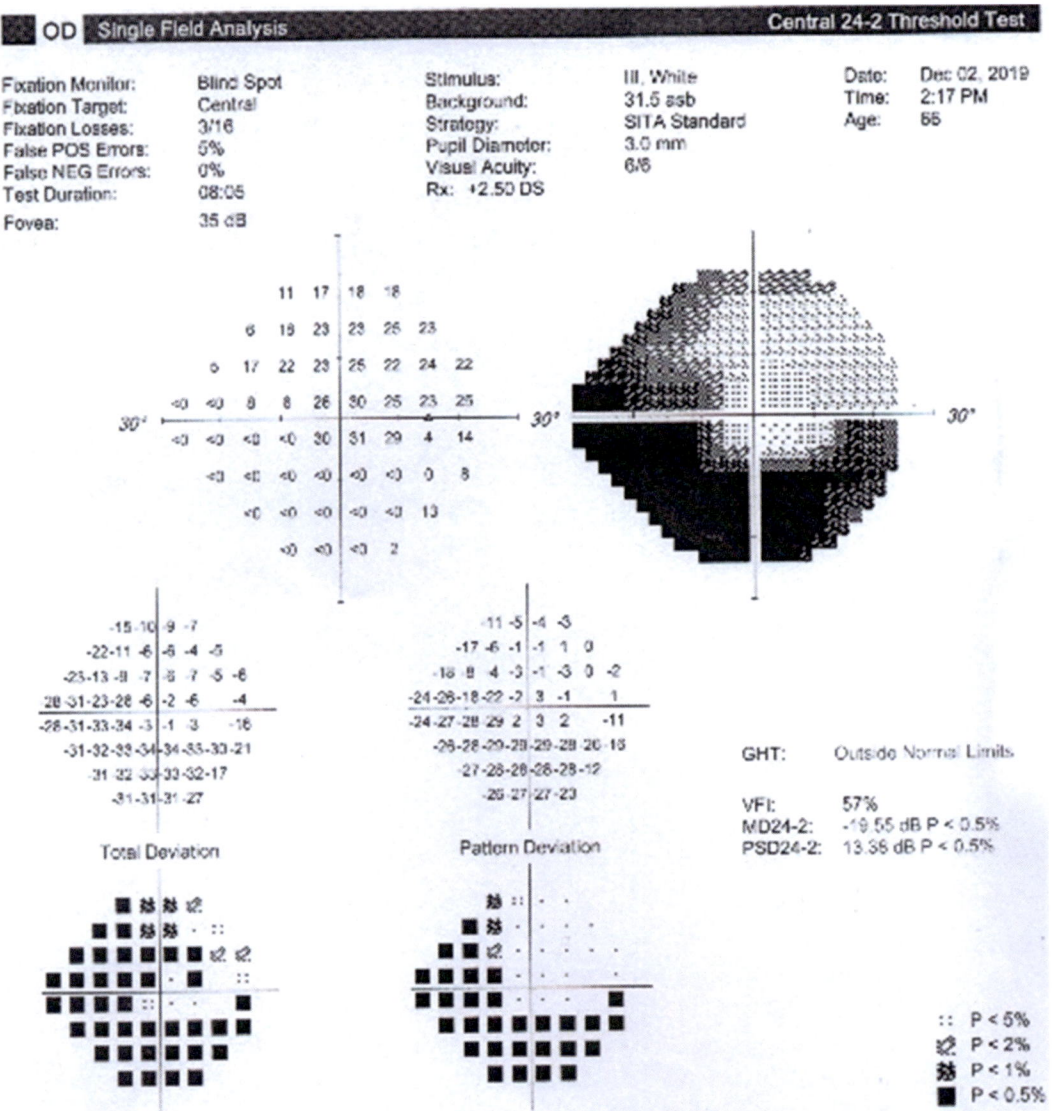

Fig. 8.24 OD double arcuate scotoma

of 0.6 with mild inferior rim thinning (Figs. 8.27 and 8.28). On probing she gave h/o closed globe injury by a wooden object to OS which was treated symptomatically 10 years back. Gonioscopy revealed angle recession of 270 degrees.

Visual fields HVF 24-2 normal in OU (Fig. 8.30). OCT showed average RNFL thickness 91:84 in OD:OS with localized thinning in inferior quadrant in OS (Fig. 8.29). *Keeping in view asymmetric IOP difference of 8 mmHg, asymmetric CDR a difference of 0.2 and OCT showing a difference of RNFL thickness 91:84 (12%) and localized thinning in inferior quadrant are suggestive of preperimetric glaucoma as shown in continuum by Weinreb that structural changes precede visual field changes in majority of the patients.*

8.3 Conclusion

Structure function correlation is integral part of glaucoma diagnosis. Visual fields are the measure of function and directly affect quality of life of the patients. However, in absence of other parameters like corresponding structural changes in optic nerve head, their value is greatly reduced

8 Structure–Function Relation in Humphrey Perimetry

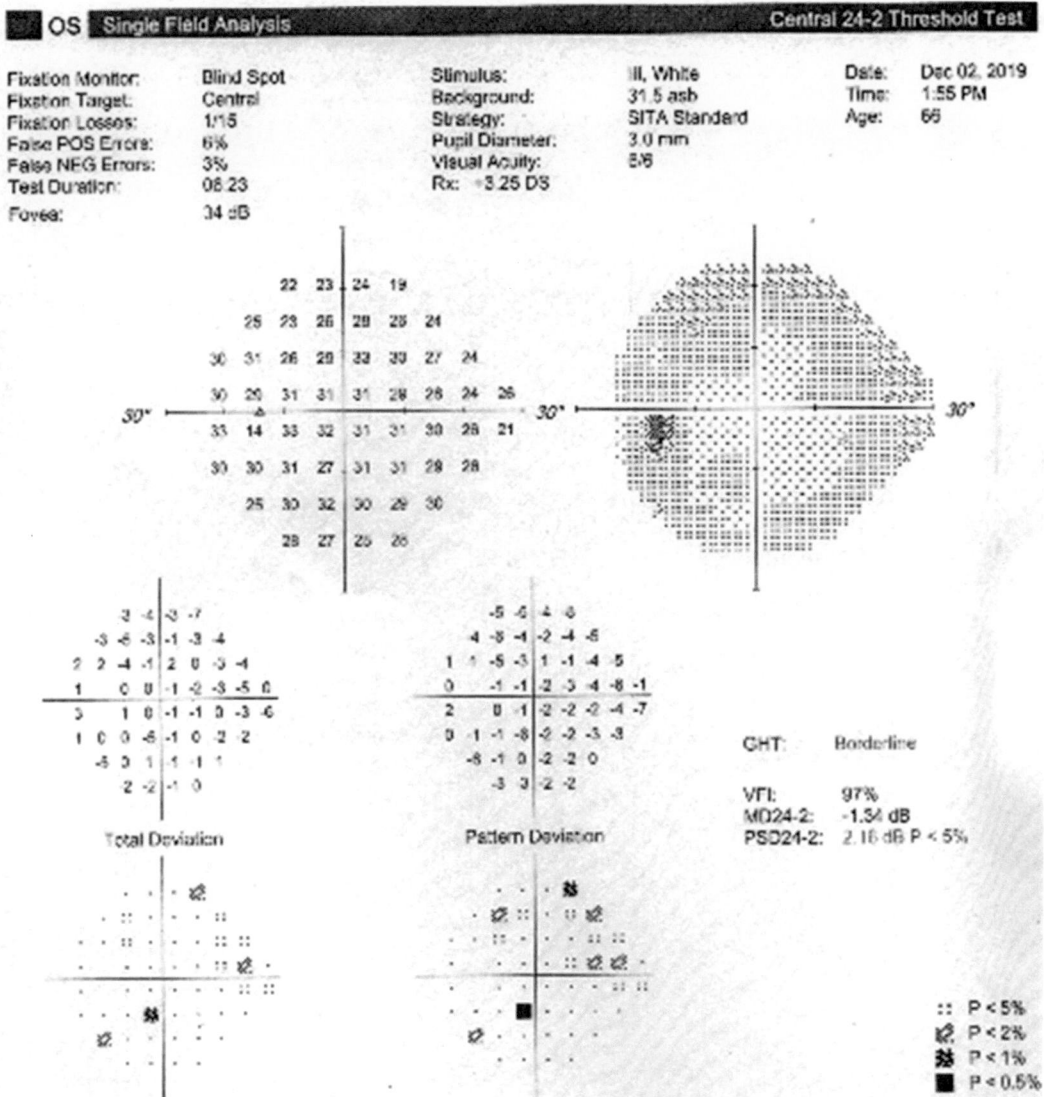

Fig. 8.25 OS normal visual field

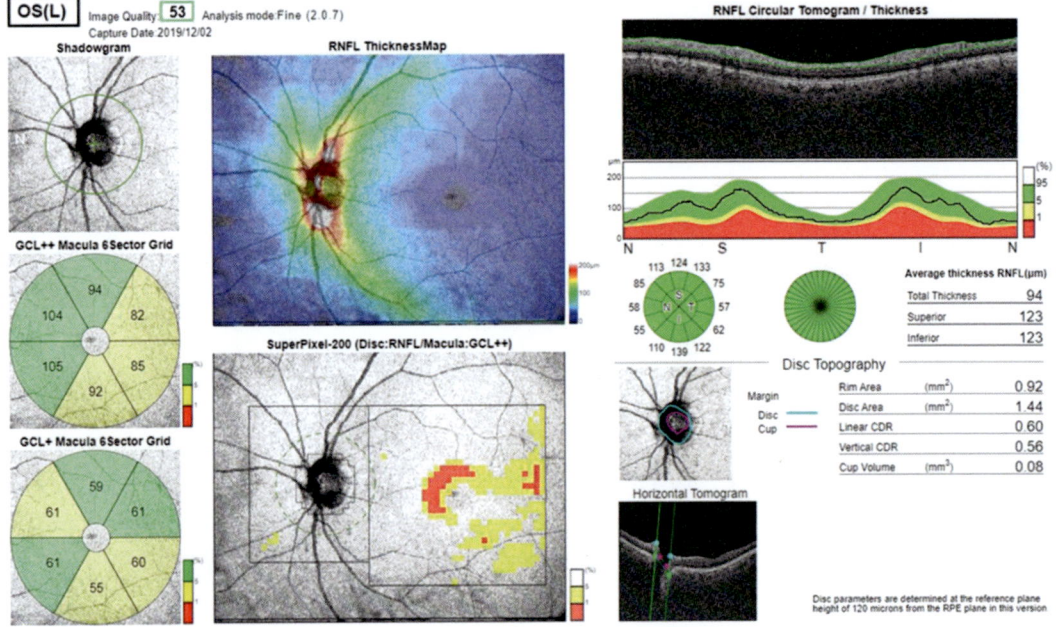

Fig. 8.26 OCT OS normal disc and RNFL GCL shows border line change

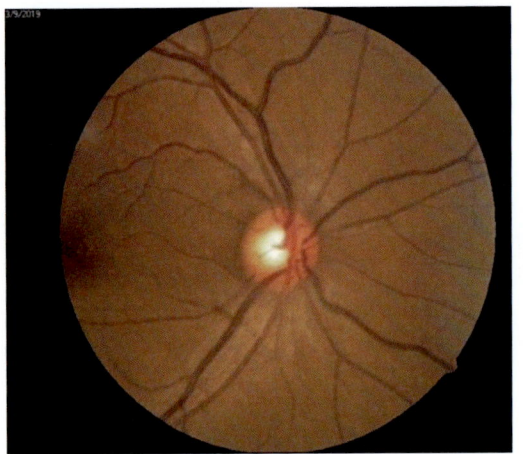

Fig. 8.27 Normal optic disc OD

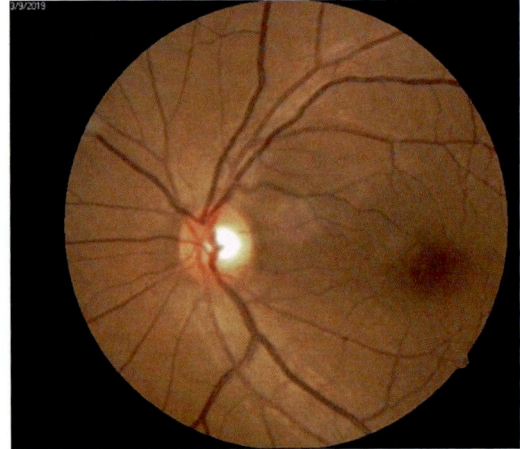

Fig. 8.28 Disc OS CDR 0.6

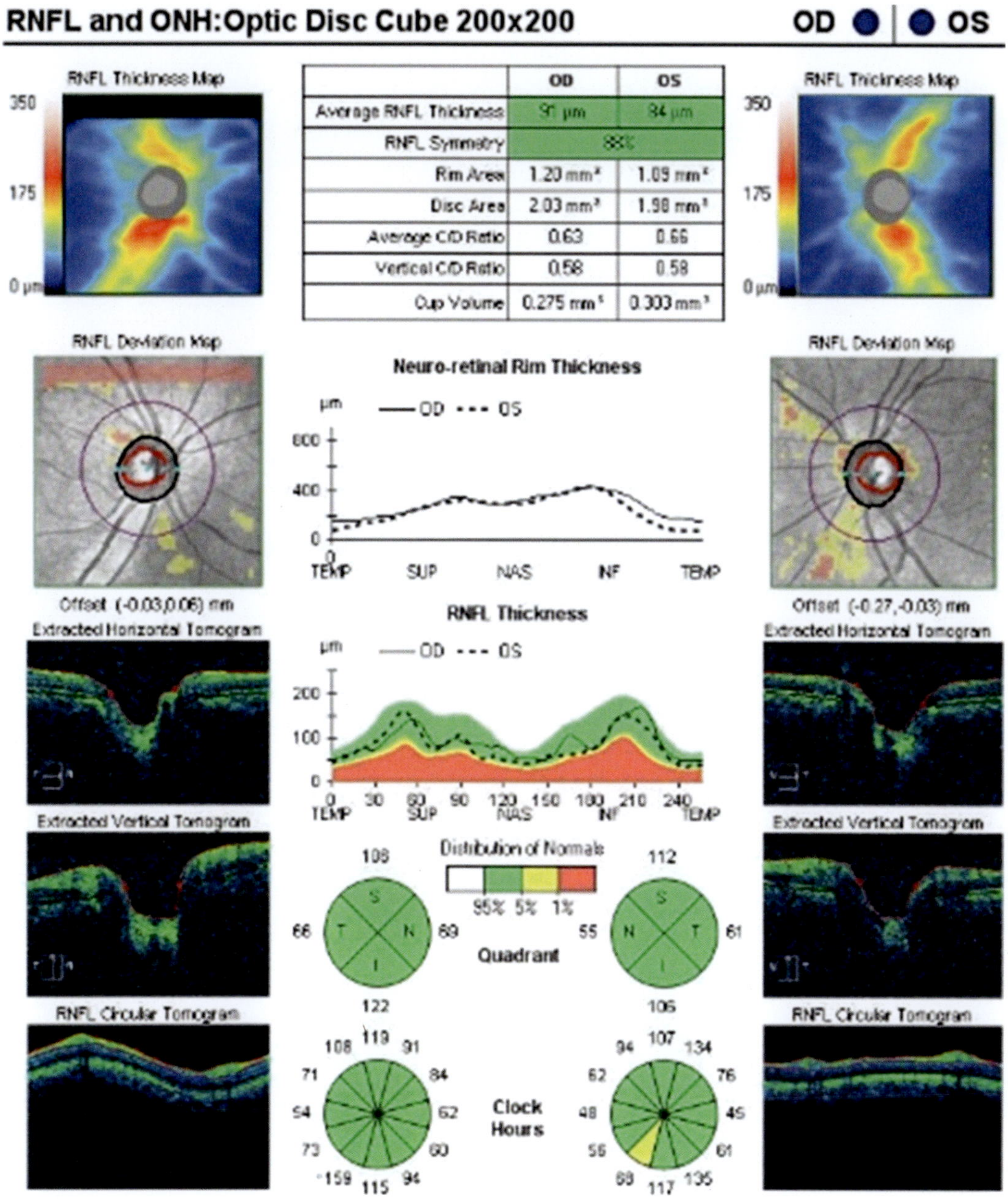

Fig. 8.29 Inferotemporal sector defect

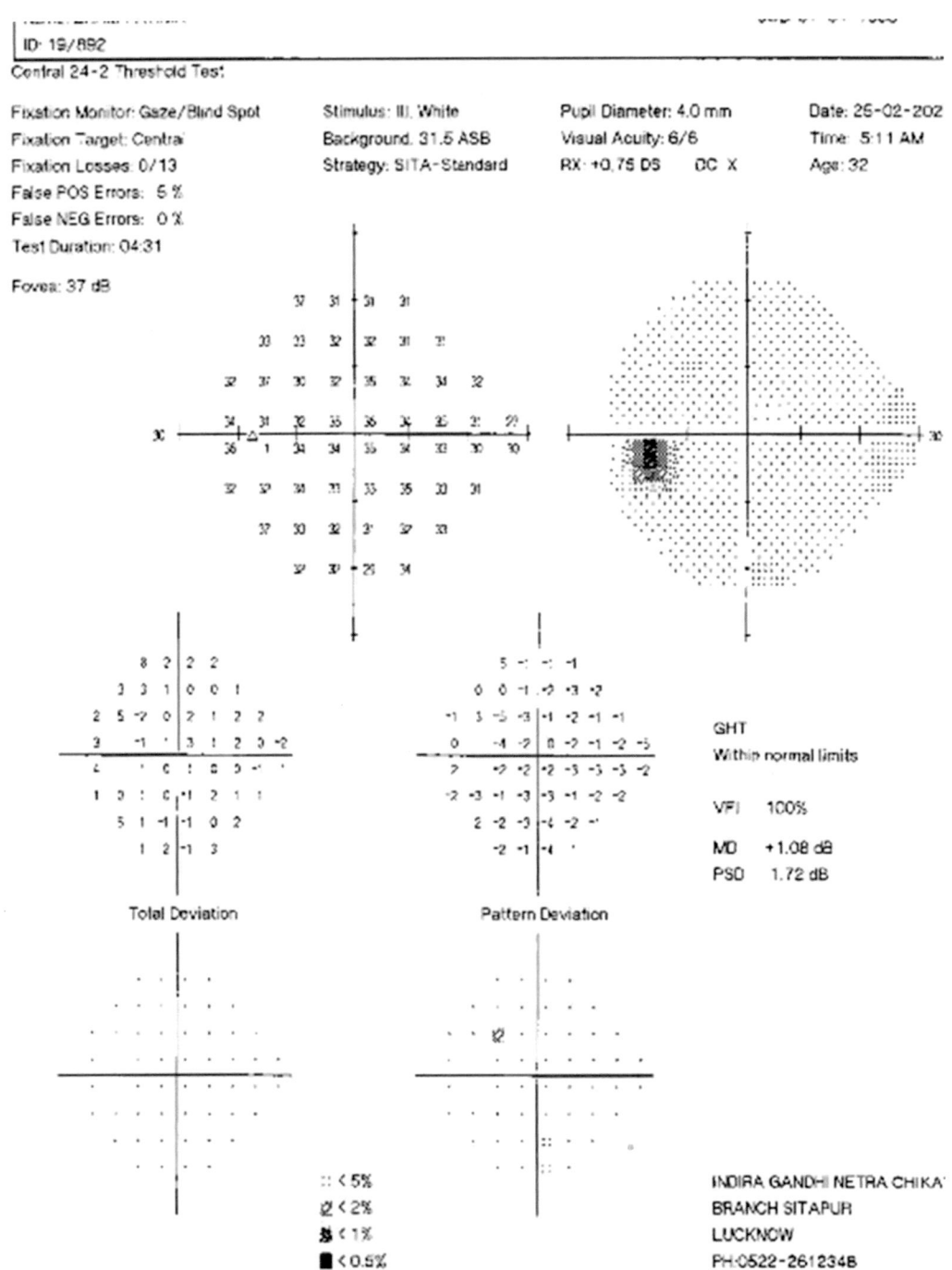

Fig. 8.30 Visual field normal

for glaucoma diagnosis as they are found in many other diseases of CNS and retina. To pinpoint the presence, degree of severity and progression a correlation with structural changes optic nerve head is mandatory. Despite the common knowledge that structural changes precede functional changes, there is sufficient evidence from OHTS and EMGS studies that visual field changes can precede structural changes in a subset of patients hence should be searched for and followed in all glaucoma suspects.

References

1. Read RM, Spaeth GL. The practical clinical appraisal of the optic disc in glaucoma: the naturalhistory of cup progression and some specific disc-field correlations. Trans Am Acad Ophthalmol Otolaryngol. 1974;78(2):OP255-74.
2. Quigley HA, Dunkelberger GR, Green WR. Retinal ganglion cell atrophy correlated with automated-perimetry in human eyes with glaucoma. Am J Ophthalmol. 1989;107(5):453–64.
3. Harwerth RS, Carter-Dawson L, Shen F, Smith EL 3rd, Crawford ML. Ganglion cell losses underlying visual field defects from experimental glaucoma. Invest Ophthalmol Vis Sci. 1999;40(10):2242–50.
4. Schlottmann PG, De Cilla S, Greenfield DS, Caprioli J, Garway-Heath DF. Relationship between visual field sensitivity and retinal nerve fiber layer thickness as measured by scanning laserpolarimetry. Invest Ophthalmol Vis Sci. 2004;45(6):1823–9.
5. Sihota R, Sony P, Gupta V, Dada T, Singh R. Diagnostic capability of optical coherence tomography in evaluating the degree of glaucomatous retinal nerve fiber damage. Invest Ophthalmol Vis Sci. 2006;47(5):2006–10.
6. Garway-Heath DF, Holder GE, Fitzke FW, Hitchings RA. Relationship between electrophysiological, psychophysical, and anatomical measurements in glaucoma. Invest Ophthalmol Vis Sci. 2002;43(7):2213–20.
7. Quigley HA, Addicks EM, Green WR. Optic nerve damage in human glaucoma. III. Quantitative correlation of nerve fiber loss and visual field defect in glaucoma, ischemic neuropathy, papilledema, and toxic neuropathy. Arch Ophthalmol. 1982;100(1):135–46.
8. Pederson JE, Anderson DR. The mode of progressive disc cupping in ocular hypertension and glaucoma. Arch Ophthalmol. 1980;98(3):490–5.
9. Yablonski ME, Zimmerman TJ, Kass MA, Becker B. Prognostic significance of optic disk cupping in ocular hypertensive patients. Am J Ophthalmol. 1980;89(4):585–92.
10. Bartz-Schmidt KU, Thumann G, Jonescu-Cuypers CP, Krieglstein GK. Quantitative morphologic and functional evaluation of the optic nerve head in chronic open-angle glaucoma. Surv Ophthalmol. 1999;44(Suppl 1):S41–53.
11. Airaksinen PJ, Drance SM, Douglas GR, Schulzer M. Neuroretinal rim areas and visual fieldindices in glaucoma. Am J Ophthalmol. 1985;99(2):107–10.
12. Jonas JB, Grundler AE. Correlation between mean visual field loss and morphometric optic diskvariables in the open-angle glaucomas. Am J Ophthalmol. 1997;124(4):488–97.
13. Shafi A, Swanson WH, Dul MW. Structure and function in patients with glaucomatous defects near fixation. Optom Vis Sci. 2011;88(1):130–9.
14. Weinreb RN, Garway-Heath DF. World Glaucoma association 2011. Progression of glaucoma. Amsterdam, the Netherlands: Kugler Publications; 2011.
15. Keltner JL, Johnson CA, Anderson DR, Levine RA, Fan J, Cello KE, et al. The association between glaucomatous visual fields and optic nerve head features in the Ocular Hypertension Treatment Study. Ophthalmology. 2006;113(9):1603–12.
16. Leske MC, Heijl A, Hussein M, Bengtsson B, Hyman L, Komaroff E. Factors for glaucoma progression and the effect of treatment: the early manifest glaucoma trial. Arch Ophthalmol. 2003;121(1):48–56.

9

Structure–Function Relation in Octopus Perimetry

N. R. Rangaraj and P. Sathyan

9.1 Introduction to Structure and Function on an Octopus Perimeter

Octopus visual field machines have undergone steady changes in the hardware, programs and strategies from the time of introduction to clinical practice in the late 1970s. Imaging on the other hand underwent an exponential change from color and red-free fundus photography to OCT spectral domain and SS OCT. Integrating the functional results with appropriate representation to compliment the data representation from the scanning devices would meet the goal of better clinical interpretation of the patient's condition at hand. Patient's quality of life depends on the functional vision. The functional vision estimated by perimetry quantifies the quality of vision in the context, for activities of daily living and driving, e.g., the Esterman binocular visual field testing for driving abilities. The structure and functional investigations compliment the diagnosis and follow-up of primary open angle glaucoma. The present chapter details the use of visual field representation in the Octopus perimeter that is useful for clinical correlation and

complimenting various imaging modalities for diagnosis and follow-up.

9.2 Octopus Perimeter Representations Useful in Diagnosis

The new Octopus EyeSuite 9 in 1 single field analysis printout provides new additional representations that help to compliment the data from imaging and clinical examination. The 9 in 1 printout (Fig. 9.1) includes the cluster and polar analysis in addition to the typical representations in the 7 in 1 printout [1].

9.2.1 Cluster Analysis

Cluster analysis is sensitive to detection of change that occurs in early glaucoma. Single test locations showing change probability is subject to considerable fluctuation. The clusters represent the tested location of the corresponding nerve fiber bundle that is grouped to calculate the local mean or the cluster MD. The 30° visual field is divided into ten clusters. Each hemifield superiorly and inferiorly has five clusters that represent the test locations in the macular, nasal step, superior arcuate, and temporal wedge. Small changes in a sector are highlighted in Fig. 9.2 that shows the superior arcuate cluster

N. R. Rangaraj (✉)
Premier Eye Care and Surgical Center, Chennai, India

P. Sathyan
Sathyan Eye Care Hospital and Coimbatore Glaucoma Foundation, Coimbatore, India

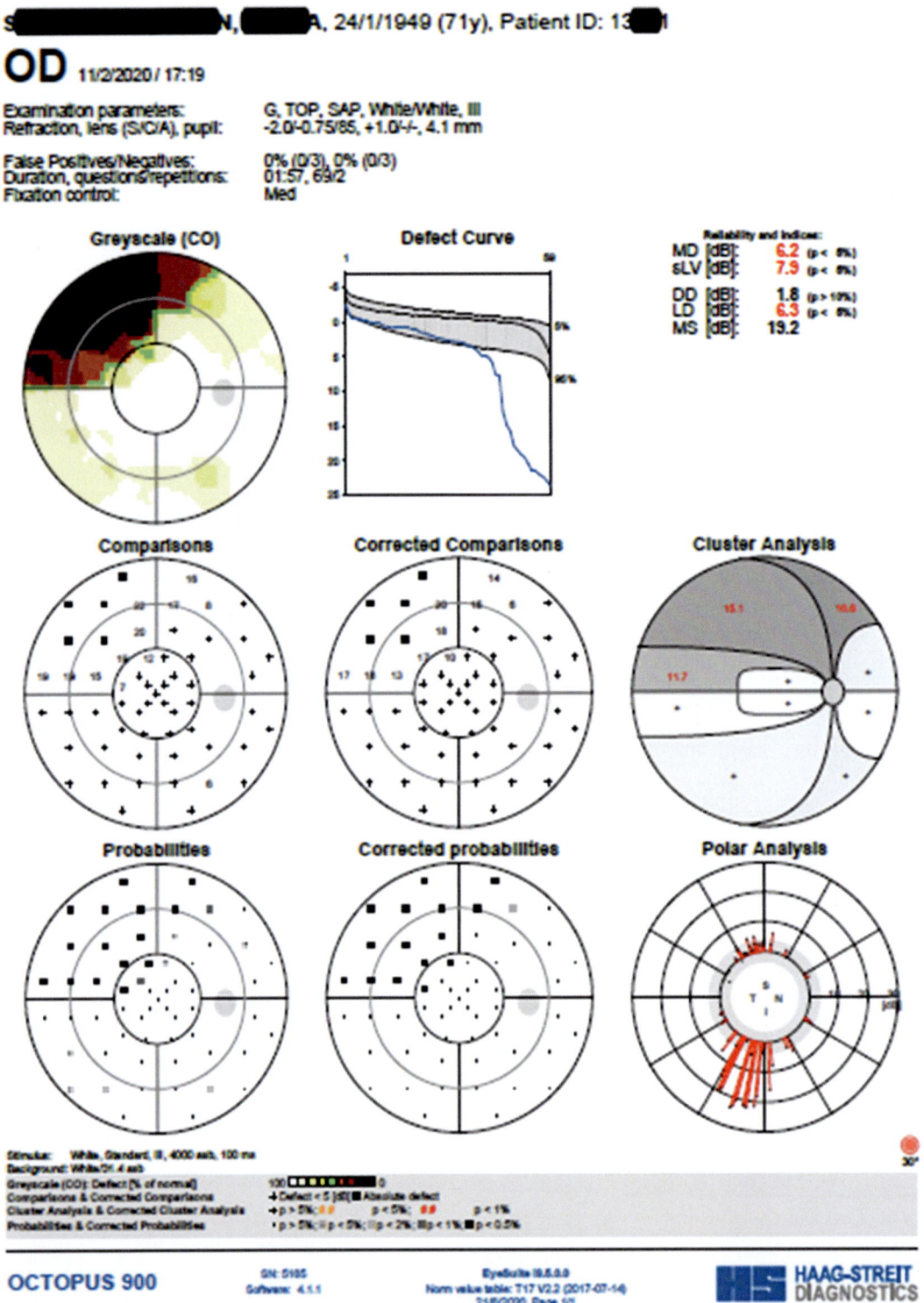

Fig. 9.1 The 9 in 1 printout with cluster and polar analysis

MD at 3.3 indicating a worsening or decrease in sensitivity at test locations clustered together that represent the corresponding nerve fiber bundles. The other clusters show a "+" sign indicating a normal value. The gray scale and defect curve almost pass of as normal for the same patient as in Fig. 9.3. The global index MD being −1.8 (<2.0 normal MD) in this patient. The clinical utility of the cluster analysis is demonstrated in the two clusters representing the superior arcuate MD at 3.3 with bold letters indicating 1% significance and nasal step MD at 1.5 with normal font indicating 5% significance. The defect curve shows a dip on the right side within the normative band. Cluster analysis highlights subtle changes which flag the clinician to look for structural changes.

9.2.2 Polar Analysis

The polar analysis display is exclusive to glaucoma in the 9 in 1 printout. The representation is the functional extrapolation of the structural changes due to glaucoma that gives a pointer to the expected structural damage on the optic nerve head. The polar analysis is based on the nerve fiber distribution; the superior visual field loss representation is flipped across the horizontal to correspond to loss in the inferior portion of the optic disc representation. The site of the test location determines the angle of entry for the polar representation. The length of the bar showing the loss of sensitivity in dB with the gray zone showing the normal values between −2.0 and +2.0.

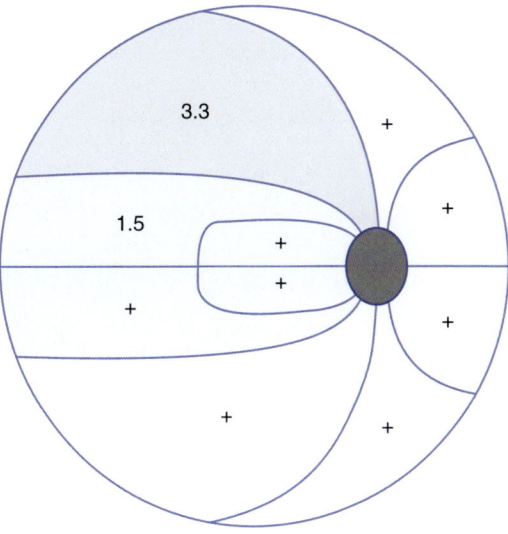

Fig. 9.2 Cluster analysis highlighting sector MD worsening

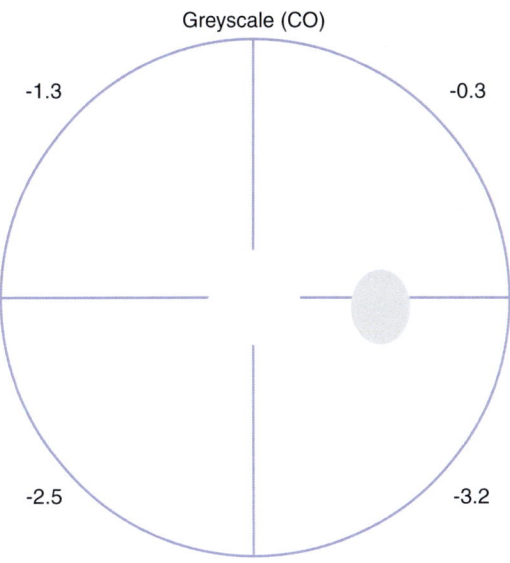

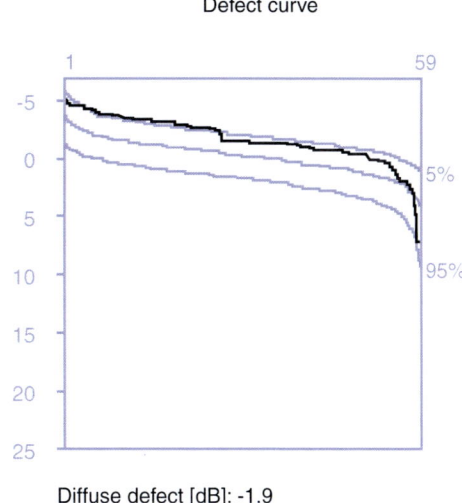

Fig. 9.3 Gray scales and defect curve show no worsening

9.3 Octopus Perimeter Representations Useful in Follow-up

The follow-up representations in Octopus EyeSuite software compliment the structural imaging. The polar and cluster trends are functional representations that highlight the structural damage in images at the optic disc and macula map in the follow-up examinations [2, 3]. The cluster and polar trends are described in Chap. 7. The function and structure correlation is best highlighted with examples.

9.3.1 Illustrative Example

59-year-old patient diagnosed to have POAG on follow-up with visual fields, fundus pictures, and OCT of the RNFL and macula map. The corrected comparisons from visual field tests done in 2015 and 2019 show subtle worsening at four tested locations situated in the superior arcuate area of the 2019 single fields. (Fig. 9.6).

The composite screenshot view of the global, cluster, and polar trends with selected visual fields performed from 2015 to 2019 is displayed in Fig. 9.7. The global index sLV is flagged (open triangle) at 5% significance indicating worsening of the focal area and not sufficient enough to affect the LD and MD. The cluster trends show the affected clusters in numerical value with polar trends showing the inferior temporal area worsening. This example alerts the clinician to worsening in the visual field. Outliers of visual fields when not conforming to clinically expected results or not trustworthy may be deselected to uncover the actual worsening.

The following below example Fig. 9.8 shows the effect of manually deselecting the outlier visual fields performed in 2017 from the above example in Fig. 9.7.

The sLV is flagged at 1% significance with local defect at 5% significance. The corrected cluster and polar trends also supplement the information on topography of the defect with probable area of damage on the optic disc (Figs. 9.9 and 9.10).

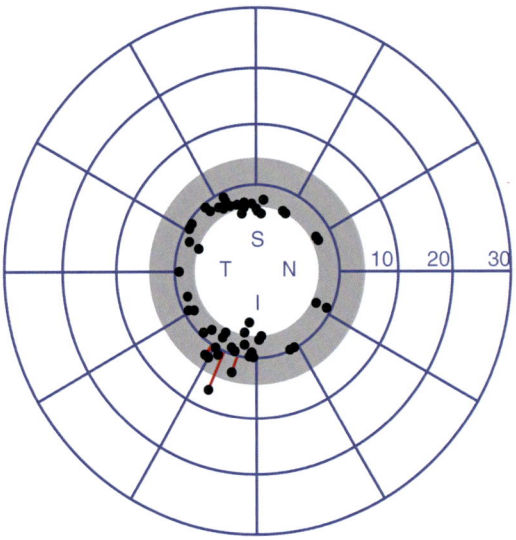

Fig. 9.4 Polar analysis

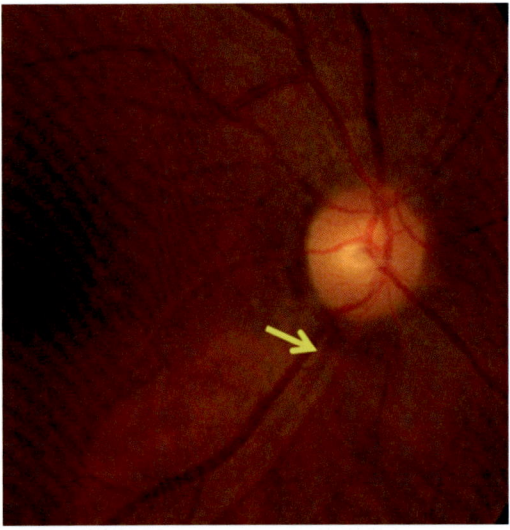

Fig. 9.5 Optic disc photo with NFL loss *inferotemporal*, yellow arrow

The polar analysis in Fig. 9.4 shows the subtle loss of sensitivity at the inferior temporal nerve fiber angle that is highlighted by the defects in the superior arcuate and the nasal step. The corresponding loss (arrow) is identified on the optic disc photograph (Fig. 9.5). The 9 in 1 printout (Fig. 9.1) displays all the representations and highlights the relevant loss of sensitivity and the pointer to look at the expected NFL loss on the optic disc.

9 Structure–Function Relation in Octopus Perimetry

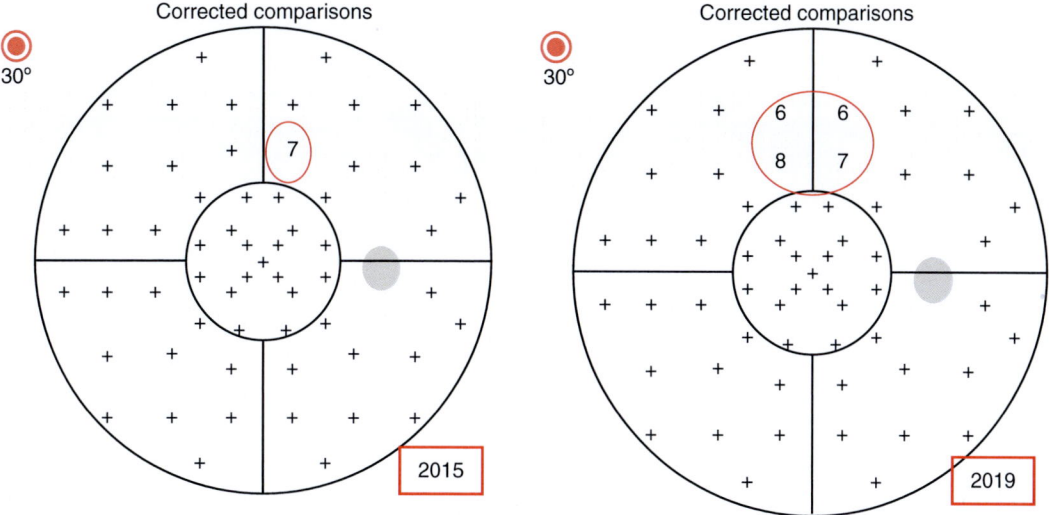

Fig. 9.6 Corrected comparisons from 2015 to 2019 showing worsening

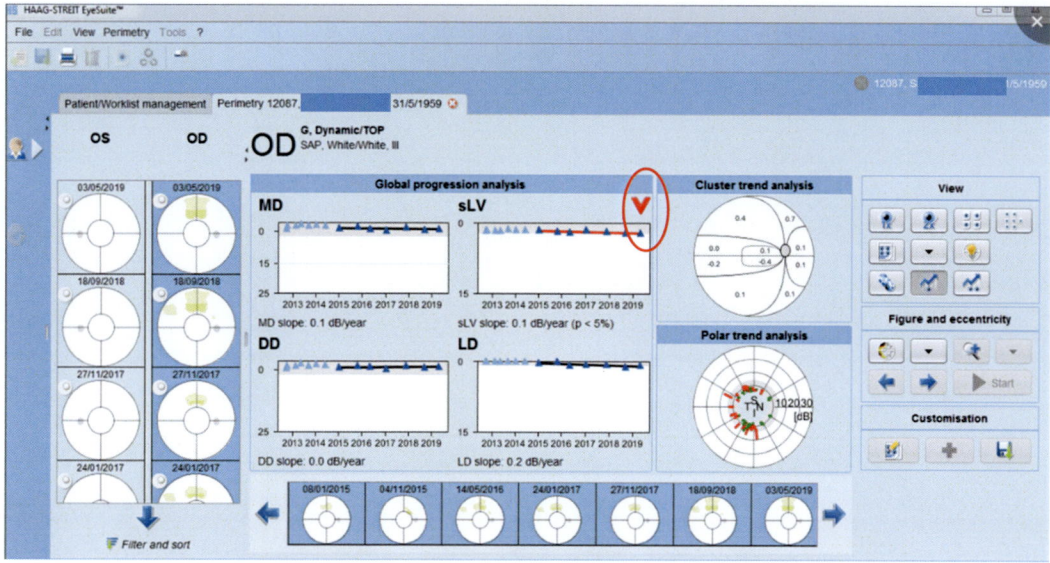

Fig. 9.7 Screenshot of serial gray scales, global indices, cluster trends, and polar trends with ten visits selected manually

The serial fundus picture of the same patient from 2015 to 2019 (Fig. 9.11) shows splinter heam on the optic disc and nerve fiber loss (NFL) in red free [4].

The serial OCT RNFL maps (difference maps) show the 12-sector optic disc analysis flagging the subtle loss of RNFL at optic disc inferior temporally with significant "*p* value" (Fig. 9.12) [5]. Sector analysis can be done as 2 sectors, 4 sectors, or 12 sectors. The 2 sectors pie chart computes the average in the upper and lower hemifield, hence may not be sensitive to small changes. The 12 sectors pie chart is sensitive to small changes hence a useful selection in this case, red arrow in the Fig. 9.12.

The OCT macula map (Fig. 9.13) though not showing a significant "*p* value," the arcuate area highlighted red on the sectorial map drawing the

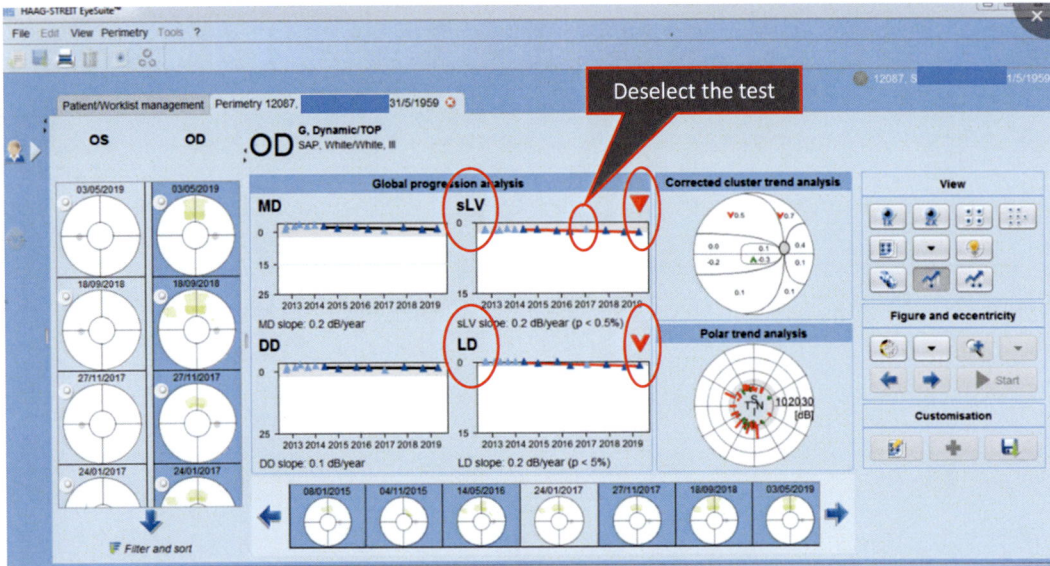

Fig. 9.8 Manual deselecting of outlier 2017 test result

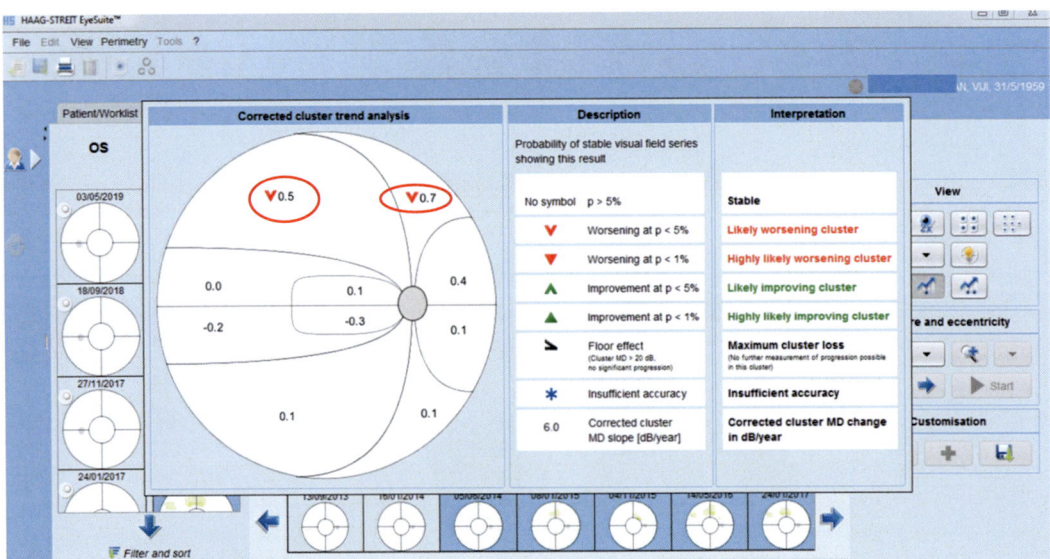

Fig. 9.9 Corrected cluster trend analysis

attention of the clinician to the worsening or thinning in that area. The difference map highlights the change in thickness measured from the baseline map.

The above case example can be summarized as follows; the base line data of the visual field was good with one outlier being deselected. Short strategy was used (G TOP) to make it patient friendly. The frequency was customized to yearly follow-up in this patient who had stable IOP. The visual fields and structure images compliment to give the clinician a good idea of the significance of the worsening over the years. The structural images with use of color and red-free images display the optic disc as it looked on follow-up. The OCT RNFL and macula map quantified the nerve fiber loss with easy-to-understand display (difference maps) to make therapeutic decisions.

9 Structure–Function Relation in Octopus Perimetry

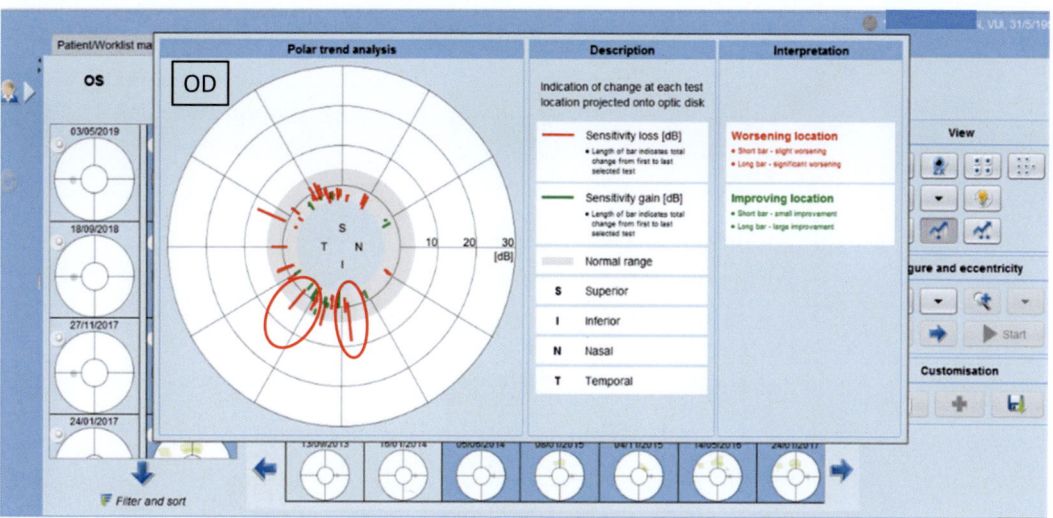

Fig. 9.10 Polar trend analysis

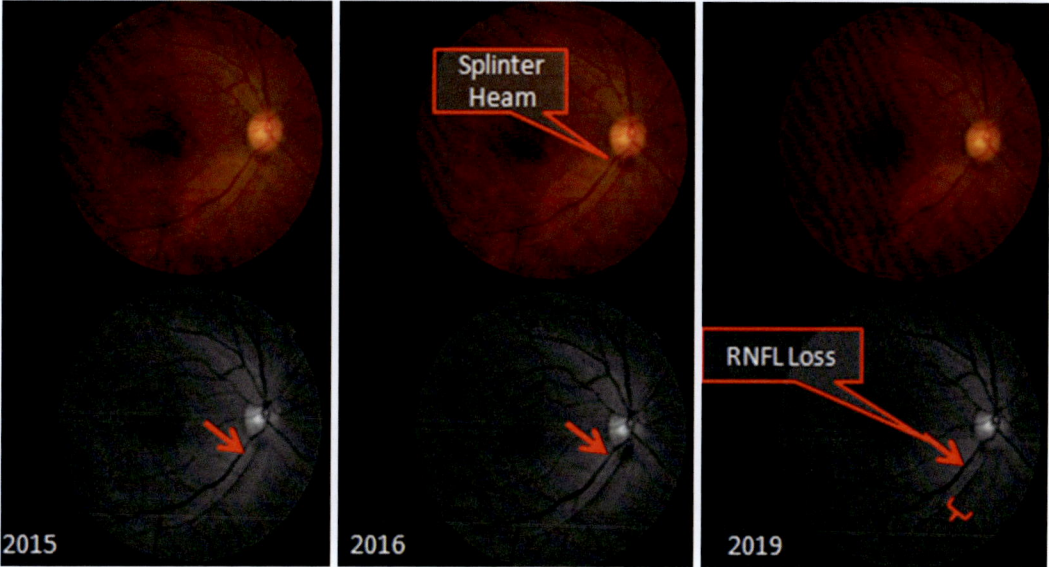

Fig. 9.11 Serial fundus photography, color and red free

9.4 Structure and Function the Current Status in Detecting Progression

Structure and function is often debated to claim superiority of one modality over the other. This debate could be abandoned now with a fresh look at using the imaging and the visual function studies to complement each other to provide the best modality for the given stage in the natural history of the disease to detect progression [6]. Studies have shown that detection of simultaneous change in structure and function occurs infrequently. Öhnell et al. study of the data from EMGT showed the correlation to be simultaneous in only 1 in 360 study eyes [7]. Ocular hypertension study showed that, eyes that progressed from ocular hypertension to

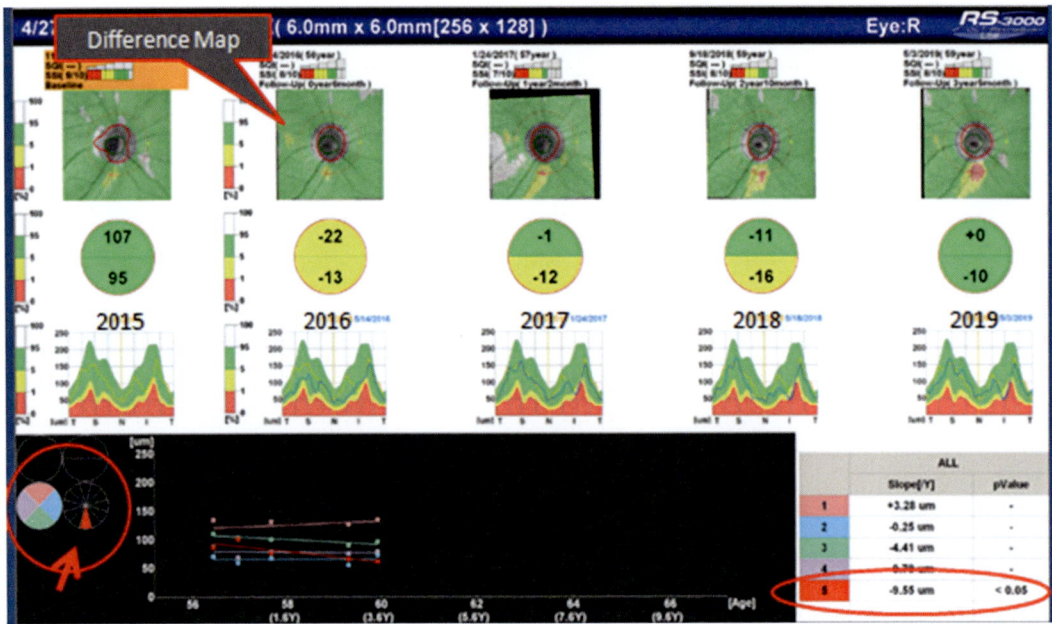

Fig. 9.12 RNFL difference map shows the baseline and subsequent changes

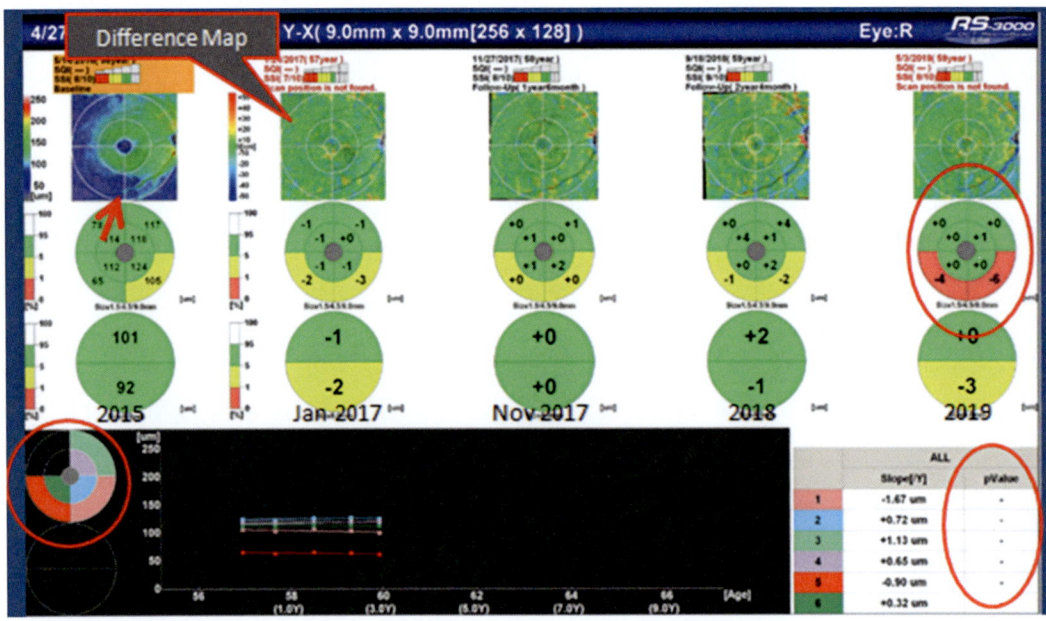

Fig. 9.13 OCT macula map (red highlight) with inferior arcuate loss in thickness

glaucoma, only 7% showed simultaneous correlation. The dynamic range of the structural changes is linear and the visual function being algorithmic. This disagreement does not indicate poor predictive ability, rather demonstrates the complimentary role of the two modalities of monitoring progression.

Imaging studies have most utility in early stages of the disease, and OCT rates of RNFL thinning at 1 μm per year was associated with two times higher risk of visual field loss over time. When patient presents with early visual field loss the perimetry seems to track changes better. The disagreements between the two modalities can be used to better arrive at decision on intervention with a little more objectivity.

References

1. Visual Field Digest 6th edition Haag-Streit AG Koniz Switzerland (ISBN 978-3-033-06001-2).
2. Liu T, Tatham AJ, Gracitelli CP, et al. Rates of retinal nerve fiber layer loss in contralateral eyes of glaucoma patients with unilateral progression by conventional methods. Ophthalmology. 2015;122:2243–51.
3. Leung CK, Liu S, Weinreb RN, et al. Evaluation of retinal nerve fiber layer progression in glaucoma a prospective analysis with neuroretinal rim and visual field progression. Ophthalmology. 2011;118:1551–7.
4. Medeiros FA, Lisboa R, Zangwill LM, et al. Evaluation of progressive neuroretinal rim loss as a surrogate end point for development of visual field loss in glaucoma. Ophthalmology. 2014;121:100–9.
5. Miki A, Medeiros FA, Weinreb RN, et al. Rates of retinal nerve fiber layer thinning in glaucoma suspect eyes. Ophthalmology. 2014;121:1350–8.
6. Chauhan BC, Nicolela MT, Artes PH. Incidence and rates of visual field progression after longitudinally measured optic disc change in glaucoma. Ophthalmology. 2009;116:2110–8.
7. Öhnell H, Heijl A, Brenner L, et al. Structural and functional progression in the Early Manifest Glaucoma Trial. Ophthalmology. 2016;123:1173–80.

10. Check–Recheck: Visual Field Dilemmas in Retinal Disorders

Ritesh Narula and Chitralekha De

Objectives Visual field testing in retinal disorders is an underutilised investigation, the potential of which needs to be realised. It is one of the most readily available functional tests. Through this case-based chapter, we would like to introduce our readers to using Humphrey visual fields for both diagnosis and prognosis of various retinal diseases.

10.1 Introduction

Retinal practice today is strongly dependent on the use of various diagnostic modalities. Most of those commonly used such as fluorescein angiography (FFA), optical coherence tomography (OCT) and ultrasonography (USG) are structural tests. These investigations give us a detailed understanding of the anatomy of the retina and its vascular supply and if any abnormality in the same but do not actually reflect upon its actual functional integrity. With more awareness amongst patients with regard their disease, very often a pretreatment functional assessment becomes necessary. Fundus reflectometry, electrophysiological tests (EOG, pattern ERG, flash ERG) and microperimetry are some of the tests of functional integrity which can be useful but are often not readily available [1].

In contrast, static perimetry using Humphrey visual field analyser can be an easily available, useful tool for assessment of retinal function though its use in practice has been limited. This traditional method of visual function testing is extremely useful to evaluate changes in visual function when visual acuity is not the best method to assess disease progression in both glaucoma and retinal disorders [2].

Some of the field changes associated with retinal disorders have been well documented. Peripheral constriction of fields is seen in patients of retinitis pigmentosa and other rod cell dysfunction [3] while macular disorders such as age-related macular degeneration (AMD) are associated with central/paracentral scotomas [4]. An absolute scotoma opposite to the quadrant of lesion is associated with retinoschisis while a relative scotoma is seen in patients with retinal detachment [5].

In spite of these well-known changes, visual field testing can be quiet confusing in patients with many retinal disorders especially if coexisting with glaucoma. At the same time, if properly done and utilised, visual field can add a lot to both the prognosis and management of patients with retinal diseases. The following illustrated case descriptions will highlight the above points in more detail.

R. Narula (✉) · C. De
Centre for Sight Eye Institute, New Delhi, India

10.2 Clinical Situation 1: Humphrey Visual Field in Retinal Detachment

10.2.1 Case 1

A 55-year-old male patient, with history of cataract surgery in both eyes 1 year back, presented to us with extensive itching in the left eye especially around lower lids with excoriation of the skin. He gave history of the left eye retinal detachment surgery (scleral buckling) 9 years back. He had been diagnosed with left eye open angle glaucoma 3 years back and was on Timolol (0.5%) + Brimonidine (0.2%) combination since then. His best corrected visual acuity was 6/6, N6 both eyes. He had a well-attached retina in both eyes with a good buckle indent seen nasally in the left eye. He had a cup disc ratio of 0.3:1 in the right eye and 0.5–0.6:1 in the left eye. Humphrey visual field (30-2) (Fig. 10.1) showed a field defect in the superotemporal quadrant of the left eye which corresponded to the borderline RNFL loss in the inferonasal quadrant (Fig. 10.2). The dilemma was triggered because the field changes were more dense in the periphery than near the optic nerve head (ONH) (as seen in arcuate scotomas due to glaucoma), and the RNFL loss did not correlate with degree of field loss. *So was this patient's field defects due to glaucoma? Should he continue his antiglaucoma medication?*

A review of records from his retinal detachment surgery showed that the patient had an old inferonasal retinal detachment, macula on secondary to lattice with holes for which a nasal buckle explant was done. The detachment corresponded to the RNFL loss and the subsequent field changes.

Sasoh et al. in their large retrospective series of 205 eyes with 10 years follow-up post scleral buckling had shown similar field defects after retinal detachment. The visual field changes improved significantly up to 1 month post-surgery, and subsequently no significant change was seen over the next 10 years. The degree of visual field loss positively correlated with extent and duration of retinal detachment [6]. Our patient who had an old inferior detachment prior to surgery had a persistent visual field defect in spite a successful attachment of retina post-surgery.

10.2.2 Case 2

This case aptly contrasts the above case and highlights the importance of timely surgical intervention. A 60-year-old male patient had undergone a scleral buckling surgery for a macula on retinal detachment 6 years ago. The interval between detachment and surgery was less than 48 hours. Post-operatively he achieved a BCVA of 6/6, N6 and the Humphrey visual field 30-2 showed minimal isolated scotomas in the quadrant of the detachment (Fig. 10.3). This further proves the positive correlation between field loss and duration of detachment.

10.2.3 Case 3: Does Pars Plana Vitrectomy Carry the Same Results in Visual Field Changes as in Scleral Buckling? Does the Extent of Retinal Detachment Affect the Field Loss?

A 57-year-old male had undergone primary vitrectomy with silicon oil injection for a 10-day-old macula off superior retinal detachment in his left eye. He subsequently underwent silicon oil removal 3 months later. At his 1-year follow-up, he had a BCVA left eye of 6/18, N12 with a well-attached retina. He had a normal cup disc ratio but complained of difficulty in reading and going down the stairs with his left eye. Humphrey visual field 30-2 showed a dense inferior field defect involving fixation (Fig. 10.4). Though the patient improved appreciably in visual acuity, the field loss did not show any significant change. *Was it due to duration of retinal detachment or was vitrectomy responsible for contributing to it?*

Visual field defects have been reported after vitrectomy in multiple studies, even in cases with pre-existing healthy peripheral retina. Generally,

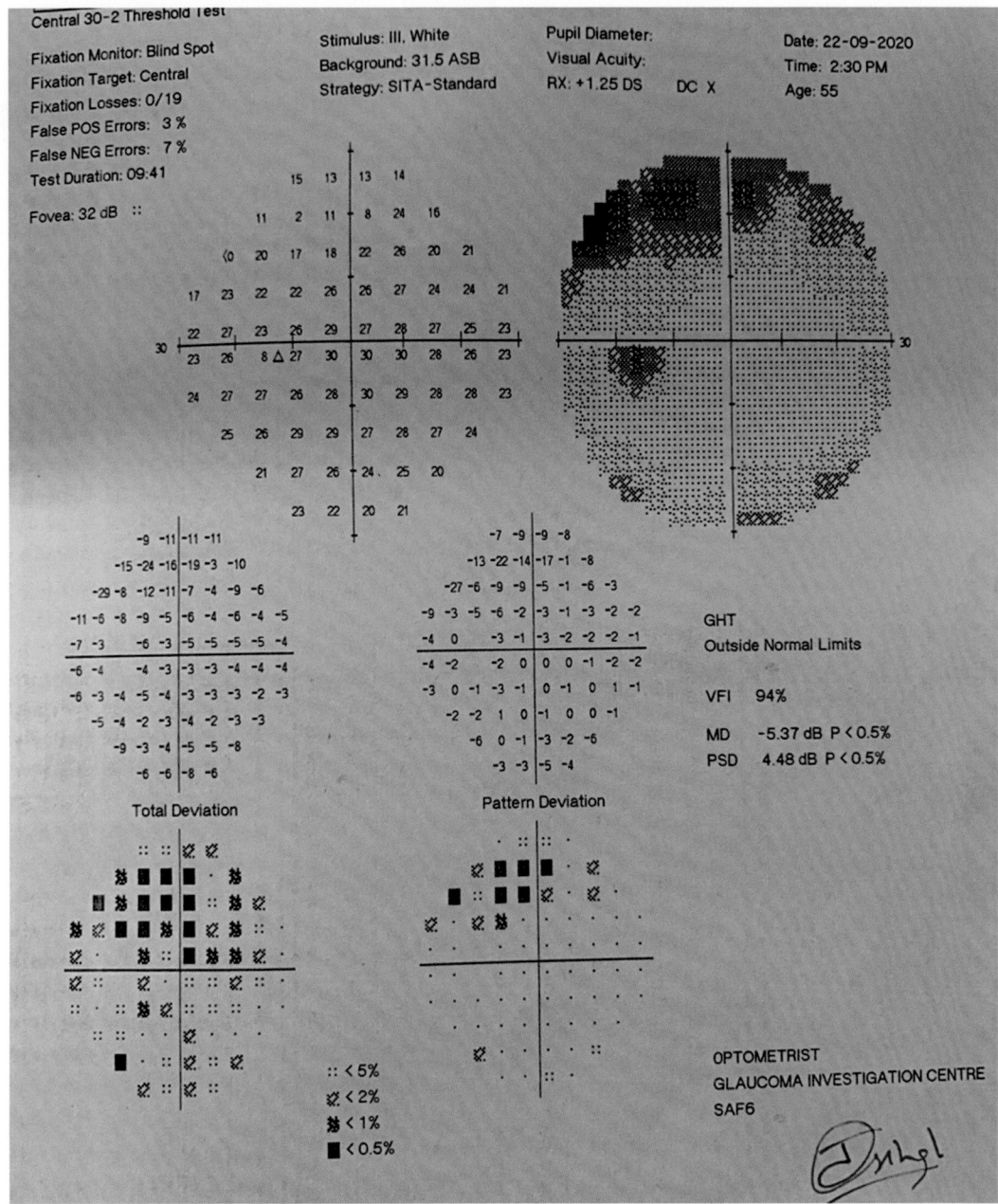

Fig. 10.1 Humphrey visual field (30-2) of the left eye showing an absolute field defect in the superotemporal quadrant of the left eye not involving the fixation

an altitudinal defect has been reported, as seen in our case. Fluid air exchange, an integral part of most vitrectomies, is the step often considered responsible for the same, though some authors have also implicated mechanical damage to the optic nerve head during PVD induction as the possible cause. The most common field defect first noted, in these eyes, was in the inferotemporal quadrant, and it was postulated that it is possible due to inferotemporal location of infusion canula causing air pressure jet towards superonasal quadrant during the air fluid exchange leading

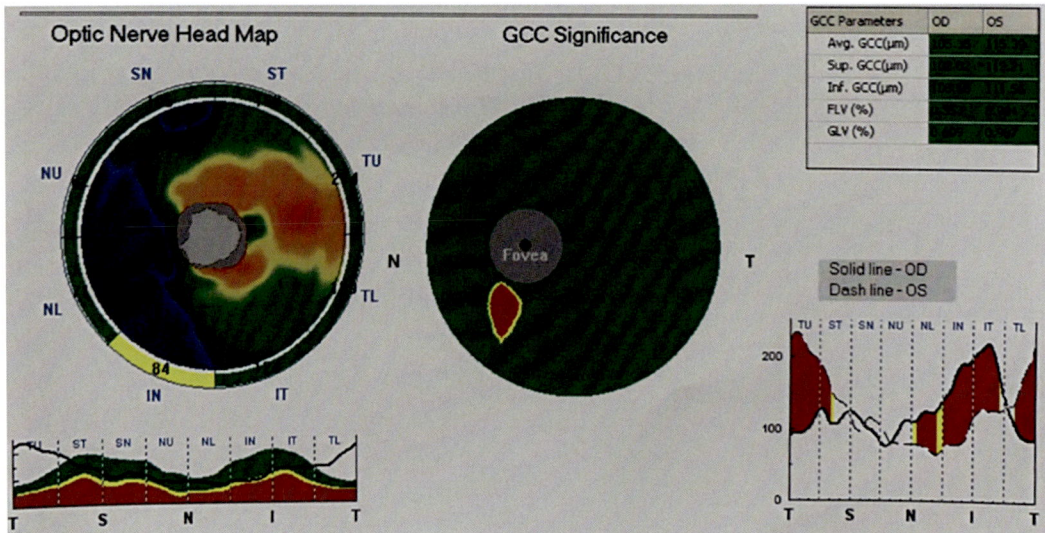

Fig. 10.2 Optical coherence tomography (OCT) of the left eye through the disc showing borderline retinal nerve fibre layer (RNFL) loss in the inferonasal quadrant along with ganglion cell (GCC) loss in the same area

to damage to the inner retinal layers [7]. But an optic nerve damage due to pressure fluctuation is now also considered a possible cause especially due to the use of newer generation vitrectomy machines with pressurised infusion system. Hirata et al. have advised to keep air infusion pressure to <30 mm of Hg during fluid air exchange, which according to them decreased the incidence of visual field defects from 24% to 4% [8].

10.3 Clinical Situation 2: Humphrey Visual Field in Retinoschisis

Retinoschisis is characterised by a split in the neurosensory retina. It can either be congenital or degenerative in aetiology. The visual field defect depends on the location of retinoschisis. Typically, a peripheral retinoschisis is characterised by an absolute scotoma in the area of retinoschisis [5].

10.3.1 Case 4: A Typical Retinoschisis

A 51-year-old female presented to us with an appreciable superior field defect in the left eye. Her BCVA was 6/6 in both eyes. Fundus examination revealed a well-demarcated inferotemporal retinoschisis with a split at the level of outer nuclear layer. There were multiple outer retinal holes also visible (Figs. 10.5 and 10.6). Humphrey visual field showed a superonasal peripheral defect away from the fixation corresponding to the area of retinoschisis (Fig. 10.7).

10.3.2 Case 5: Retinoschisis with Glaucoma

A 14-year-old presented to us diagnosed as open angle congenital glaucoma with advanced cupping and pallor. He had been on prostaglandin analogues for the last few years and was referred to retina specialist for treatment of prostaglandin-induced cystoid macular oedema (Fig. 10.8). The optical coherence tomography revealed a split in the neurosensory retina at the level of outer nuclear layer throughout the macula with foveal thinning (Fig. 10.9). This was seen on fundus examination as a cartwheel appearance of fovea (Fig. 10.8). His BCVA in both eyes were 6/18. The child could perform a reliable field in only the right eye, which showed a

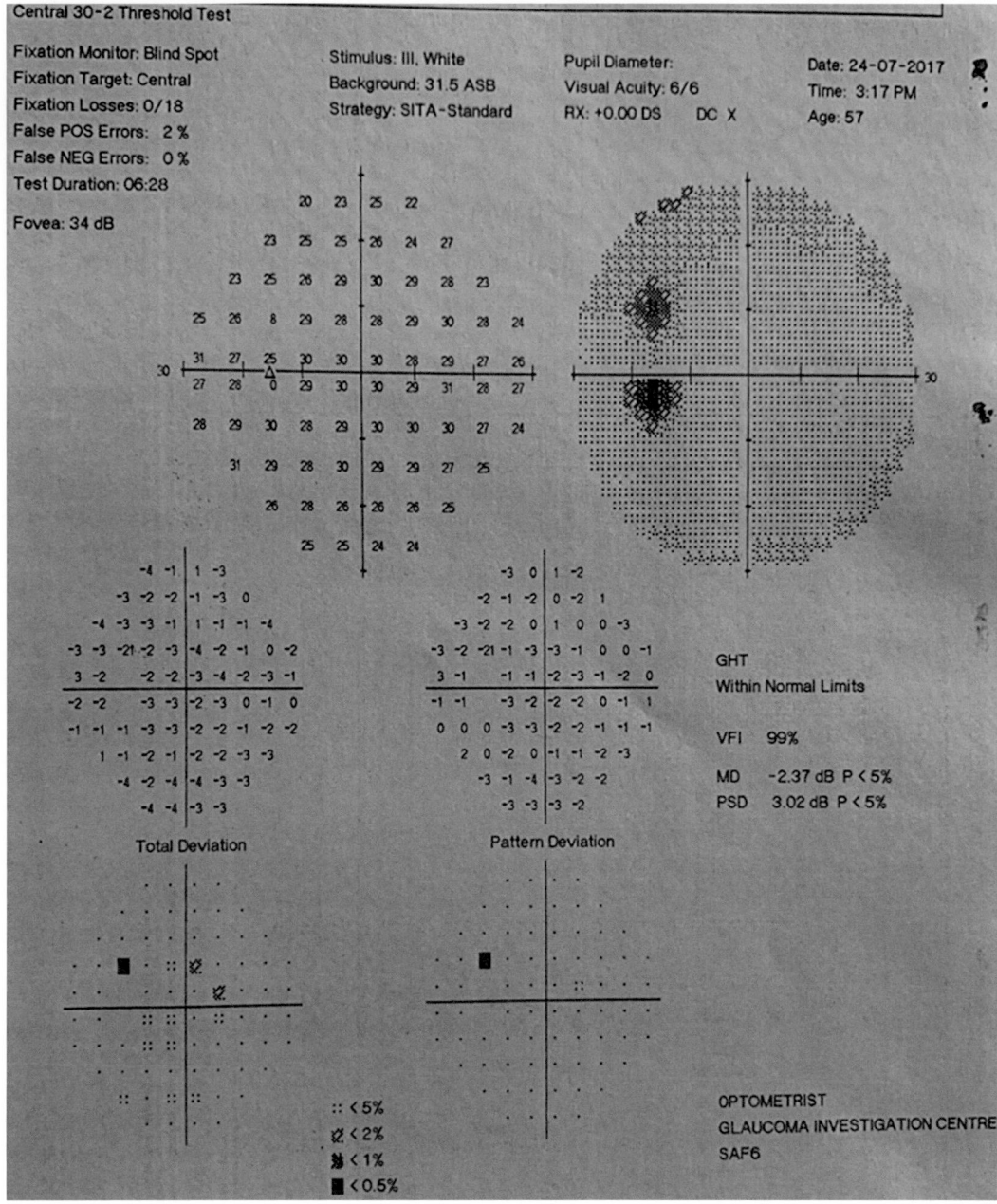

Fig. 10.3 Humphrey visual field 30-2 of the left eye post scleral buckling surgery showed essentially a normal visual field with minimal isolated scotomas in the quadrant of the detachment

consistent superotemporal field defect, stable over a year (Fig. 10.10). *Were these field changes due to congenital glaucoma?*

A detailed evaluation of the fundus periphery showed a shallow dome-shaped retinoschisis in the inferonasal quadrant in both the eyes. The

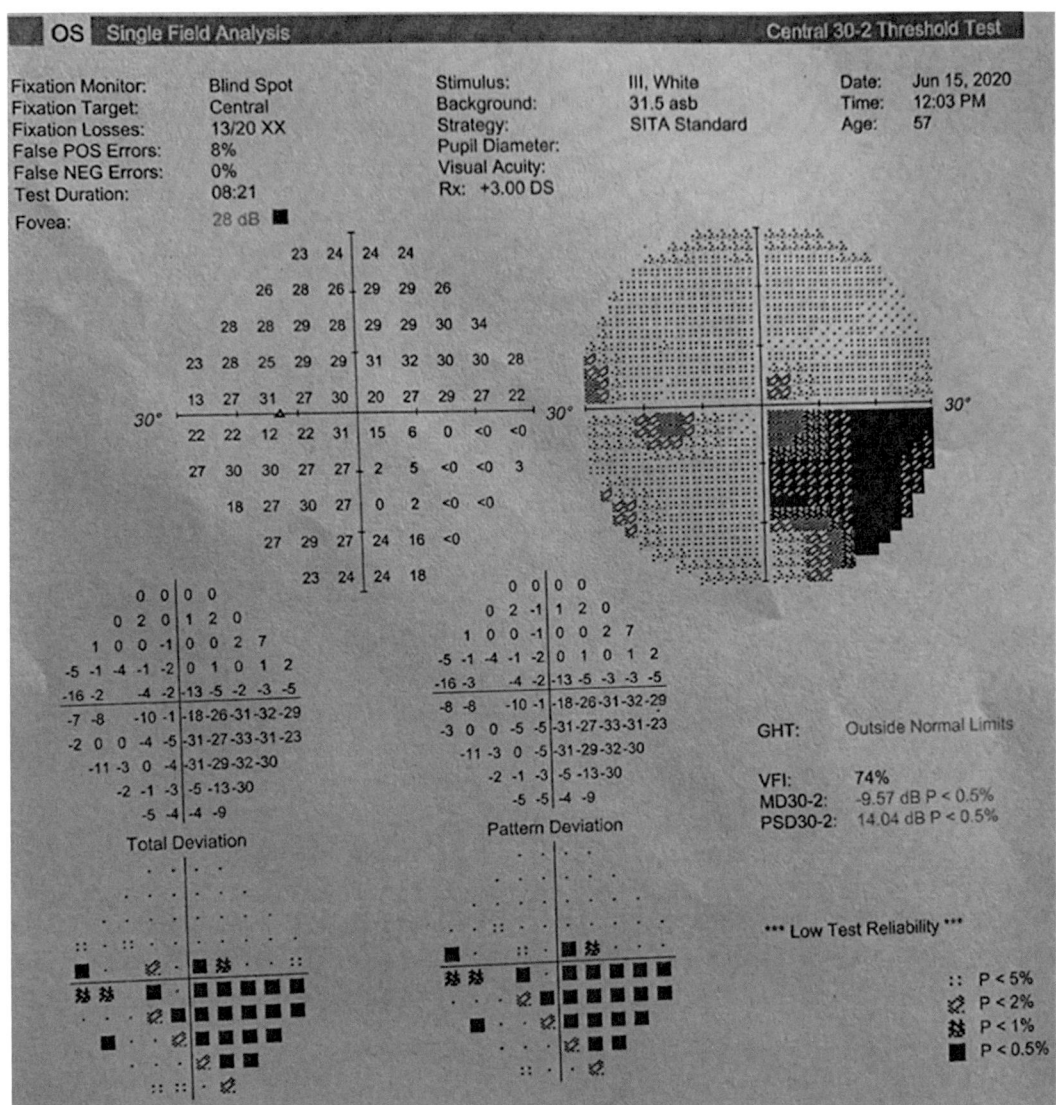

Fig. 10.4 Humphrey visual field 30-2 of the left eye post vitrectomy with silicon oil for a retinal detachment showed a dense inferior field defect involving fixation

visual field changes seen correlated exactly with the area of peripheral retinoschisis.

10.4 Clinical Situation 3: Humphrey Visual Field in Age-Related Macular Degeneration (ARMD)

ARMD is a disease typically affecting the central macular region and hence is also responsible for mostly field changes in the central 10°. A most basic form of field testing in these patients is done using home Amsler's test, which is very useful in assessing the metamorphopsia and relative scotomas induced by the macular lesion. A typical central scotoma with scalloped margin has been reported in ARMD by Nazemi et al. using a computer-automated visual field test [9]. The authors also documented a steep slope of the scotoma corresponded to a nonexudative AMD while a shallow slope was seen in exudative

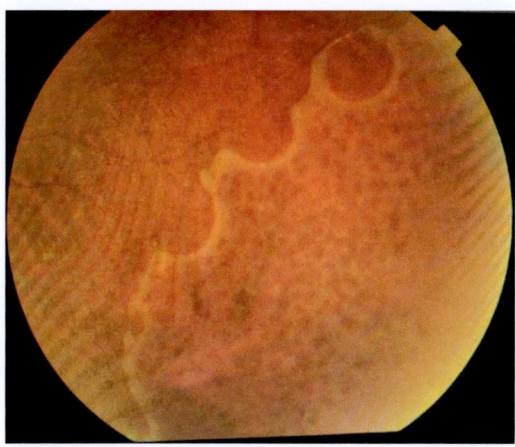

Fig. 10.5 Fundus photograph of the left eye revealed a well-demarcated inferotemporal retinoschisis with multiple outer retinal holes visible

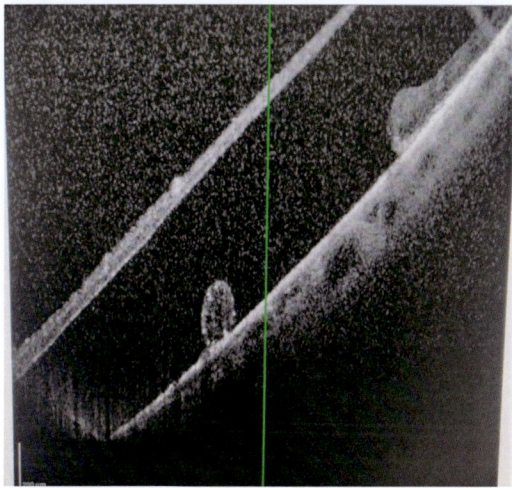

Fig. 10.6 OCT line scan through the retinoschisis showing a split at the level of outer nuclear layer with multiple outer retinal layer defects corresponding to the holes

visual field and its improvement on antiVEGF therapy as a reliable marker of functional outcome [10].

10.4.1 Case 6: Correlation Between Humphrey Visual Field and Optical Coherence Tomography

A 65-year-old female presented to us for second opinion regarding her glaucoma medications for the left eye, started on basis of her Humphrey visual field changes. She was a known case of exudative AMD (with polypoidal transformation) and had received multiple antiVEGFs since 2016. Her BCVA in the left eye was 6/12p, N8. Her Humphrey visual fields 24-2 showed a paracentral superonasal scotoma involving the fixation (Fig. 10.11), which had been the basis of starting her antiglaucoma medications while there was no RNFL loss seen on disc OCT (Fig. 10.12).

So, Is It Possible to Correlate the Field Change with Structural Changes on OCT?

Kiranmayi et al. have reported a correlation between Humphrey visual field patterns and OCT patterns in ARMD [11]. They observed that visual field defects correlated with areas of neurosensory retinal thinning seen on the structural OCT scans. In our patient, though the area of active disease (fibrovascular PED and exudation) was seen superior to fovea but the overlying neurosensory retina was normal in thickness. Inferotemporal to fovea was a well-defined area of atrophy with thinning of neurosensory retina which corresponded to the field defect superonasal to fovea (Fig. 10.13).

AMD with the area of shallow slope corresponded to the area of neovascularisation. Humphrey visual fields using a 10-2 protocol or a macular threshold protocol to document these scotomas is a very useful tool to assess the functional outcomes in this disease and to prognosticate the patients. Lavinsky et al. have shown in their paper the benefits of using decibel loss on the macular threshold protocol of Humphrey

10.4.2 Case 7: Humphrey Visual Field to Aid in Rehabilitation of Advanced ARMD Patient

An 85-year-old retired businessman presented to us with chief complaints of difficulty in face identification and reading work. He was diagnosed as both eye scarred CNVM. His uncor-

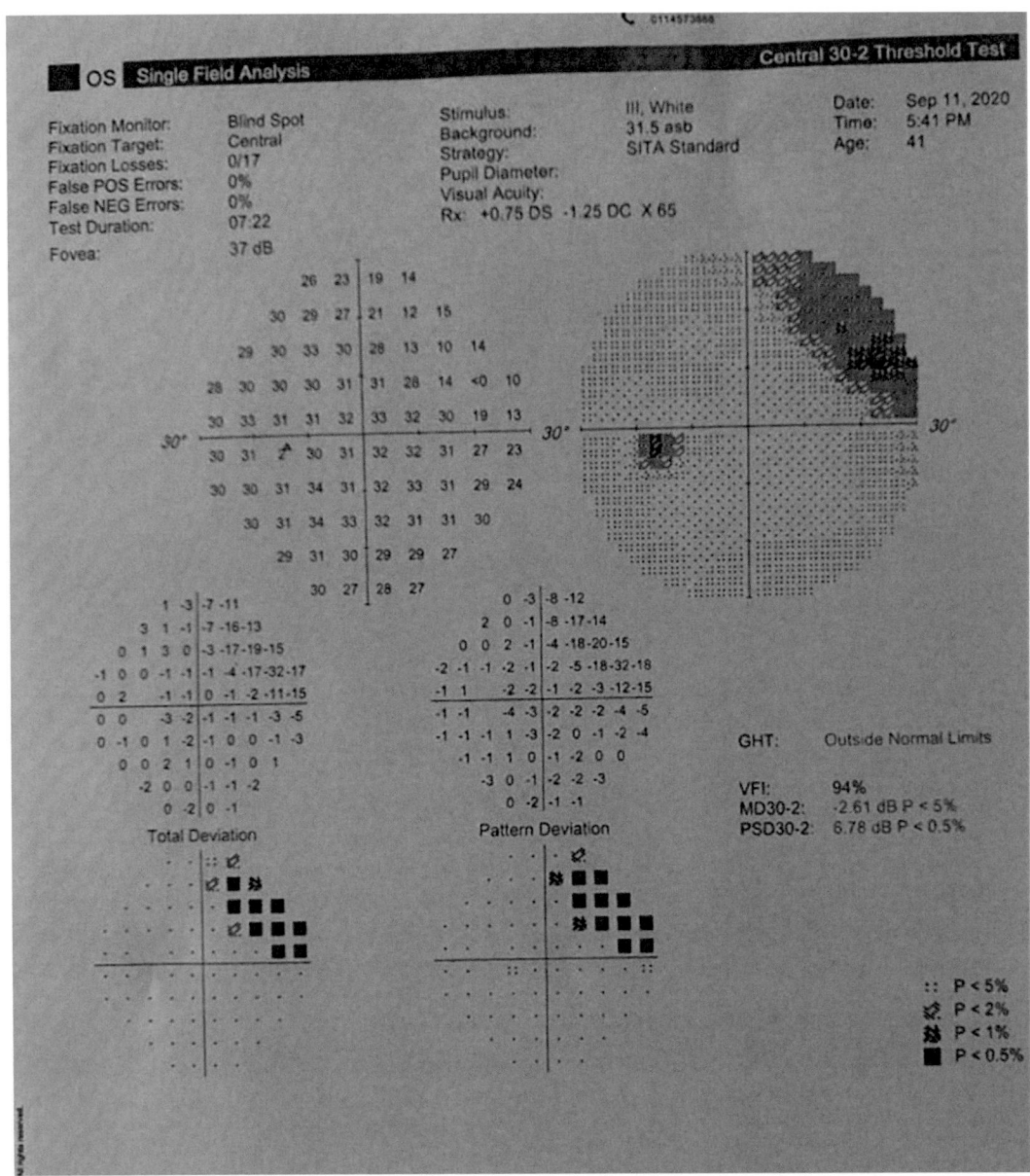

Fig. 10.7 Humphrey visual field 30-2 of the left eye showing a superonasal peripheral defect away from the fixation corresponding to the area of retinoschisis

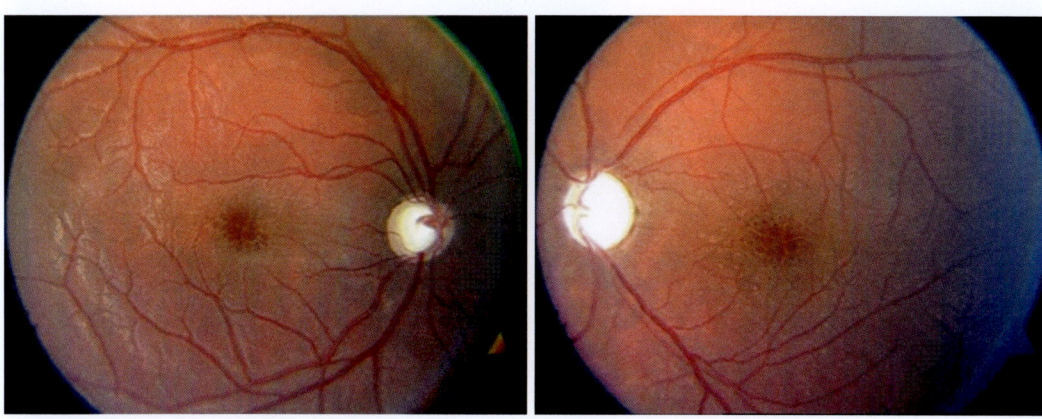

Fig. 10.8 Fundus examination of both eyes showing a typical cart wheel appearance of fovea in patient of juvenile retinoschisis

rected visual acuity was 20/200 in the right eye improving to 20/120 with −4.5DS; 20/120p LE improving to 20/80 with +1.5 DS. His fundus examination revealed a scarred CNVM in both eyes with geographic atrophy patch involving the fovea (Fig. 10.14). *Though atrophy appeared involving fovea in both eyes, does Humphrey visual field explain a better vision in left eye?*

Humphrey visual filed 10-2 revealed a central scotoma, more dense temporally in the right eye and nasally in the left eye with fixation spared in the left eye (Fig. 10.15). This was responsible for a slightly better visual acuity in the left eye. Macular threshold protocol showed a more dense field loss temporal to fixation in the right eye and nasal to fixation in the left eye. Foveal threshold was 27 db in the right eye and 26 db in the left eye (Fig. 10.16). This was suggestive of a more denser field loss to the right side of fixation. A trial of 2.1 x SEE TV with slight right-head turn improve his binocular vision to 20/40. This case nicely highlights that Humphrey visual field can be a really useful functional tool to guide in the rehabilitation of patients with macular disorders. If properly done, it can be really useful to understand the eye which can be used for preferential fixation or like microperimetry to map the area of the macula which can be used for fixation in either eyes. The low visual acuity does raise concerns over the validity of visual fields in these patients. But Markowitz et al. have shown in their study that macular perimetry in the presence of residual vision of 20/200 or better should be viewed as valid as an acceptable fixation maintenance is possible, and it can be useful to map scotomas and look for loci of eccentric fixation [12].

10.5 Clinical Situation 4: The Vascular Occlusions

Both arterial and venular obstruction in the retina can result in perimetric changes. Many of the changes may mimic glaucomatous field defects and hence the importance of a complete retinal examination cannot be overemphasised. All central retinal vein occlusions produce central scotoma while the peripheral field changes vary according to ischaemic and non-ischaemic variants and are picked up better by Goldman Perimetry [13]. Sensitivities and specificities of visual field findings are almost as good as those of ERG in differentiating ischemic from non-ischemic CRVO during the first year after the onset of CRVO [13]

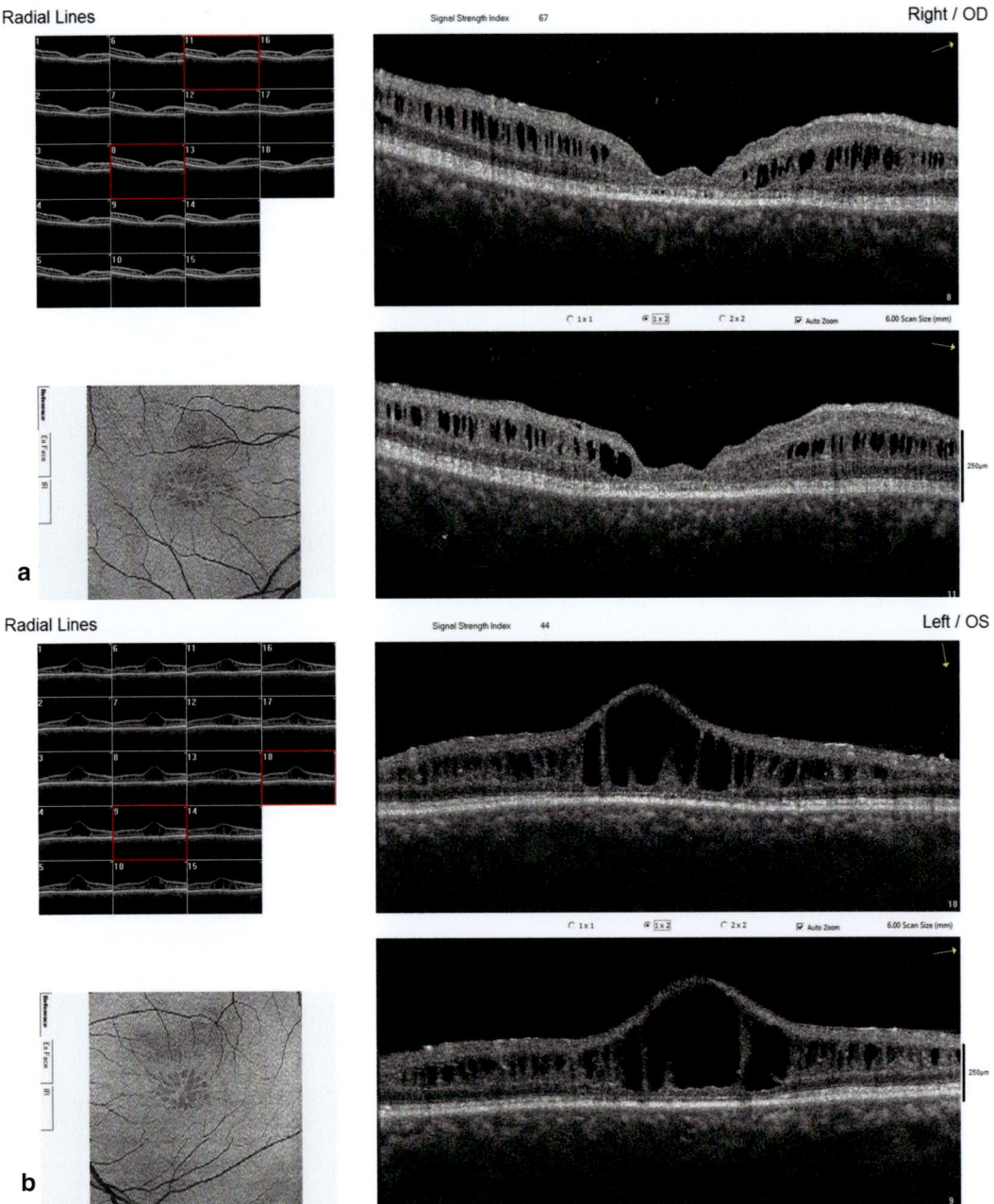

Fig. 10.9 Optical coherence tomography revealed a split in the neurosensory retina at the level of outer nuclear layer throughout the macula with foveal thinning

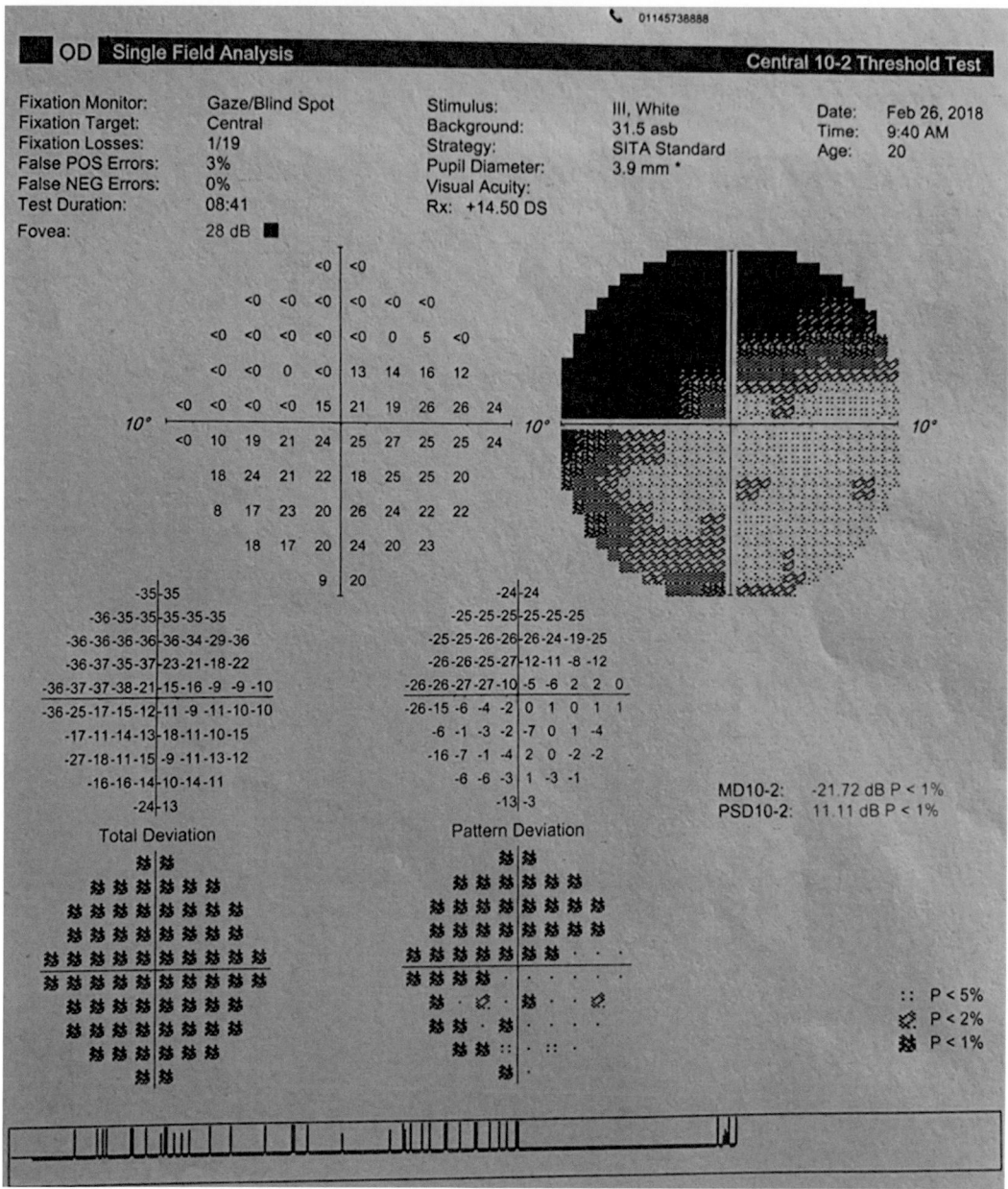

Fig. 10.10 Humphrey visual field 30-2 of the right eye showing a consistent dense supero temporal field defect

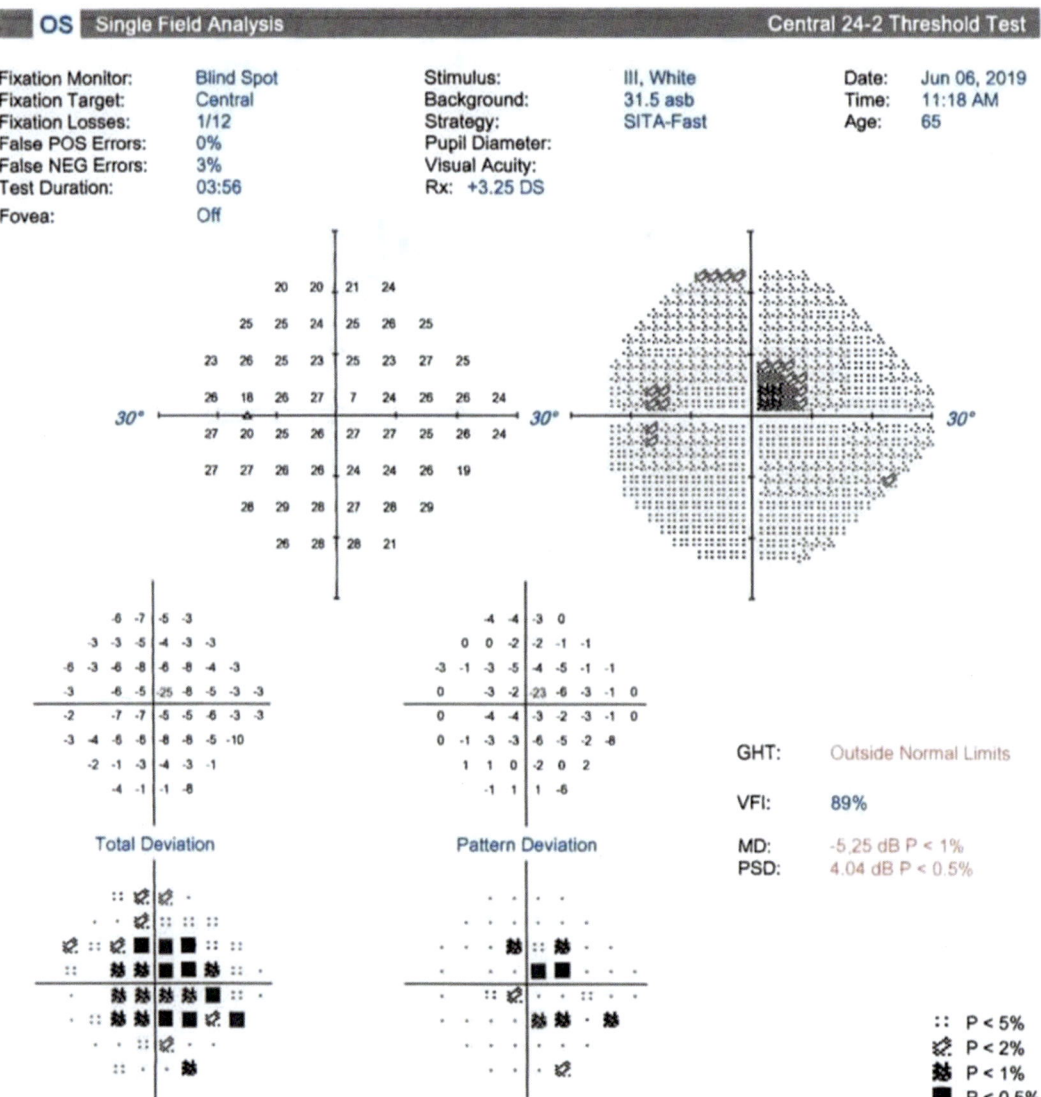

Fig. 10.11 Humphrey visual fields 24-2 of the left eye showing a paracentral superonasal scotoma involving the fixation

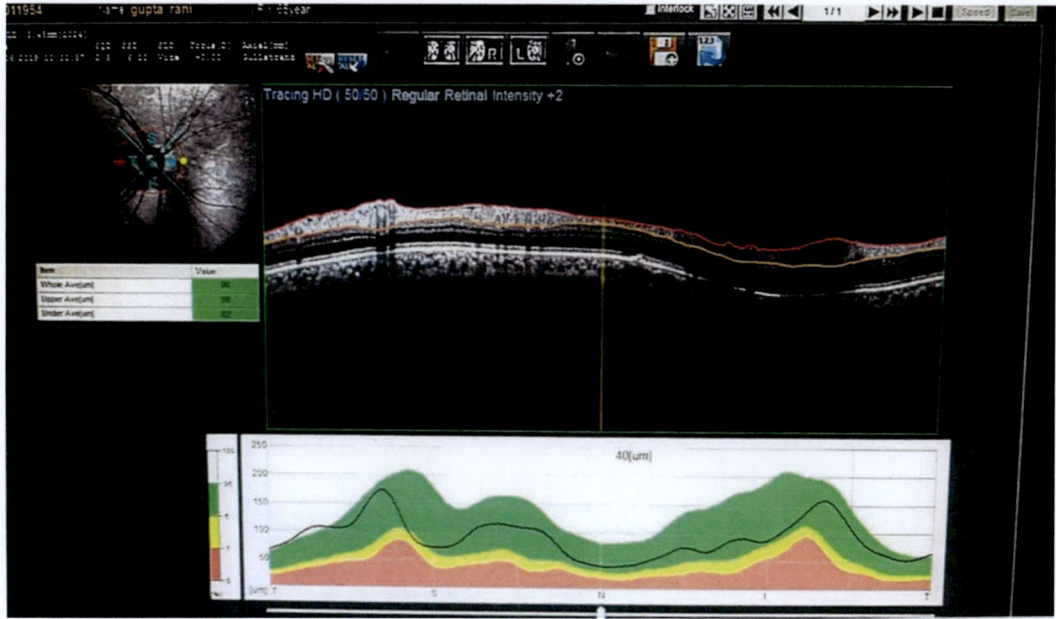

Fig. 10.12 Optical coherence tomography (OCT) of left eye through the disc showing normal retinal nerve fibre layer (RNFL) thickness

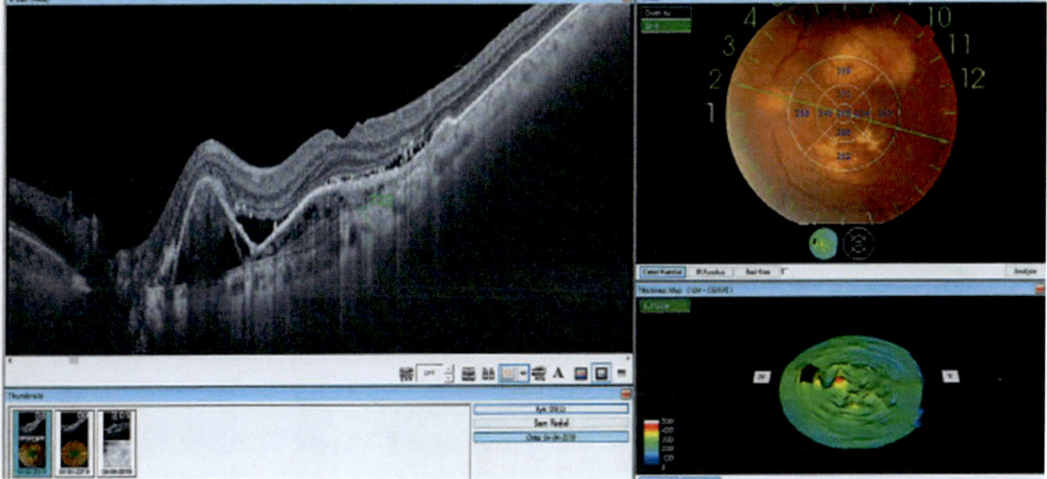

Fig. 10.13 Fundus photo along with OCT showing an area of active disease (fibrovascular PED and exudation) seen superior to fovea with the overlying normal thickness neurosensory retina. Inferotemporal to fovea was a well-defined area of atrophy with thinning of neurosensory retina which corresponded to the field defect superonasal to fovea

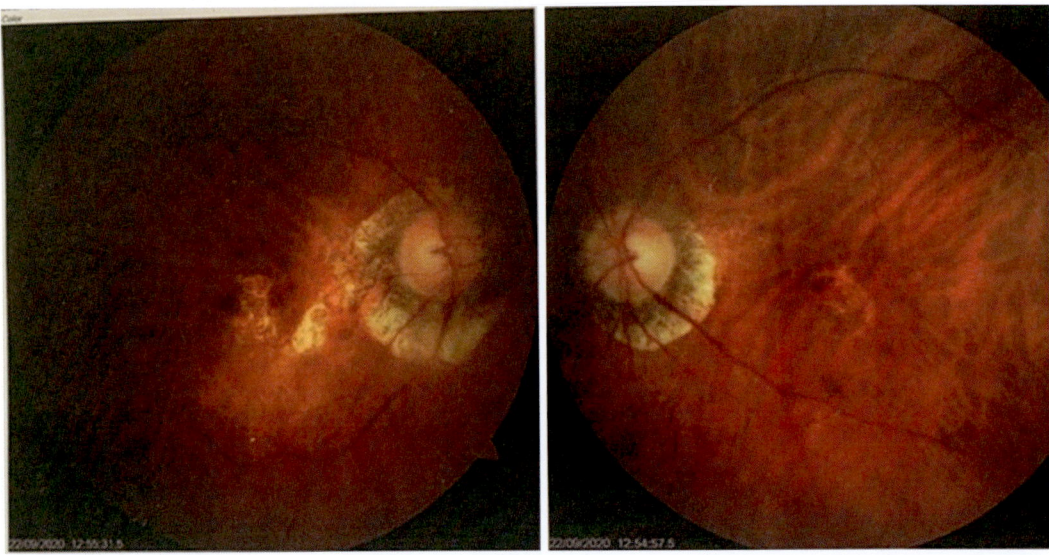

Fig. 10.14 Fundus photo of both eyes showing a scarred CNVM with geographic atrophy patch involving the fovea

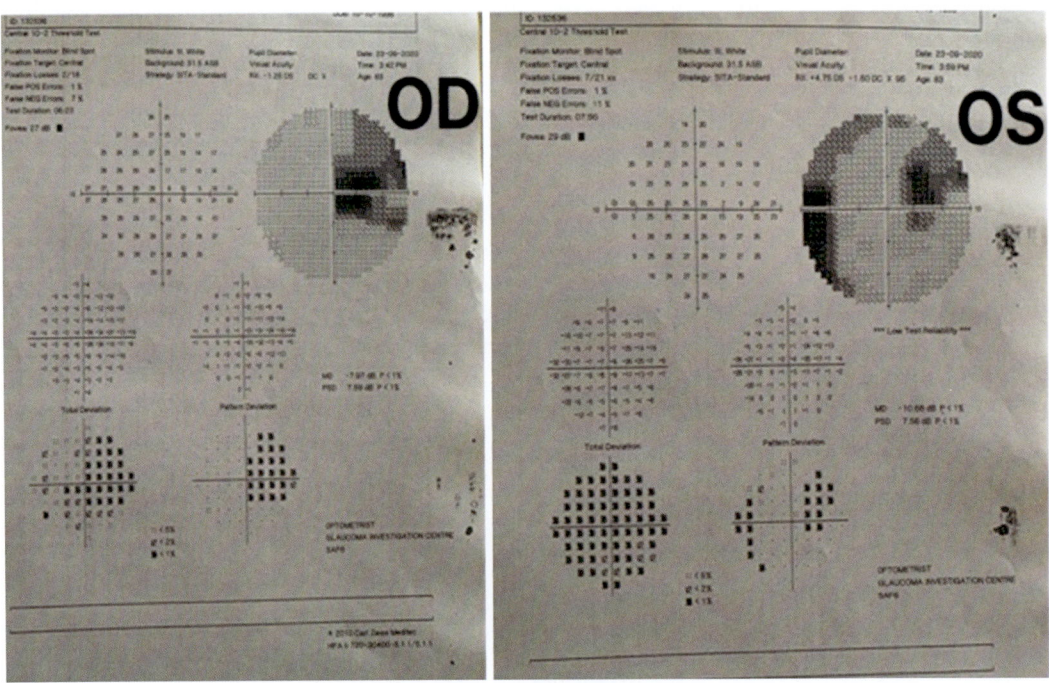

Fig. 10.15 Humphrey visual files 10-2 of both eyes revealed a central scotoma, more dense temporally in the right eye and nasally in the left eye with fixation spared in the left eye

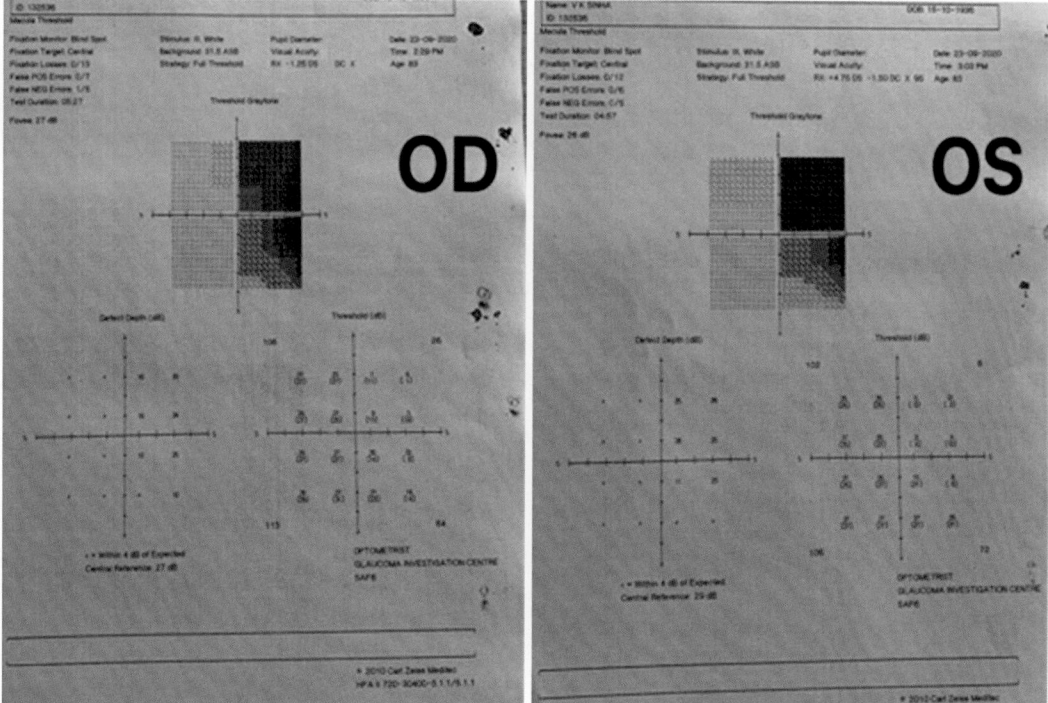

Fig. 10.16 Macular threshold protocol showed a more dense field loss temporal to fixation in the right eye and nasal to fixation in the left eye. Foveal threshold was 27 db in the right eye and 26 db in the left eye

10.5.1 Case 8: Hemi-Central Retinal Vein Occlusion

A 59 years old male presented with blurred vision in the right eye. His BCVA was 6/24, N18 in the affected eye. Fundus examination revealed a superior hemi-central retinal vein occlusion with a corresponding central and inferior defect in his Humphrey visual field.

Dilemma: These defects mimic the arcuate defects associated with glaucomatous damage. However, in this case, the visual field changes corelated with the distribution of the retinal vein occlusion.

10.5.2 Case 9: Old Lasered Branch Retinal Vein Occlusion

A 60 years old male patient was referred for second opinion for glaucoma. His BCVA was 6/12. N8 with normal intraocular pressure in the left eye. His Humphreys visual field revealed a superior arcuate defect. Fundus examination revealed an old inferior branch retinal vein occlusion with laser scars. The field defect noted was in the area of distribution of the retinal vein occlusion, and hence the patient was advised periodic visual fields instead of antiglaucoma medications.

Dilemma: Arcuate perimetric defects are seen in glaucomatous damage too, so all other cause of arcuate field defects need to be ruled out by the clinician after a comprehensive ocular examination.

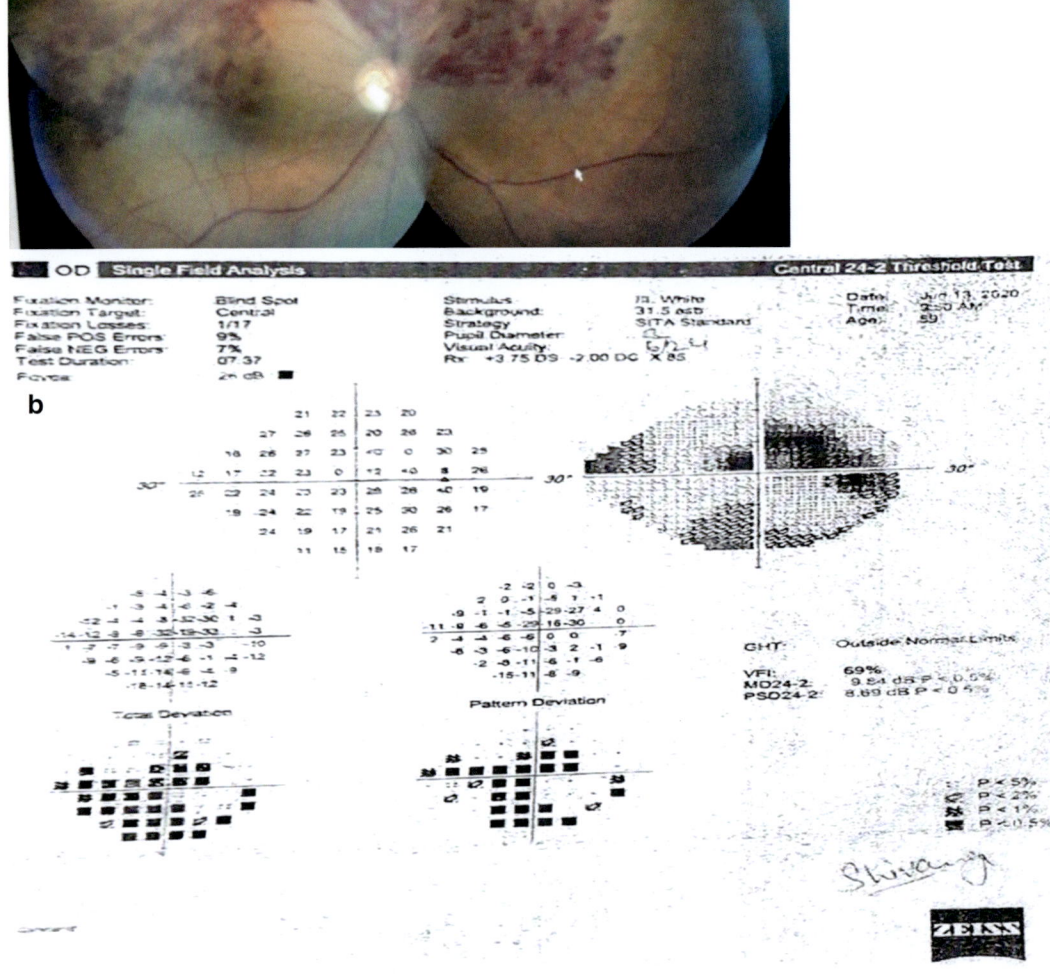

Fig. 10.17 (a) Colour fundus photo of the right eye showing superior hemi-central retinal vein occlusion. (b) The corresponding Humphrey field defect showing a predominantly inferior defect along with central defect

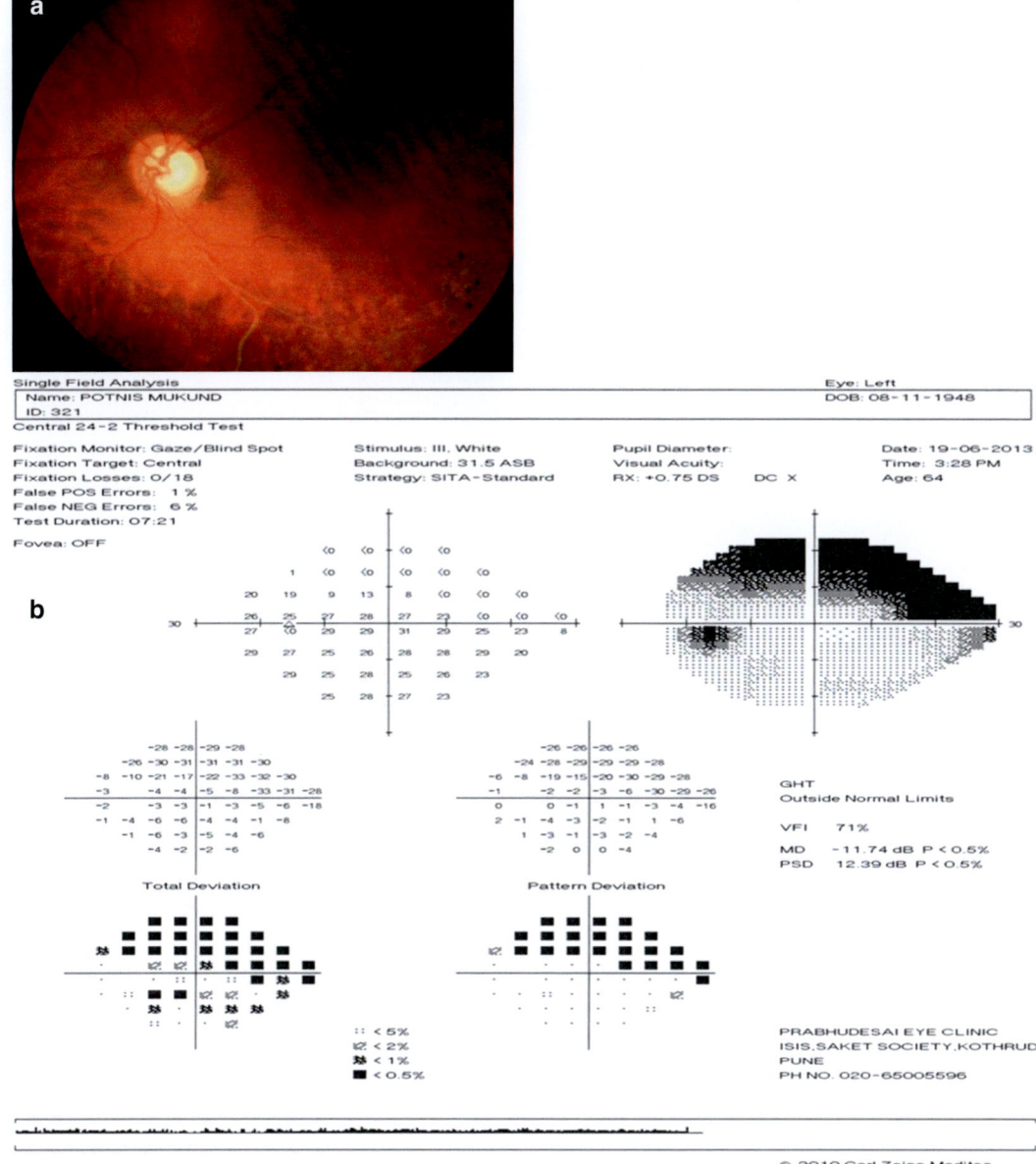

Fig. 10.18 (**a**) Old inferotemporal branch retinal vein occlusion (lasered). (**b**) Humphreys visual field shows a superior arcuate defect

10.6 Clinical Situation 5: The Neurosensory Detachments

10.6.1 Case 10: Central Serous Chorioretinopathy or Glaucoma?

Blue-on-yellow perimetry is more sensitive than achromatic perimetry to reveal the central sensitivity loss in central serous chorioretinopathy [14]. Also, eyes with CSC showed significantly lower retinal sensitivity not only at the central but also in the paracentral area as determined by microperimetry [15]. Hence, a field defect in CSCR may create a dilemma for the treatment of glaucoma.

A 43 years old male was referred for second opinion to our Glaucoma department for starting antiglaucoma medications. His Humphreys visual field showed a small superior paracentral defect which persisted on repeated field tests. However, his fundus examination did not reveal any corresponding RNFL defect. Optical coherence tomography was then done in the corresponding macular area which revealed the presence of shallow subretinal fluid in the temporal macula thus explaining the paracentral visual field defect. The patient was diagnosed with CSCR and was thus spared the burden of unnecessary antiglaucoma medication.

10.6.2 Case 11: Sudden Onset Visual Defect!

Retinal detachment gives rise to the development of a relative scotoma which is generally described by patients as a dim curtain falling across the field of vision [16]. A through history taking will elicit the occurrence of pre-existing flashes and floaters too [17].

A 56 years old male patient reported to the emergency late night with acute onset visual defect in the left eye. The patient was evaluated by our resident who decided on a Humphreys

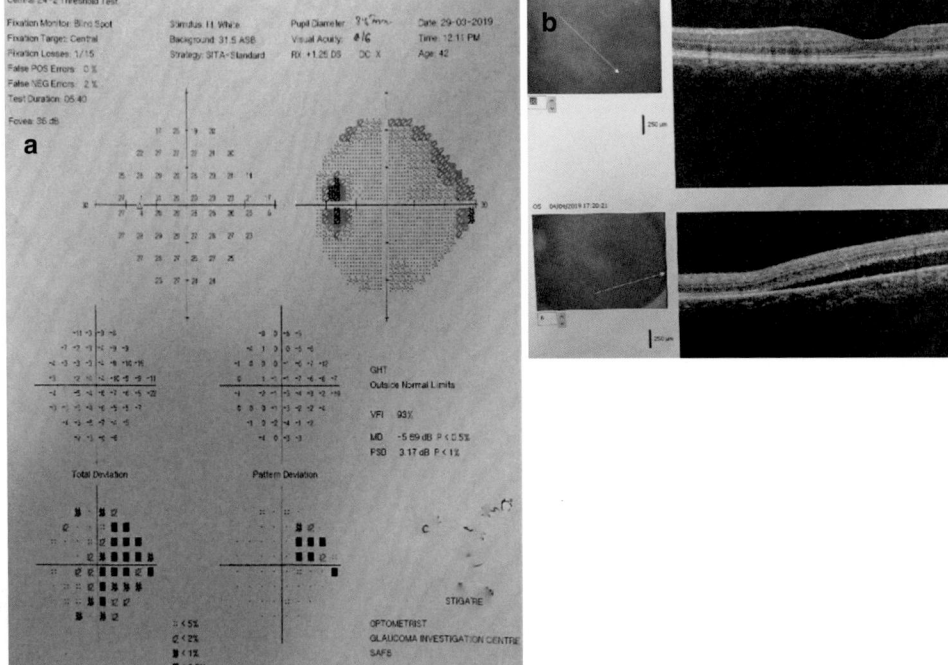

Fig. 10.19 (a) Humphreys visual field with paracentral field defect in the left eye. (b) OCT showing neurosensory detachment in inferotemporal macula in the left eye

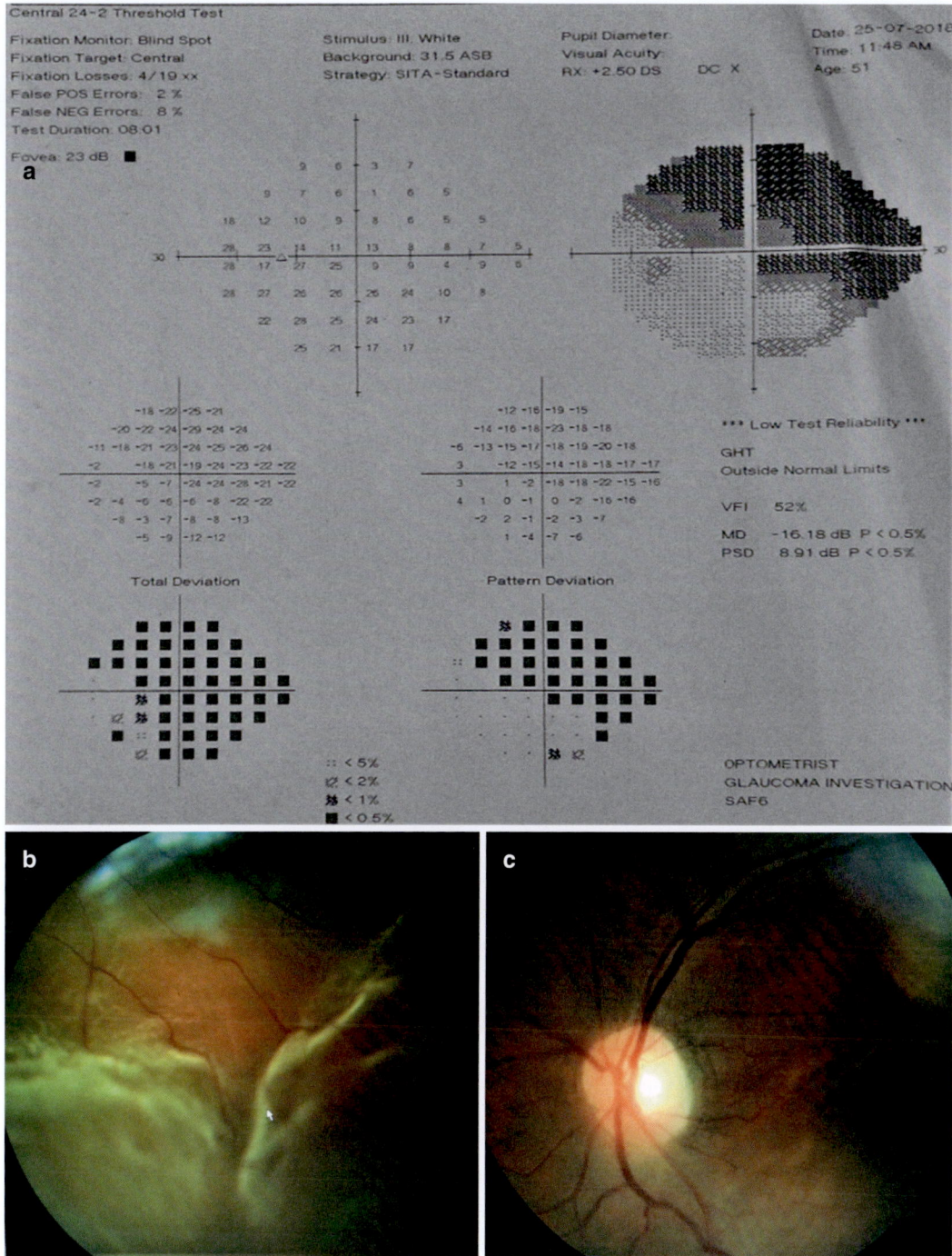

Fig. 10.20 (a) Humphreys visual field with large superotemporal field defect. (b, c) Inferior retinal detachment bisecting fovea in the left eye

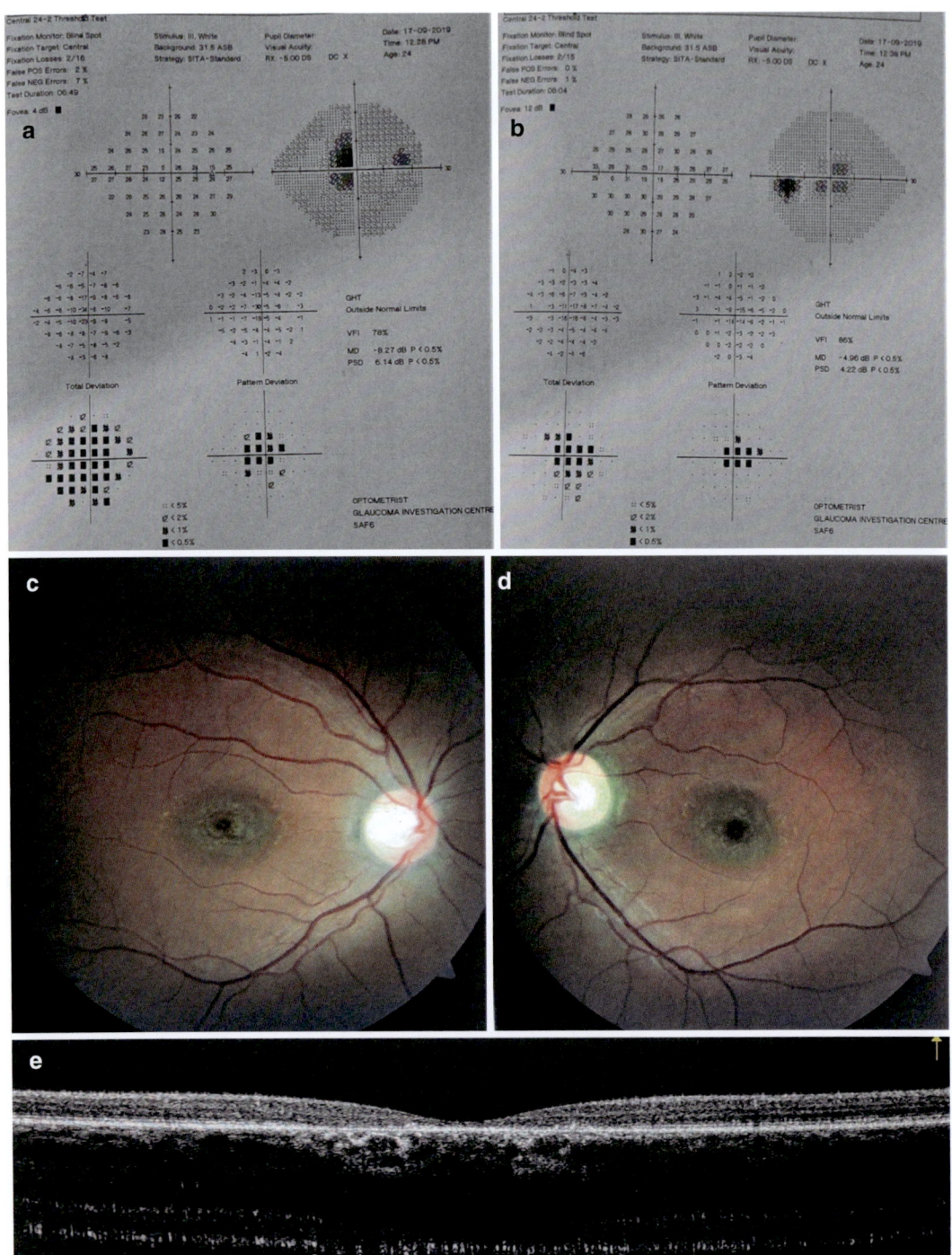

Fig. 10.21 (**a**, **b**) Humphrey visual field with central field defects in the right and left eyes. (**c**, **d**): Fundus images with macular dystrophy (Stargardts) in the right and left eyes. (**e**, **f**) OCT images with foveal atrophy in the right and left eyes

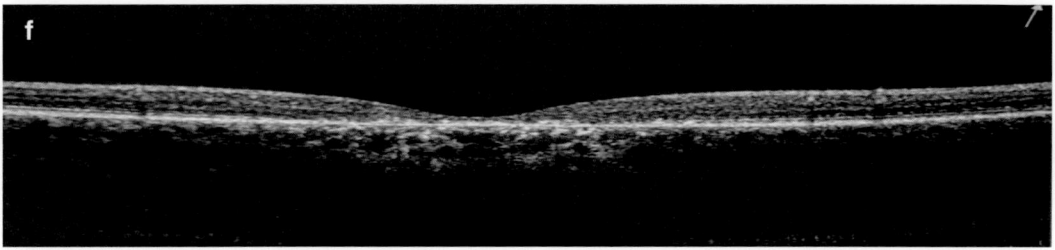

Fig. 10.21 (continued)

visual field test for the patient. The test revealed presence of extensive superior field defect so the patient was referred for a dilated fundus examination. Fundus examination diagnosed an inferior rhegmatogenous retinal detachment abutting the fovea. The patient was then taken for an urgent surgical procedure for the retinal detachment.

This case emphasizes the importance of history in cases of sudden onset field defect wherein the presence of flashes, floaters and progression should point us in the direction of rhegmatogenous retinal detachment.

10.7 Clinical Situation 6: Macular Dystrophy and Visual Field Defect

10.7.1 Case 12: Central Scotomas

Macular dystrophies cause central scotomas or fixation sparing scotomas. Visual field testing misses small scotomas and is often complicated by unstable fixation in macular diseases. Microperimetry allows mapping of light sensitivity of the macula and provides topographic information on visual function beyond visual acuity in macular diseases. In Stargardts disease, microperimetric mean sensitivity was lower in the fovea than in the peripheral macula [18]. Advanced disease will throw up central scotomas in automated visual field tests.

Our patient of probable Stargardts (not tested for ABCA4 gene mutation) [19] presented with bilateral low vision of 20/200 which was slowly progressive in nature. Automated perimetry revealed central scotomas in both eyes with corresponding macular changes in the fundus of both eyes. There was no evidence of glaucomatous optic disc changes. The patient underwent optical coherence tomography which showed gross foveal thinning with loss of outer retinal layers at the fovea (foveal atrophy).

References

1. Albert, Daniel M., Joan W. Miller, and Dimitri T. Azar. 2008. Albert & Jakobiec's principles and practice of ophthalmology. 3rd edition. Chapter 124.
2. Hawkins AS, Szlyk JR, Ardickas Z, Alexander KR, Wilensky JJ. Comparison of contrast sensitivity, visual acuity and humprey visual field testing in patients with glaucoma. J Glaucoma. 2003;12:134–8.
3. Grover S, Fishman GA, Brown J. Patterns of visual field progression in patients with retinitis pigmentosa. Ophthalmology. 1998;105(6):1069–75.
4. Nazemi PP, Fink W, Lim J, Sadun A. Scotomas of age related macular degeneration detected and characterized by means of a novel three dimensional computer automated visual field test. Retina. 2005;25(4):446–53.
5. Klystra JA, Holdren DN. Indirect ophthalmoscope perimetry in patients with retinal detachment or retinoschisis. Am J Ophthalmol. 1995;119(4):521–2.
6. Sasoh M, Ito Y, Wakiteni Y, Matsutara H, Matsunga K, Uji Y. 10 year follow up of visual function in patients who underwent scleral buckling. Retina. 2005;25:965–71.
7. Takenaka H, Maeno T, Mano T, et al. Causes of visual field defect after vitrectomy. J Jpn Ophthalmol Soc. 1999;103:399–403.
8. Hirata A, Yonemura N, Hasumura T, Murata Y, Negi A. Effect of infusion air pressure on visual field defects after macular hole surgery. Am J Ophthalmol. 2000;130:611–6.

9. Nazemi P, Fink W, Lim J, Sadun A. Scotomas of age releated macular degeneration detected and charaterized by means of novel three dimensional computer automated visual field test. Retina. 2005;25:446–53.
10. Lavinsky F, Tolentino M, Lavinsky J. The macular threshold protocol of the Humphrey visual filed analyzer: a superior functional outcome of intravitreal bevacizumab for treatment of neovascular age related macular degeneration. Arq Bras Oftalmol. 2010;73(2):111–5.
11. Kiranmayi VSD, Bharathi NR, Prasad K, Raju RSN, Raju RS. Correlation between Humphrey visual field patterns and optical coherence tomography patterns in age related macular degeneration. J.Evolution Med. Dent. Sci. 2017;6(10):753–6.
12. Markowitz SN, Muller C. Macular perimetry in low vision. Can J Ophthalmol. 2004;39(1):56–60.
13. Hayreh SS. Retinal vein occlusion. Indian J Ophthalmol. 1994;42:109–32.
14. Afrashi F, Erakgun T, Uzunel D, Mentes J, Kose S, Akkin C. Comparison of achromatic and blue-on-yellow perimetry in patients with resolved central serous chorioretinopathy. Ophthalmologica. 2005;219:202–5.
15. Ozdemir H, Senturk F, Karacorlu M, Arf Karacorlu S, Uysal O. Macular sensitivity in eyes with central serous chorioretinopathy. Eur J Ophthalmol. 2008;18(5):799–804.
16. Michels RG, Wilkinson CP, Rice TA, Hengst TC. Retinal detachment. St. Louis: Mosby; 1990. p. 952–3.
17. Dayan MR, Jayamanne DG, Andrews RM, Griffiths PG. Flashes and floaters as predictors of vitreoretinal pathology: is follow-up necessary for posterior vitreous detachment? Eye (Lond). 1996;10(Pt 4):456–8.
18. Schönbach EM, Wolfson Y, Strauss RW, et al. Macular sensitivity measured with microperimetry in stargardt disease in the progression of atrophy secondary to stargardt disease (ProgStar) study: report no. 7. JAMA Ophthalmol. 2017;135(7):696–703. https://doi.org/10.1001/jamaophthalmol.2017.1162.
19. Tanna P, Strauss RW, Fujinami K, Michaelides M. Stargardt disease: clinical features, molecular genetics, animal models and therapeutic options. Br J Ophthalmol. 2017;101(1):25–30.

Perimetry in Neurological Disorders

11

Sumit Monga

11.1 Introduction

Visual fields are extremely useful when evaluating patients complaining of visual loss (especially when the cause of visual loss is not obvious after ophthalmic examination) or patients with neurologic disorders that may affect the intracranial visual pathways (e.g., space occupying lesions, cerebrovascular attack, and head/eye trauma). Visual field examination allows localization by correlating the pattern of defects to the abnormal portion of the visual pathways [1]. The improvement or worsening of the disease process can also be charted by serial visual field testing [1].

11.2 Points to Ponder

It is imperative that visual fields be interpreted, keeping certain points in mind [2]:
- *Is the visual field reliable enough?* The reliability is often judged by the reliability parameters on the automated perimetry printout, and its repeatability.
- *Is the visual field loss, unilateral or bilateral?* Unilateral field defects are more often caused by lesions of anterior visual pathway (ocular, orbit and cavernous sinus region), while bilateral lesions are hallmark of posterior visual pathway (optic chiasma and beyond).
- *Does the visual field defect respect the vertical meridian or not?*
  Respecting the vertical meridian is considered the hallmark of visual pathway lesions involving chiasma and beyond, owing to the phenomenon of crossover of optic nerve fibers in the chiasma.
- *What are the patterns of the visual field defect?*
  Some common patterns are hemianopia, quadrantanopia, arcuate defects, altitudinal defect, etc., which help to localize the site of the lesion.
- *If bilateral, is the visual field defect homonymous?*
  Field defects, lying on same side of the vertical midline, are labeled homonymous hemianopias, typically caused by retro-chasmal lesions. A bitemporal hemianopia is theoretically heteronymous, but characteristic of chiasmal lesions.
- *If bilateral and homonymous, which side of the field is affected?*
  For example, right homonymous hemianopia is suggestive of left-sided brain pathology, and vice versa.
- *Is the visual field defect congruous?*
  Congruity (same size and shape of visual field defects) is more typical of posterior visual pathway lesions (parieto-occipital region lesions).

S. Monga (✉)
Senior Consultant, Pediatric Ophthalmology, Strabismus and Neuro-Ophthalmology Services, Centre for Sight Group of Eye Hospitals, New Delhi, India

The idea of this chapter is to facilitate the reader to utilize the information from the visual field test to crack the clinical cases, and not just theoretically enumerate the possible visual field defects.

Some of the management pearls to solve the clinical dilemmas, aided by clues from visual fields, are illustrated below:

11.3 Scenario 1: Orientation of the Visual Field Printouts for Interpretation

A cropped digital image (Fig. 11.1a, b) of the visual fields was shared by a colleague, for opinion. A cursory look reveals a bi-nasal hemianopia pattern, which is an unusual field defect,

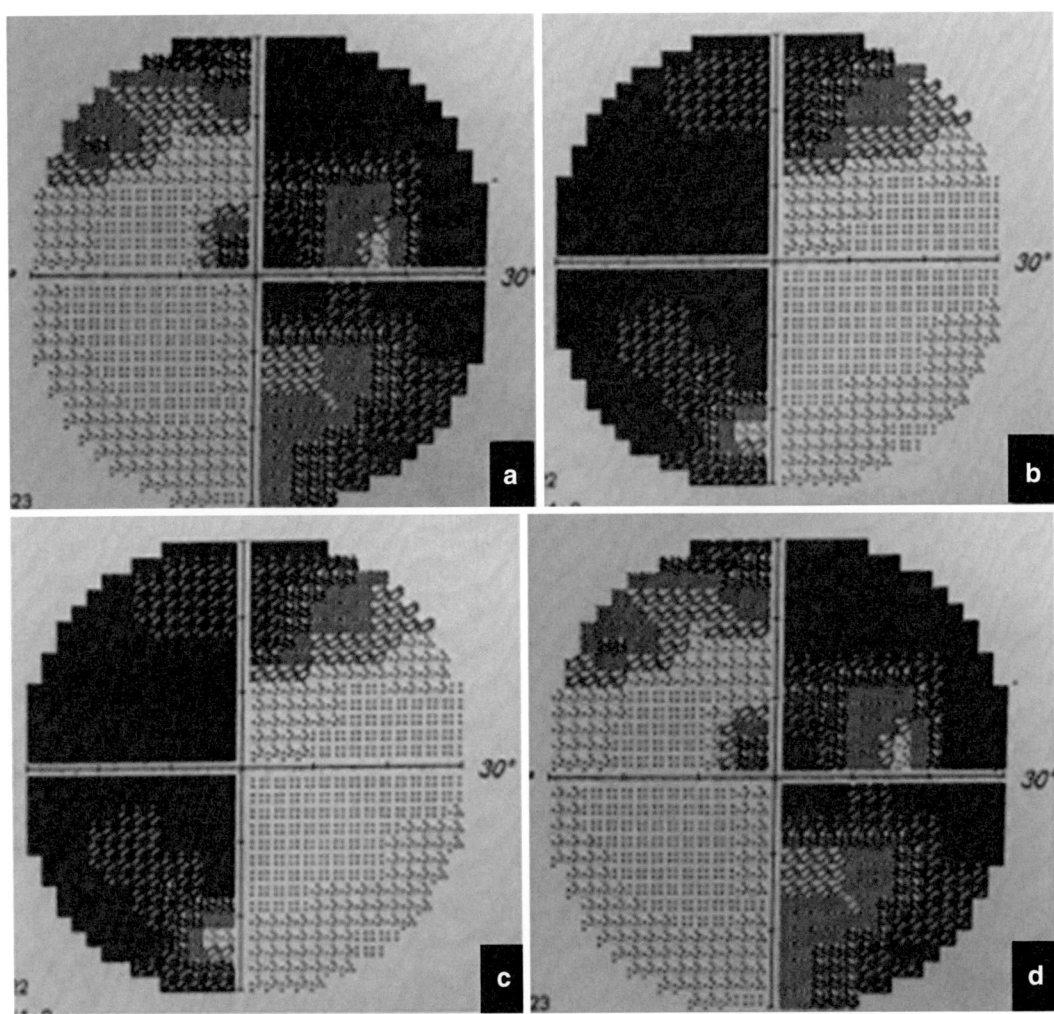

Fig. 11.1 Orientation of visual fields: bilateral nasal hemianopia, when right visual field is placed on left (**a**) and left visual field is placed on right (**b**); on correct placement of visual fields (left field on left side—**c**; right field on right side—**d**), bitemporal hemianopia was unraveled

often caused by either ocular causes or compression of temporal fibers at the chiasm (e.g., by an internal carotid malformation). However, a careful look reveals that Fig. 11.1a, b are right eye field and left eye fields, respectively (the blind spots are camouflaged by the temporal hemifield defect of each eye). *The first rule for simultaneous binocular field interpretation is that the patient's left eye visual field should be kept in examiner's left hand, and patient's right eye visual field in examiner's right hand* [1]. The correct placement of the above visual fields revealed that the patient had a bitemporal visual field defect (Fig. 11.1c, d). Correct interpretation, ultimately, led to the diagnosis of chasmal compression by a pituitary tumor.

11.4 Scenario 2: Interpreting the Visual Field Test

11.4.1 Gray Zone Versus Pattern Standard Deviation Plot

For most of the neurological field defects, both the gray scale and pattern standard deviation plot (PSD) are often used interchangeably. On the one hand, the gray scale representation of the visual field provides a gross picture of the size and severity of the visual defect. While on the other hand, the pattern deviation plot helps to highlight the exact focal abnormalities of the visual field [2]. Figure 11.2a depicts that the gray scale is similar to the pattern of field defect on pattern

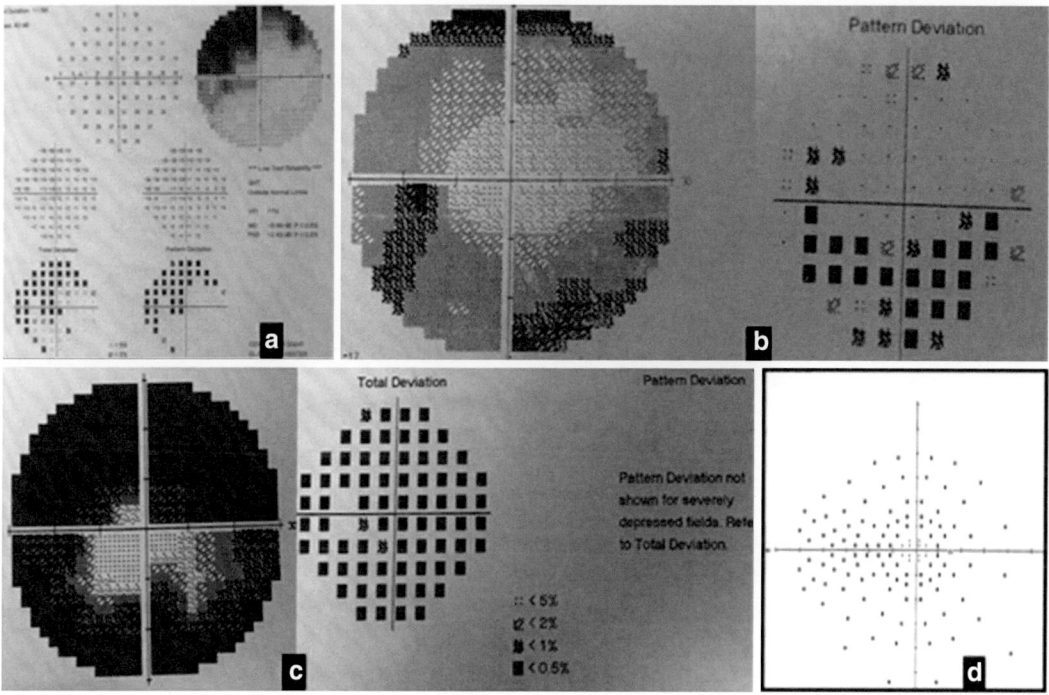

Fig. 11.2 Visual field plots: identical left superotemporal quadratic defect in both gray zone and PSD plots (**a**); right altitudinal field defect better discerned on PSD, rather than gray zone (**b**); advanced visual field defect on gray zone, even when PSD plot is not generated (**c**); and 120 point neurological screening test to delineate the extent of peripheral visual field defect in a case of retinitis pigmentosa (**d**)

standard plot (superotemporal quadratic field defect). However, there are situations, like in Fig. 11.2b, where the pattern of field defect is better discerned on the PSD. Conversely, in severely advanced fields on gray scale (Fig. 11.2c), the PSD may not be generated by the computer program. *Hence, it is equally important to look at both the zones (gray scale and PSD) to decipher the pattern of visual field defect.* And only if they mirror each other, then either can be used to interpret the visual fields. *For most neurological visual field defects, a 30-degree visual field (30_2 program) is good enough* [3]. However, the advanced, peripheral defects are better ascertained on 120 point screening test strategy [3] (Fig. 11.2d).

11.5 Scenario 3: Correlation of Visual Fields with Patient's Clinical Findings

A 30-year-old married lady presented to us with decreased vision in her left eye, since 1 week (visual acuity OD 6/9, OS PL negative). Her right eye visual field test revealed high false-positive errors and showed gross constriction of visual field (Fig. 11.3a1). Before her referral to our cen-

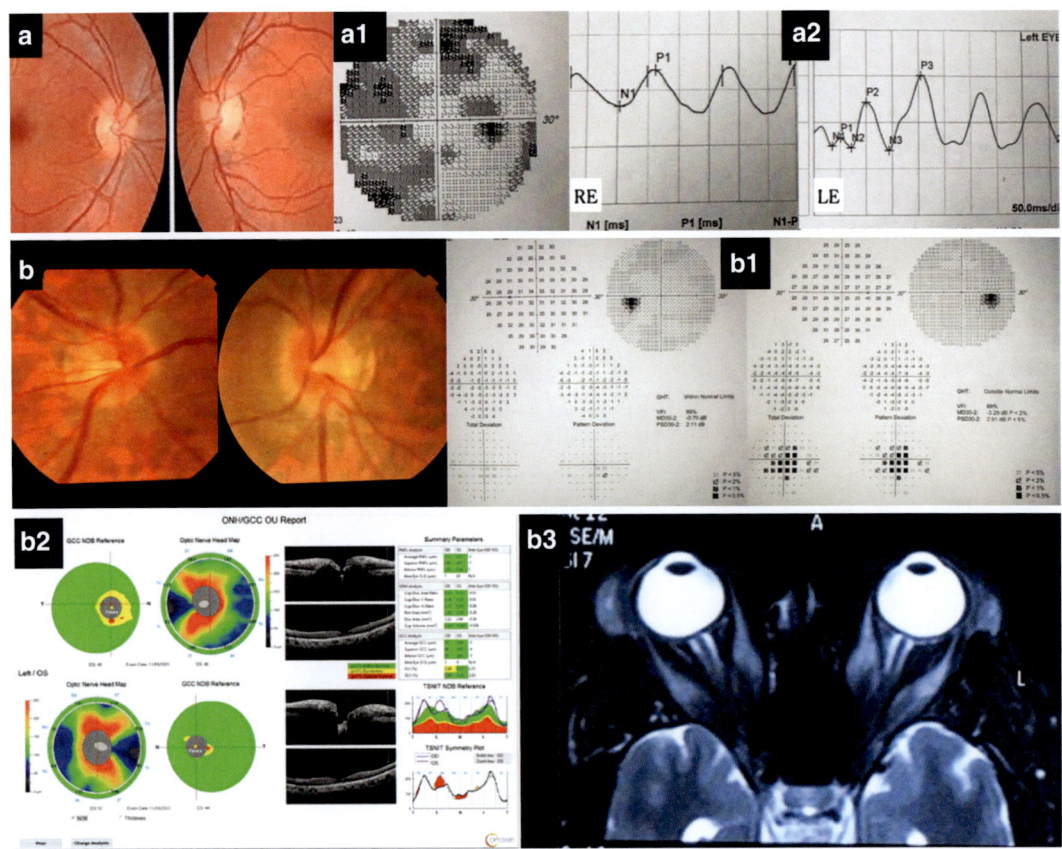

Fig. 11.3 Correlation of patient's clinical findings with visual fields (VF): A 30 yr lady with OU normal fundi OU (**a**), high false-positive errors on VF (**a1**), OU normal latency and amplitudes on VEP exam (**a2**)—case of malingering falsely presumed to be retrobulbar optic neuritis (**a**). Case of thyroid orbitopathy with bilateral optic disc edema (**b**)—depressed central field in the right eye confirmed optic nerve compression (**b1**), Normal RNFL and GCC thicknesses on OCT (**b2**) and MRI orbit showing grossly swollen extraocular muscles with crowding at the orbital apices (**b3**)

ter, she had been provisionally diagnosed as bilateral retro bulbar optic neuritis (L ≫ R), elsewhere. Her brain MRI did not show any pathology. She had been administered intravenous methyl-prednisolone therapy (IVMP; 1 g/day for 3 days) and was started on oral steroids. We discovered that her clinical examination was essentially normal in both eyes (including normal pupillary reactions—No RAPD; 36/36 color vision in her right eye, normal fundi OU). Her visual evoked potential (flash VEP) showed symmetrical wave response in both eyes with good amplitudes (Fig. 11.3a2), indicating good bilateral optic nerve conduction. Our suspicion was confirmed, when we did tests of malingering. On inadvertent fogging of each eye, patient had 6/6 visual acuity OU! On probing, severe psychological stress owing to marital discord was revealed. The patient was appropriately referred for psychological counseling. *The learning was that if your patient's subjective response (including visual fields) does not match your objective findings (clinical and investigations), then probe further and rule out malingering.*

In another case, a 36-year-old physician patient complained of blurred vision in her right eye. She was a known case of thyroid eye disease, maintained on intermittent steroid therapy for her orbitopathy. Her aided vision was recorded as 6/6 OU, normal color vision, no apparent RAPD on clinical, and normal anterior segment exam. She had edema of nasal optic disc margin in both eyes (Fig. 11.3b). Her work up for papilledema did not reveal any intracranial pathology (normal MRI brain imaging, normal MR venogram, and normal CSF opening pressure on lumbar puncture). However, there was no decrease in retinal nerve fiber thickness (RNFL) and ganglion cell complex (GCC) thickness on optical coherence tomography (OCT; Fig. 11.3b2). Her visual fields, however, revealed a reproducible, fairly dense central scotoma in her right eye (on PSD plot only; not even on gray scale printout; Fig. 11.3b1). The mean deviation was reduced on the right side (−3.28 dB), compared to the left side (−0.75 dB). This was suggestive of early compressive optic neuropathy. An orbital scan confirmed enlarged extra ocular muscles (EOM) bilaterally, extensive soft tissue stranding at the intraconal lateral orbits with resultant soft tissue crowding at the orbital apices (Fig. 11.3b3). The patient was counseled for pulse steroid therapy, followed by possible decompression surgery of orbit. Visual field testing has been found to be sensitive marker for compressive optic neuropathy, in thyroid eye disease [4].

The learning from these cases is that never ignore patient's symptoms. Investigate thoroughly and rule out whether there is an objective defect correlating with patient's complaints.

11.5.1 Localization of Lesions

One should have a working knowledge of the visual pathway, as the fibers traverse from retina to optic nerve, then partially crossover in the chiasma, and traverse as optic tract and optic radiations to the occipital lobe cortex (Fig. 11.4).

The visual field and retina have an inverted and reversed relationship, relative to the point of fixation (Fig. 11.5). The upper visual field falls on the inferior retina (below the fovea). The lower visual field falls on the superior retina (above the fovea) [5]. The nasal visual field falls on the temporal retina. The temporal visual field falls on the nasal retina. The nasal fibers of the ipsilateral eye (53% of all fibers) cross in the chiasm to join the uncrossed temporal fibers (47% of all fibers) of the contralateral eye [5]. They form the optic tract, which synapses in the lateral geniculate nucleus to form the optic radiations, which terminate in the visual cortex (area 17) of the occipital lobe. Because more fibers in the optic tract come from the opposite eye (crossed fibers), a relative afferent pupillary defect

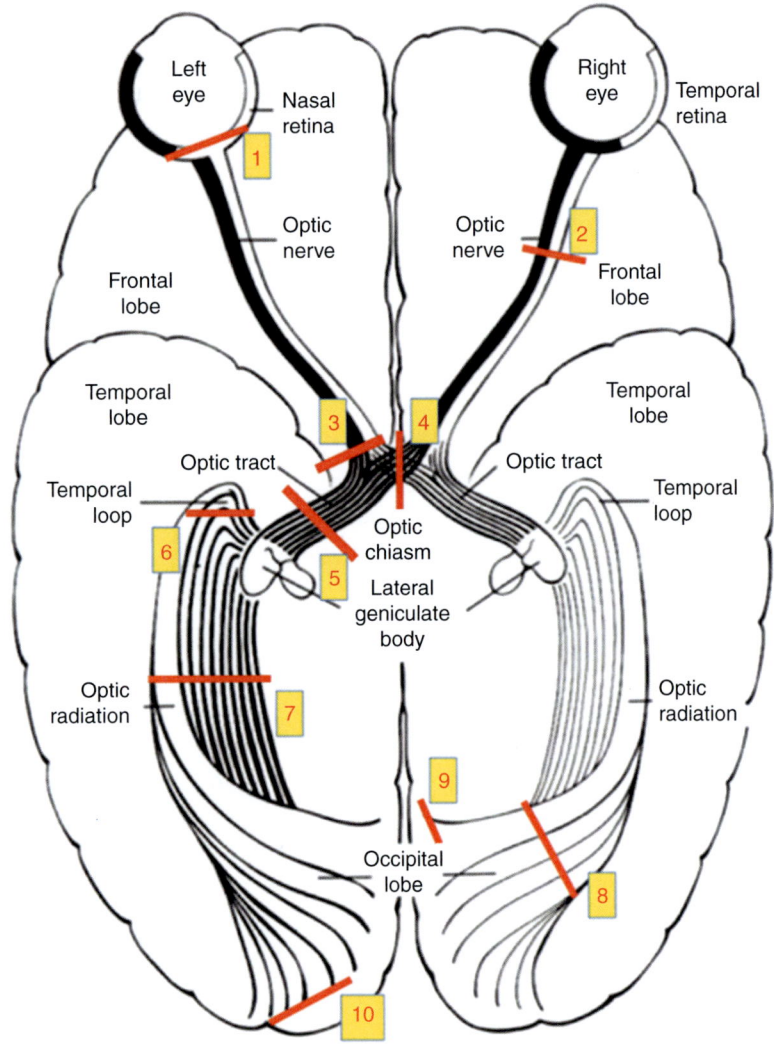

Fig. 11.4 Pathologies at different sites along the visual pathway (1–10) cause specific pattern of visual field defects. Optic nerve head (1), intra orbital optic nerve (2), pre-chiasmal region (3), chiasma (4), optic tract (5), Meyer's loop (temporal lobe) (6), optic radiations in parieto-occipital lobe (7), occipital lobe (8), para-sagittal lobe (9), occipital lobe tip (10)

(RAPD) is often observed in the eye contralateral to an optic tract lesion [2, 5]. At the level of the chiasm, the crossing inferonasal fibers travel anteriorly toward the contralateral optic nerve before passing into the optic tract. This is termed Von-Willebrand's knee and is responsible for the "junctional scotoma" in lesions of the posterior optic nerve [2, 5]. Although the anatomical presence of Willebrand's knee is debated, junctional scotomas are observed clinically. The visual field of each eye overlaps centrally [2, 5]. The normal visual field in each eye is approximately 60° superiorly, 70° to 75° inferiorly, 60° nasally, and 100° to 110° temporally [2]. The physiologic blind spot corresponds to the optic disc (no overlying photoreceptors) and is located approximately 15° temporally in each eye [2]. As of now, visual field testing remains a subjective test and is prone to errors. Nonetheless, it is an extremely useful tool to localize the lesions of the visual pathway, based on the characteristic pattern of visual field defects, as illustrated below.

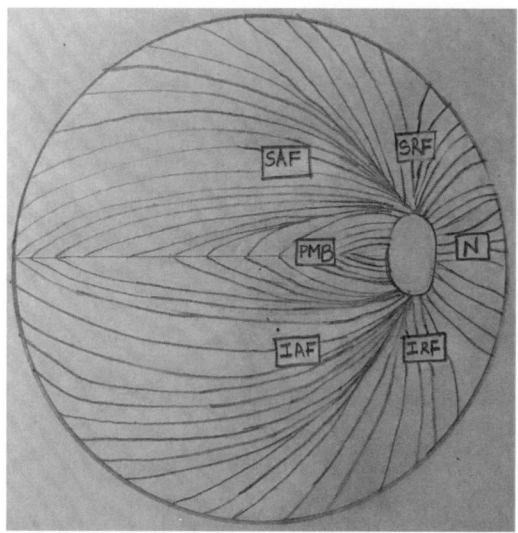

Fig. 11.5 Schematic drawing of the retinal nerve fiber axon arrangement: superior arcuate fibers (SAF) and inferior arcuate fibers (IAF), running temporally; papillomacular bundle (PMB) centrally; superior radiating fibers (SRF), nasal (N), and inferior radiating fibers (IRF) in the nasal quadrant

11.6 Scenario 4: Lesions Involving the Optic Nerve

11.6.1 Case 5A

A 21-year-old female presented with history chronic headaches and visual obscuration in both eyes. Her best corrected visual acuity was 6/6 OU, and color vision intact in both eyes. On examination, she had *florid papilledema* in both eyes (Fig. 11.6a1). She was evaluated by doing MRI imaging, MR venogram, and lumbar puncture. The visual field had *enlarged blind spots* (Fig. 11.6a2), corresponding to the swollen optic nerve heads [6]. The final diagnosis was *idiopathic intracranial hypertension,* after due investigations. Her papilledema resolved with acetazolamide therapy.

Localization of lesion due to visual field defect: both eyes optic nerve head (ONH; Fig. 11.4).

11.6.2 Case 5B

A 62-year-old diabetic and hypertensive female came with diminution of vision in both eyes. BCVA was 6/24p in the right eye and 6/60, PR accurate in the left eye. She had mild cataracts (nuclear grade 2 OU) but those were not commensurating with the vision. Fundus exam revealed that there was partial optic atrophy in the left eye and the right eye showed pale disc edema with a streak hemorrhage at the right disc margin (Fig. 11.6b1). On sharing the clinical findings, the patient got panicky and enquired whether neuro-imaging is required. The visual fields settled the debate. They demonstrated the inferior *altitudinal field defects* in both eyes (Fig. 11.6b2). The final diagnosis was *non-arteritic ischemic optic neuropathy (NAION)* in both eyes (right acute episode, left eye old sequelae), which did not require any neuroimaging per se. The altitudinal field defect (damage to superior or inferior visual field, respecting the horizontal meridian) occurs as a result of vascular damage to the retina or the optic nerve [7]. The optic nerve head is supplied by the paraoptic branches of short posterior ciliary vessels, the arrangement of which is in the form of two semicircles, separated at the horizontal meridian [3, 7]. Hence, optic disc hypoperfusion and infarction results in an altitudinal pattern of visual field defect [7].

Localization of lesion due to visual field defect: Both eyes superior retinal fibers (Fig. 11.5).

11.6.3 Case 5C

A 24-year-old female presented with the right eye ocular discomfort since 4 days. She had pain on ocular movements and blurred vision in her right eye. On exam, her visual acuity was 6/60 in the right eye, and 6/6 in the left eye. She had RAPD in her right eye, and fundus exam revealed right eye swollen and hyperemic disc (Fig. 11.6c1). Her visual fields showed generalized depression

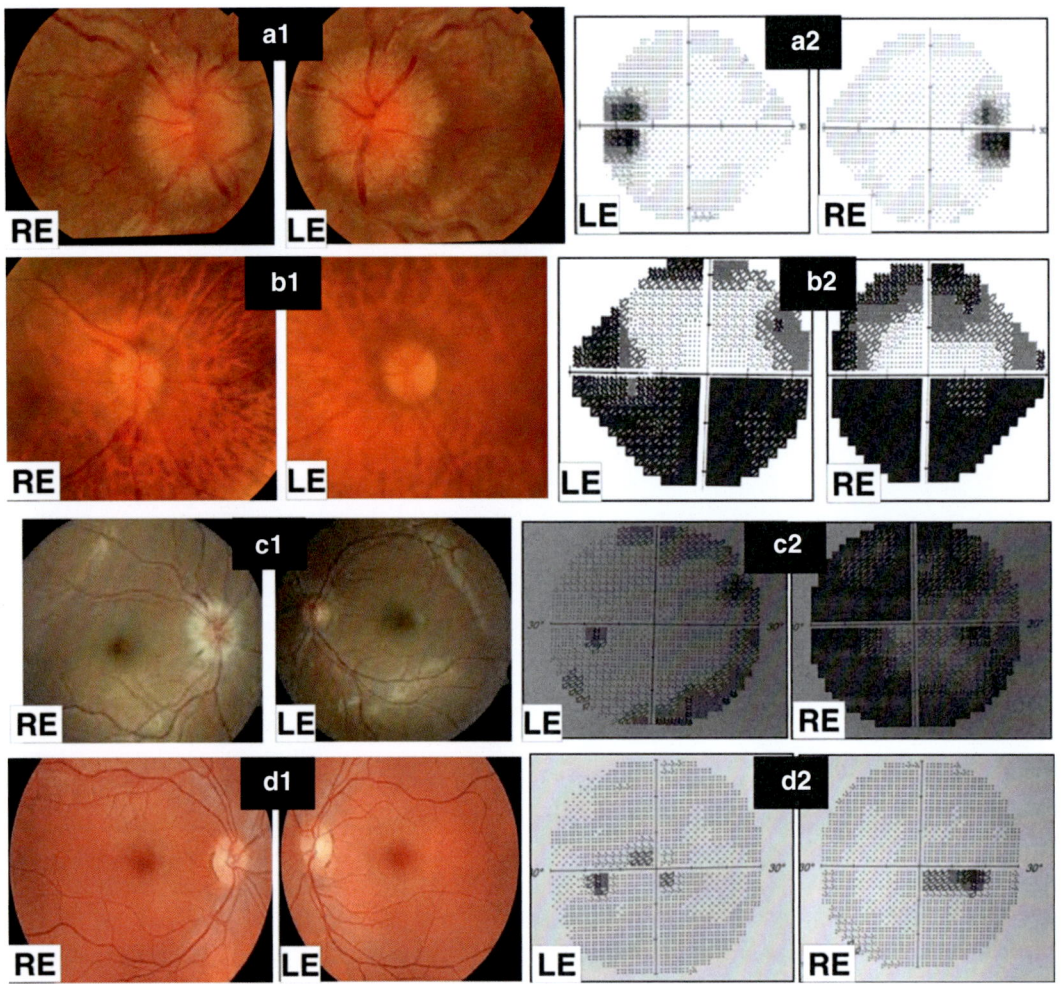

Fig. 11.6 Pattern of field defect in optic nerve head pathologies: papilledema of IIH causing enlarged blind spots (**a1**, **a2**), altitudinal field defects due to bilateral NAION (**b1**, **b2**), right papillitis causing advanced depression of field (**c1**, **c2**), and bilateral toxic optic neuropathy due to ethambutol causing centrocecal scotomas (**d1**, **d2**)

and *advanced scotoma* (Fig. 11.6c2) in her right eye, while the left eye field was unremarkable. The clinical profile hinted towards right optic neuritis [8]. It is known that the optic neuritis can present with virtually any type of visual field defects—central/centrocecal scotomas, altitudinal field defect, hemianopia field defect, etc. [8]. The VEP test and neuroimaging confirmed the diagnosis of right *demyelinating acute optic neuritis* (isolated). She was immediately referred for IVMP therapy followed by oral steroid therapy, as per recommended protocol.

Localization of lesion due to visual field defect: Right eye optic nerve head and optic nerve (Site 1 and 2; Fig. 11.4).

11.6.4 Case 5D

A 46-year-old male came with foggy vision in his eyes since 1 month. The patient was documented to have best corrected visual acuity of 6/9p elsewhere, with apparent normal eye exam, and started on lubricants. However, patient wanted a second opinion. Meanwhile, he had got a neuroimaging also done, on advice of a neurologist. The MRI imaging was unremarkable. The patient was categorical that he could not see books or mobile, clearly enough, as before. On probing, it was revealed that the patient was on antituberculous drugs (4 drug regimen) since 5 months, for pulmonary Koch's and chest-wise stable. His ocular examination was indeed unremarkable (normal fundi OU, Fig. 11.6d1). However, we insisted on getting a visual field done, which showed characteristic *centrocecal scotomas* in both eyes (R > L; Fig. 11.6d2). These were suggestive of ensuing *toxic optic neuropathy*, and he was immediately advised physician review, for stopping the potentially toxic drug ethambutol. He subsequently recovered in visual function, after stopping ethambutol and had normal visual fields, on examination after 3 months. In toxic optic neuropathy and nutritional optic neuropathies, the papillomacular bundle is preferentially involved, due to its high energy requirement. As a result, centrocecal scotomas are common in these pathologies [9].

Localization of lesion due to visual field defect: Both eyes papillomacular bundle (PMB; Fig. 11.5).

11.7 Scenario 5: Is it Glaucoma or Neuro-Ophthalmic-Related Field Damage?

11.7.1 Case 6.1

A 38-year-old lady presented with history of decreased near vision for few months. After examination elsewhere, she was diagnosed to optic disc cupping (cup disc ratio 0.55:1 in the right eye and 0.45:1 in her left eye). Intraocular pressure was documented to be 21 mm Hg in both eyes, and she was already on timolol 0.5% eyedrops OU. Her BCVA was 6/12p, N6 in the right eye and 6/9p, N6 in the left eye. On careful examination, she was found out to have bilateral temporal pallor of optic discs (Fig. 11.7a; pallor > cupping). Her OCT evaluation revealed decreased RFNL thickness in

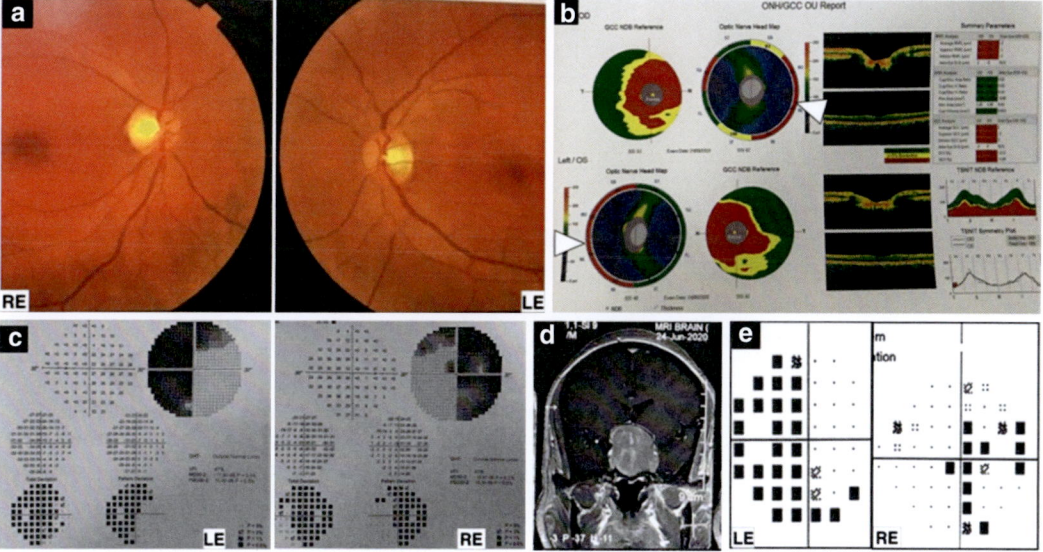

Fig. 11.7 Optic chiasmal lesion, misdiagnosed as glaucoma: bitemporal optic disc pallor simulating optic disc cupping (**a**); reduced RFNL thickness in temporal quadrants (**b**, white arrows); bitemporal hemianopia, with extension of defect into the superonasal quadrant in the left eye (**c**); pituitary gland macro adenoma causing chasmal compression (**d**); and partial resolution of the visual field defects, postsurgical excision of the pituitary mass (**e**)

nasal quadrant in both eyes and decreased macular ganglion cell thickness (Fig. 11.7b). Corresponding to the bi-nasal decreased RNFL thickness, her visual fields revealed *bitemporal hemianopia*, spilling over to the nasal quadrants, in superior quadrants (Fig. 11.7c). An urgent neuroimaging was requested and showed the inevitable—a *pituitary macroadenoma*, impinging on the chiasma (Fig. 11.7d). The patient was initially reluctant for surgical excision, due to the COVID pandemic. But finally agreed, and surgical excision led to partial resolution of the visual field deficit (Fig. 11.7e). The bilateral, symmetric temporal visual field defect (respecting the vertical meridian) is due to the compression of the crossing nasal fibers, at the chiasm, of the two optic nerves [10]. The nasal fibers, from each optic nerve, represent the temporal field of each side. Pituitary tumor leads to a denser visual field defect in superotemporal quadrant, initially, since the compression of the chiasm is from inferior aspect. Eventually of course, the unabated compression leads the scotoma to spill over into inferotemporal and nasal quadrants.

Localization of lesion due to visual field defect: Optic chiasma [9] *(Site 4; Fig. 11.4).*

11.7.2 Case 6.2

A 50-year-old female was being followed up in glaucoma clinic, since past 3 months. She was diagnosed as having open angle glaucoma OU. She had IOP recordings of 24 mm Hg OU on brinzolamide 1% eyedrops. She was referred to neuro-ophthalmology service for occasional "headaches." As per "routine protocol," her fundus findings were rereviewed. Both eyes had small sized discs; cup disc ratio (CDR) of 0.7:1 (inferior rim < superior rim) in the right eye, CDR of 0.55–0.6 in the left eye (with inferior notch); no disc pallor in either eye (Fig. 11.8a). Her visual fields showed a relatively advanced constriction of visual field in her left eye, with dense attitudinal scotoma in the superior quadrant (Fig. 11.8b). While in the right eye, it showed a superotemporal field defect (outside the arcuate area) in the periphery, possibly respecting the vertical meridian and possibly an evolving nasal step (on PSD plot) as well (Fig. 11.8b). On her OCT analysis, she had thinning of RFNL (predominantly nasal and inferior in the right eye and marked inferior thinning in the left eye; Fig. 11.8c). Her GCC thickness was grossly reduced in both eyes (Fig. 11.8c). No doubt, on first look her disc findings fitted in the glaucoma diagnosis, but somehow we believed that the pattern of her visual loss did not "fit in." So, we insisted on a neuroimaging with fine-cut sections through the chasmal region, in view of bilateral field defect (an advanced field defect in the left eye and possible junctional scotoma in the right eye). The patient luckily complied and we discovered a tubercular sella meningioma, compressing both optic nerves (L > R) and displacing the chiasma and internal carotid arteries (Fig. 11.8d).

It is not uncommon to misdiagnose certain cases as glaucoma, in cases of compressive optic neuropathy [11]. A quick revision can help to correlate our patient's visual field defect, with her investigation findings. The left eye optic nerve (in the pre-chasmal region) was more compressed (inferior >superior; Fig. 11.8d). In this region, the inferonasal and inferotemporal optic nerve fibers come to lie in the inferior quadrant, which is different from fiber arrangement at the optic disc (Fig. 11.8e). Hence, any optic nerve compression, in pre-chiasmal area, from beneath will lead to superior quadrant field defect (as seen in the left eye visual field in our case) [1, 2]. Due to the increasing compression, the field defect can gradually extend into advanced field defect (which was found in our case). We know that a pre-chiasmal pathology is also known to compress the optic nerve fibers comprising the anterior Von-Willebrand's knee [2]. These are crossing fibers from inferonasal retina of the fellow eye, and thus tend to cause a superotemporal field defect in the other eye (as was seen in the right eye visual field in our case) [2]. We believe that glaucomatous visual field defects also coexisted in this patient. In the left eye, the glaucomatous pattern may have got camouflaged into the predominant field defect due to optic nerve compres-

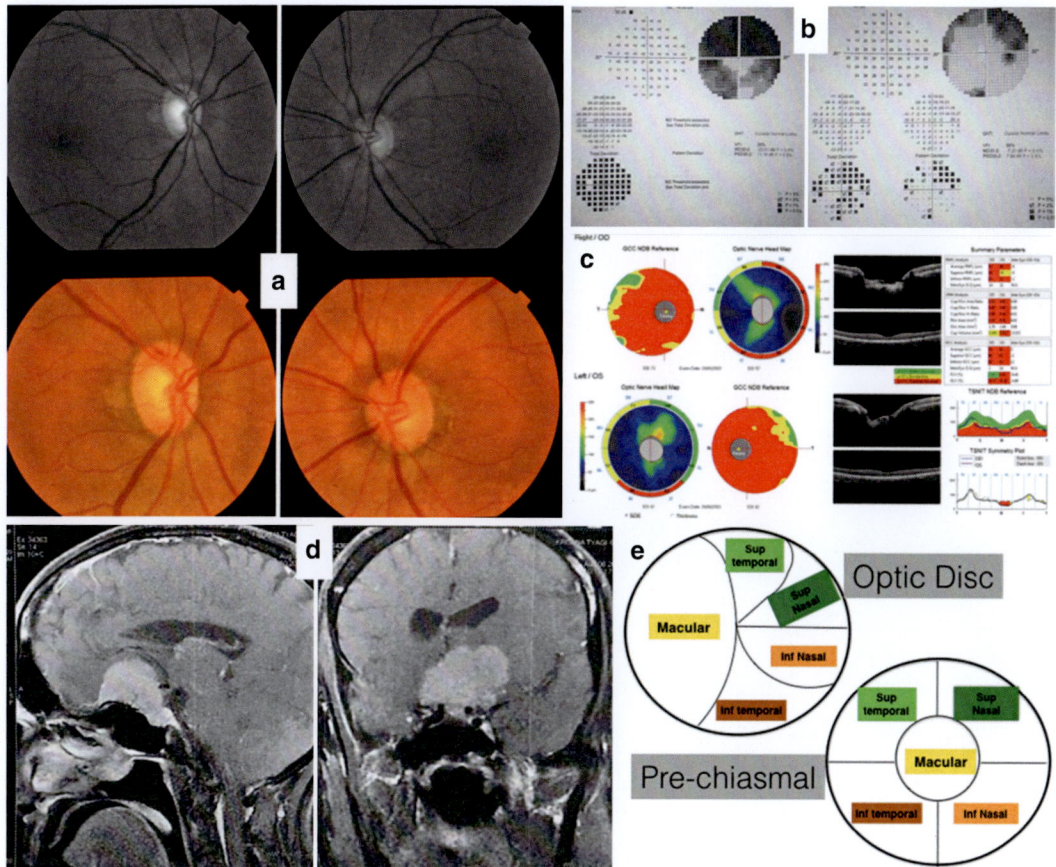

Fig. 11.8 Compressive optic neuropathy simulating glaucoma: glaucoma suspect OU (**a**); advanced field defect, denser in upper quadrant, in the left eye, right superotemporal quadratic defect (**b**); extensive RFNL and GCC thickness reduction in both eyes (**c**); tubercular sella meningioma causing pre-chiasmal compression of optic nerves and causing chasmal displacement (**d**); and arrangement of axonal nerve fibers at optic disc and pre-chiasmal levels (**e**)

sion (Fig. 11.8b). While in the right eye (particularly in PSD plot), a nasal step may be evolving (Fig. 11.8b). Hence, we decided to continue the appropriate antiglaucoma management. An urgent neurosurgeon review was sought for the intracranial pathology, and a prompt surgical excision of the tumor was recommended (considering the compression of sensitive structures). Altitudinal field defect, apart from ischemic optic neuropathy, is known to be caused by compressive lesions [12].

This challenging case beautifully highlights the importance of visual field in decision-making.

Localization of lesion due to visual field defect: Pre-chiasmal region (compressive pathology) and retina (glaucomatous pathology) (Site 1 and 3; Fig. 11.4).

11.8 Scenario 6: Visual Pathway Lesions

11.8.1 Case 7.1

A 42-year-old female came for treatment of her eye deviation. She indeed had an exodeviation, 40 prism diopters. Her visual acuity was 6/9 in her right eye and finger counting 1 m, PR accurate in the left eye. The left eye RAPD was present. Fundus examination revealed partial optic atrophy OU (L ≫ R; Fig. 11.9a). On probing, she popped out a previously done CT scan head, which did not show any intracranial pathology (Fig. 11.9d). It took some effort to convince the patient for further investigations. Flash VEP revealed grossly subnormal waveform in the left eye, while moderate amplitude waveform was present in the right eye (Fig. 11.9c). Somehow, the VEP findings did not exactly match the picture of demyelinating optic neuritis. A visual field of the right eye was done, which revealed a supero-temporal field defect (Fig. 11.9b). Confrontation field in the left eye was not very accurately elicited, possibly because of advance visual field constriction. Clinically, the visual field pattern—advanced visual field defect (assumed) of the left eye and the right eye junctional scotoma—was suggestive of a pre-chiasmal compression. A junctional scotoma (of

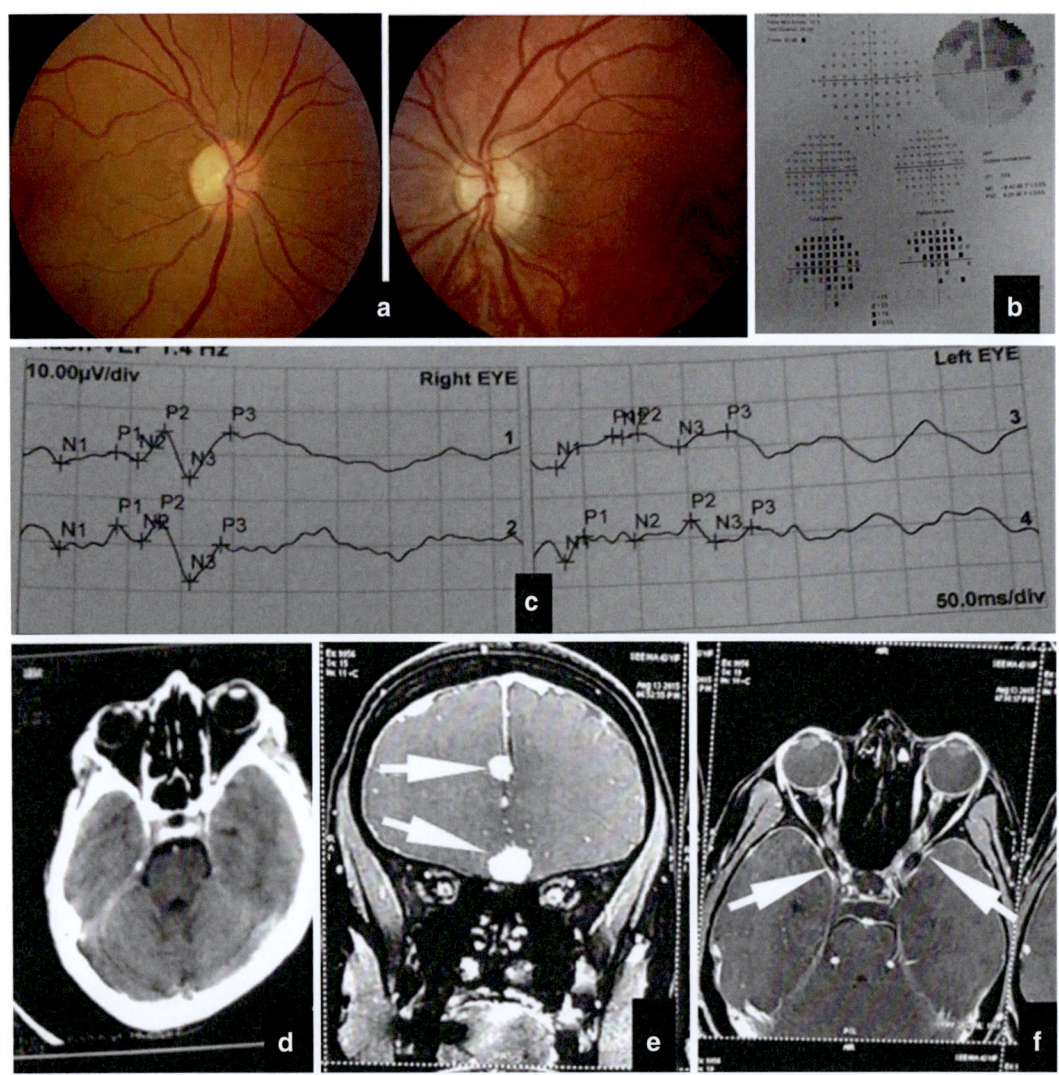

Fig. 11.9 Compressive optic neuropathy: both eyes partial optic atrophy, L ≫ R (**a**); right superotemporal quadrantic defect—junctional scotoma (**b**); flash VEP showing reduction in amplitudes, L ≫ R (**c**); CT scan brain with no gross pathology (**d**); MRI brain showing multiple meningioma lesions (**e**); and meningioma lesions causing pre-chiasmal compression and infiltration of optic nerves (**f**)

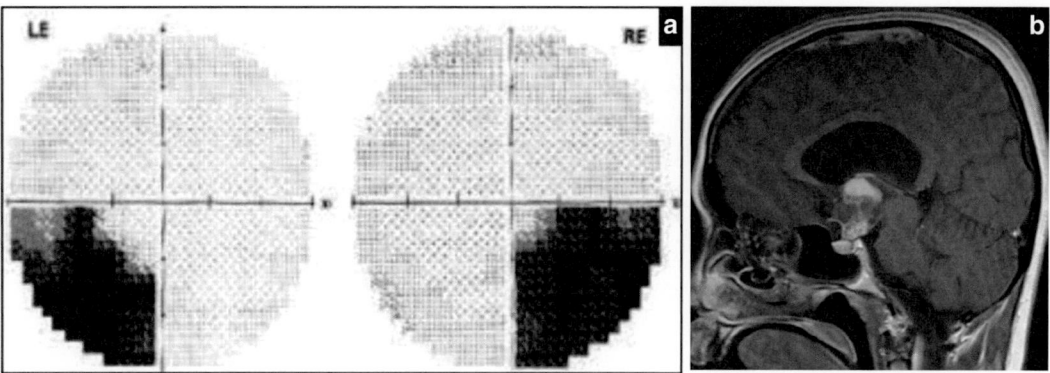

Fig. 11.10 Chiasmal compression: partial bitemporal hemianopia affecting the inferior quadrants (**a**) and suprasellar lesion causing chasmal compression (**b**)

Traquair) is a visual field defect that arises from damage to the junction of the optic nerve and the optic chiasm [2]. A compressive pathology in the pre-seller region compresses an optic nerve, causing ipsilateral central scotoma or advanced visual field defect and also causing the superotemporal quadrantanopia on the contralateral side (due to compression of fibers of Von-Willebrand's knee) [2]. Our doubts were confirmed on neuroimaging (MRI brain with contrast), the patient had multiple meningiomas—some involving falx cerebri, and another involving pre-sellar region, seemingly extending to cisternal optic nerves (Fig. 11.9e,f). Ironically, the neurosurgeons disagreed with our view of optic nerve compression, and the patient was advised conservative management. However, in view of the characteristic visual field pattern, we insisted her to take another opinion, to salvage the right eye optic nerve. She landed up with a neurosurgeon in Chennai, who operated her. In a personal communication, the neurosurgeon called few days later, to inform that per-operatively he discovered that the pre-sellar meningioma had infiltrated the optic nerves (left more than right) and would have definitely irreversibly damaged their right nerve, if left unoperated. *Our stand, which had stemmed, from the visual field pattern, was vindicated!*

Localization of lesion due to visual field defect: Pre-chiasmal region (Site 3; Fig. 11.4).

11.8.2 Case 7.2

A 10-year-old boy had been brought for inability to see the blackboard. His BCVA was recorded as 6/12 in both eyes, which was provisionally labeled as meridional amblyopia, secondary to astigmatic refractive errors. However, on careful exam, the child also had temporal pallor of both eyes. He was cajoled to do a visual field, which showed an incomplete bitemporal hemianopia pattern (in fact the field defect was confined to the inferotemporal quadrants on both sides; Fig. 11.10a). A subsequent neuroimaging confirmed the fear of a suprasellar lesion (craniopharyngioma) compressing the chiasma, from above (Fig. 11.10b). The compression of crossing nasal fibers led to the characteristic field defect, respecting the vertical meridian [10]. The child was urgently referred to the neurosurgeon.

Localization of lesion due to visual field defect: Chiasma (Site 4; Fig. 11.4).

11.8.3 Case 8.1

A 28-year-old known patient of multiple sclerosis, presented with inability to see to her left side, since a week. Her BCVA was 6/9p in both eyes. Her VEP showed comparative latencies compared to her previous records (no apparent gross decrease in conduction in the anterior visual pathway). But her visual fields revealed an incongruent left hemianopia (Fig. 11.11a). The correlation was clear on neuroimaging—she had developed a demyelinating lesion of her right optic tract region (Fig. 11.11a). The optic tract lesions are known to cause incongruent (asymmetric) hemianopia [11]. Again, in this case, the visual fields were handy in discovering a new demyelinating lesion, even though the VEP was stable. The patient was immediately sent to the neurologist for appropriate management.

Localization of lesion due to visual field defect: Optic tract (Site 5; Fig. 11.4).

11.8.4 Case 8.2

A 66-year-old gentleman came with a specific problem of reading and discomfort while climbing down the stairs. His vascular risk factors had been deranged for about a month. There was no specific limb weakness and speech or hearing defects. He had BCVA of 6/6p, N6 OU. His ocular exam (including ocular motility) was unremarkable, except for early cataracts. A visual field was requested and it solved the mystery—the patient had developed a left inferior quadrantopia (pie in the floor field defect, Fig. 11.11b). Neuroimaging revealed a subtle, localized fresh infarct in the parietal-occipital junction. An immediate neurology reference was sought. Superior optic radiations pass through the parietal lobe, and hence its lesion causes a contralateral inferior homonymous hemianopia (pie in the floor field defect) [12].

Localization of lesion due to visual field defect: Superior optic radiation at level of parietal lobe (Site 7; Fig. 11.4).

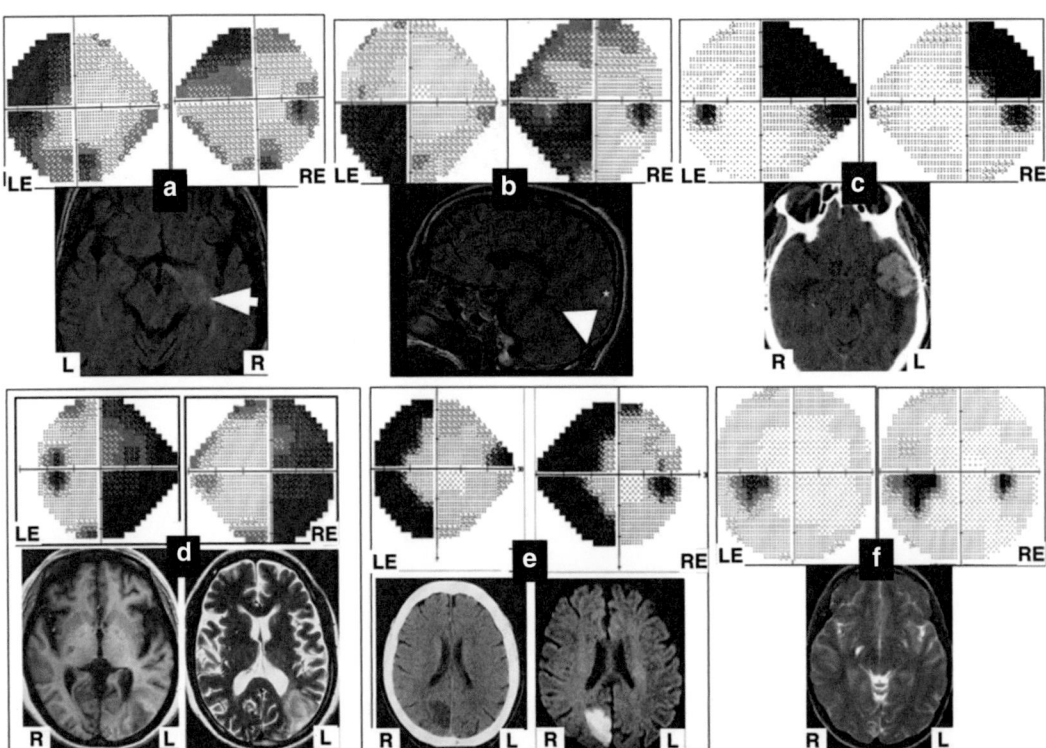

Fig. 11.11 Retro-chiasmal lesions: demyelinating lesion of right optic tract causing left hemianopia (**a**); left "pie on the floor" quadrantic field defect, caused by right parieto-occipital lobe infarct (**b**); right "pie in the sky" quadrantic field defect caused by temporal lobe hematoma (**c**); right hemianopia caused by occipital lobe infarct in an SLE patient (**d**); left hemianopia with macular sparing in right para-sagittal occipital lobe infarction (**e**); and left focal homonymous hemianopia due to infarction of right occipital lobe tip (**f**)

11.8.5 Case 8.3

A 48-year-old driver had met with an accident. He was conscious, oriented, and been kept under observation by the emergency team. He was referred for fundus exam, which was essentially normal. However, we decided to obtain a baseline visual field. The visual field showed a characteristic "pie in the sky lesion" (right upper quadrantopia, Fig. 11.11c). An emergency CT scan confirmed hematoma in the left temporal lobe. Inferior optic radiations (also called Meyer's loop) carry information from inferior retinal quadrants. These pass through the temporal lobe. Hence, a temporal lobe lesion can disrupt the Meyer's loop pathway and cause contralateral superior homonymous hemianopia (pie in the sky field defect) [13].

Localization of lesion due to visual field defect: Inferior optic radiation at level of temporal lobe (Site 6; Fig. 11.4).

11.8.6 Case 8.4

A 31-year-old, intelligent lady complained "some abnormality in vision." She was a known case of systemic lupus erythematous (SLE) since past 15 years and was on immunosuppressive therapy for her nephropathy component. Presumably, she appeared distressed due to her prolonged treatment. Her BCVA in each eye was 6/6 p, with normal color vision and reasonably brisk pupillary reactions. Her fundus findings were unremarkable. A thought came to my mind that she is seemingly ok and just perturbed and anxious. But then a counter thought reasoned to investigate objectively, considering her multisystem disease. A pattern VEP exam showed normal conduction in both eyes, but a visual field demonstrated a characteristic right hemianopia lesion (Fig. 11.11d). She had a neuroimaging done 2 years back, which was documented to be normal. But on insisting, a repeat neuroimaging was done which revealed a chronic infarct of left parasagittal occipital lobe, with adjoining rim of subacute ischemia (Fig. 11.11d). Small multifocal ischemic areas were also found in other parts of brain. The neurologist confirmed the ischemic infracts and made an impression of SLE-induced vasculitis (leading to infarcts) in the brain. It meant exacerbation of her SLE disease and required more aggressive immunosuppression. Hence, a visual field test was instrumental in reaching a crucial decision and helped in the patient management.

Localization of lesion due to visual field defect: Occipital lobe [13] (Site 8; Fig. 11.4).

11.8.7 Case 8.5

A 54-year-old diabetic male had been diagnosed with stroke involving the posterior cerebral artery circulation, 2 weeks back. He had presented to the casualty with some weakness of the right side of body and some blurriness in vision. An emergency CT and MRI scan had already confirmed left occipital lobe infarction. He was discharged after conservative treatment and was referred for perimetry to us. His visual fields revealed a right homonymous hemianopia with macular sparing (Fig. 11.11e). His BCVA was indeed 6/6p in both eyes, with normal fundi OU. Posterior visual pathway lesion involving the occipital lobe is known to cause homonymous hemianopia. It is believed that sparing of the macula may be encountered in these cases, due to the collateral vascular supply to the macular region or by the very large macular representation in the occipital cortex; additionally, bilateral representation of macular vision has been suspected [14]. The exact cause for macular sparing is still not clear.

Localization of lesion due to visual field defect: Occipital lobe (Site 8; Fig. 11.4).

11.8.8 Case 8.6

A 62-year-old was being worked up for his cataract management. His BCVA was 6/18p in both eyes, which correlated with his grade of cataracts, in each eye. However, he mentioned in passing that he had foggy vision since long, after he had recovered from a road traffic accident in his teens. That prompted us to obtain visual fields, in spite of normal fundi OU. The field showed a bilateral, homonymous, focal left hemianopic field defect (Fig. 11.11f). Neuroimaging revealed that the patient had encephalomalacia involving the tip of his right occipital lobe. This was possibly sustained due to head trauma decades back.

Localization of lesion due to visual field defect: Occipital lobe [14, 15] *(Site 10; Fig. 11.4).*

11.9 Scenario 7: Visual Field Defect Due to Raised Intracranial Pressure

11.9.1 Case 9

A 30-year-old lady came with bilateral visual loss, since 2 weeks. She had previous history of "migraines," for which she used to take occasional analgesics. Her BCVA was found to be 6/24p in the right eye and 6/36 in the left eye. The positive conspicuous exam finding was florid optic disc edema with partial macular star formation in both eyes (Fig. 11.9a). She was extensively investigated, as per our papilledema protocol, and a final impression of Idiopathic intracranial hypertension (fulminant variety) was made. Her visual fields, at presentation, showed constriction in both eyes (Fig. 11.12a). She was aggressively treated with 5 days of IVMP treatment (to facilitate optic nerve salvage) and high dose acetazolamide therapy, tapered over 3 months. After about 3 months, the optic disc edema gradually resolved with residual gliosis and partial optic atrophy (Fig. 11.12b). The visual fields improved, compared to presentation, but residual central scotomas remained (Fig. 11.12b). This corroborated with the deceased macular GCC complex, in spite of relatively normal RNFL thickness in both eyes (false reading possibly due to previously swollen peripapillary nerve fibers, Fig. 11.12c). Raised intracranial pressures, due to any cause, are known to cause optic neuropathy of various grades, and visual field testing serves as a valuable resource to document the optic nerve function [16].

As illustrated by some of the examples given above, visual field testing constitutes an extremely important armamentarium in evaluation afferent visual pathway disorders, not only of pathologies within the eye but also of disruptions of the optic nerve fibers, as they course in the brain to finally terminate in the visual cortex. Although the test has its limitation, in being subjective, but often provides very valuable information in most cases. Another point to remember is that visual field findings need to be always correlated with the clinical profile of the patient.

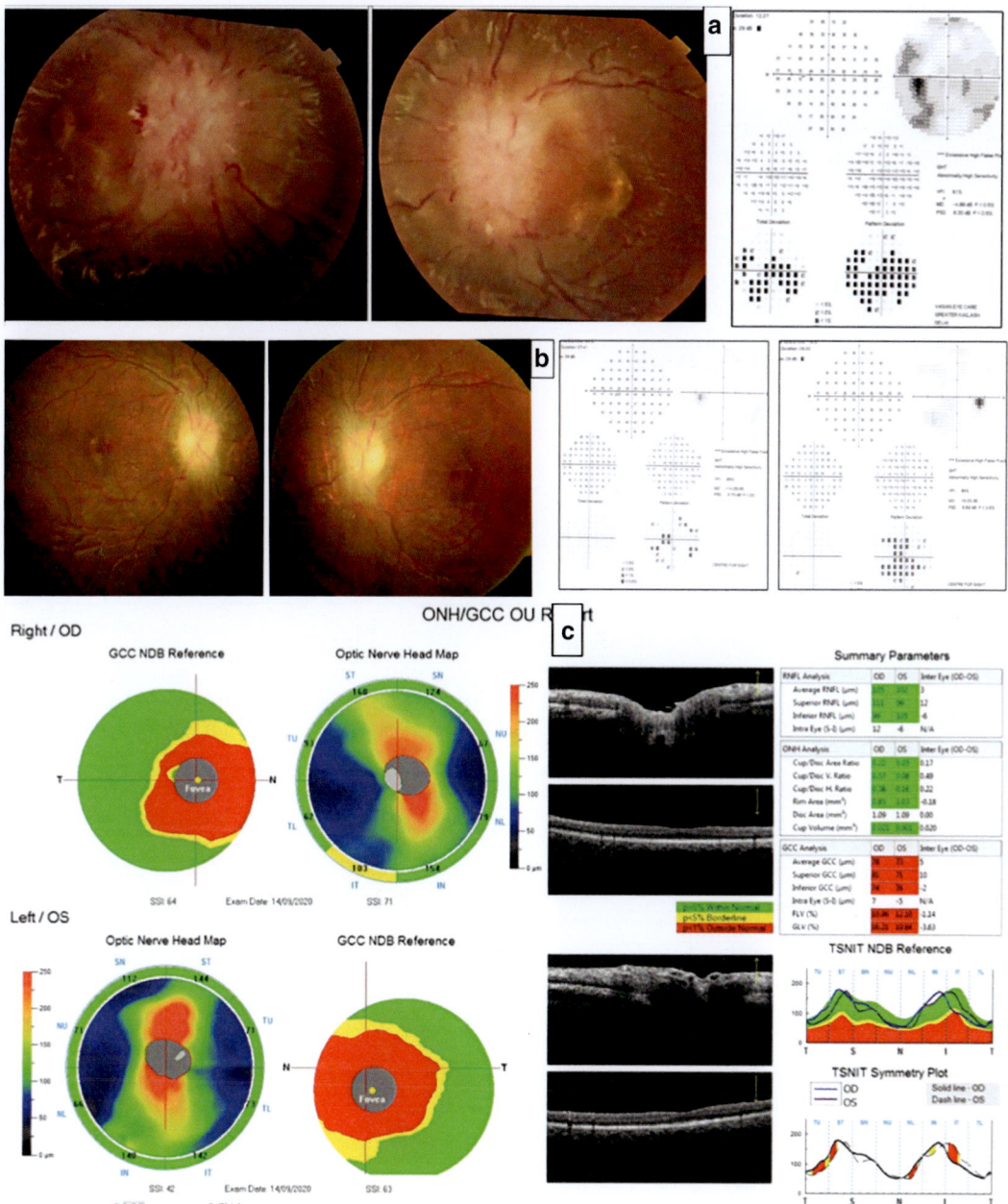

Fig. 11.12 Case of idiopathic intracranial hypertension with florid papilledema and advanced visual field depression both eyes (**a**); improvement in visual fields, as papilledema resolves with partial optic atrophy (**b**); and relatively normal RFNL thickness, with gross reduction in GCC thickness, due to partial optic atrophy (**c**)

References

1. Kedar S, Ghate D, Corbett JJ. Visual fields in neuro-ophthalmology. Indian J Ophthalmol. 2011;59:103–9.
2. Biousse V, Newman NJ. Neuro-ophthalmology illustrated. 3rd ed. New York, NY: Thieme Medical Publishers, Inc; 2020. p. 45–78.
3. Wirtschafter JD, Hard-Boberg AL, Coffman SM. Evaluating the usefulness in neuro-ophthalmology of visual field examinations peripheral to 30 degrees. Trans Am Ophthalmol Soc. 1984;82:329–57.
4. Kauh CY, Gupta S, Douglas RS, et al. Compressive optic neuropathy and repeat orbital decompression: a case series. Ophthalmic Plast Reconstr Surg. 2015;31(5):385–90.
5. Gupta M, Bordoni B. Neuroanatomy, visual pathway. In: StatPearls [internet]. Treasure Island, FL: StatPearls Publishing; 2020.
6. Corbett JJ, Savino PJ, Thompson HS, Kansu T, Schatz NJ, Orr LS, et al. Visual loss in pseudotumor cerebri. Follow-up of 57 patients from five to 41 years and a profile of 14 patients with permanent severe visual loss. Arch Neurol. 1982;39:461–74.
7. Hayreh SS, Zimmerman B. Visual field abnormalities in nonarteritic anterior ischemic optic neuropathy: their pattern and prevalence at initial examination. Arch Ophthalmol. 2005;123:1554–62.
8. Keltner JL, Johnson CA, Spurr JO, Beck RW. Visual field profile of optic neuritis. One-year follow-up in the Optic Neuritis Treatment Trial. Arch Ophthalmol. 1994;112:946–53.
9. Kahana LM. Toxic ocular effects of ethambutol. CMAJ. 1987;137:213–6.
10. Fujimoto N, Saeki N, Miyauchi O, Adachi-Usami E. Criteria for early detection of temporal hemianopia in asymptomatic pituitary tumor. Eye (Lond). 2002;16:731–8.
11. Choudhari NS, Neog A, Fudnawala V, George R. Cupped disc with normal intraocular pressure: the long road to avoid misdiagnosis. Indian J Ophthalmol. 2011;59:491–7.
12. Shapey J, Danesh-Meyer HV, Kaye AH. Suprasellar meningioma presenting with an altitudinal field defect. J Clin Neurosci. 2012;19(1):155–8.
13. Wall M, Johnson CA, Kutzko KE, Nguyen R, Brito C, Keltner JL. Long- and short-term variability of automated perimetry results in patients with optic neuritis and healthy subjects. Arch Ophthalmol. 1998;116:53–61.
14. Zhang X, Kedar S, Lynn MJ, Newman NJ, Biousse V. Natural history of homonymous hemianopia. Neurology. 2006;66:901–5.
15. Wall M, Punke SG, Stickney TL, Brito CF, Withrow KR, Kardon RH. SITA standard in optic neuropathies and hemianopias: a comparison with full threshold testing. Invest Ophthalmol Vis Sci. 2001;42:528–37.
16. Friedman DI, Jacobson DM. Diagnostic criteria for idiopathic intracranial hypertension. Neurology. 2002;59:1492–5.

Effect of Media Opacities on Perimetry: A Vexing Clinical Problem

12

Tulika Chauhan and Mithun Thulasidas

The visual field broadly refers to the area in which a stimulus can be visually detected. From the point of fixation, the monocular visual field of a normal human observer extends approximately 50° superiorly, 70° inferiorly, 60° nasally, and 100° temporally [1]. The visual field can be measured using a variety of perimetric techniques. The extent and shape of the visual field vary with stimulus parameters such as stimulus size [2]. In clinical practice, standard automated perimetry (SAP) is the common method of assessing the visual field since the 1970s and 1980s [3, 4]. As visual field results can provide clues regarding the location of the anatomy along the visual pathway, it is an instrumental component of the ocular examination [5, 6].

Opacities in the cornea cause a defect in the visual field on the same side, whereas opacities situated in the posterior layers of the crystalline lens cause a defect in the visual field on the opposite side (Fig. 12.1) [7]. Asymmetrical opacities of the optical media can cause asymmetrical defects in the visual field if they are present in the visual axis.

Diseases of the cornea often leave permanent opacities of varying density, extend and pattern.

Homogeneous opacities of the cornea can produce a generalized reduction of sensitivity to approximately one-third of the normal sensitivity. Inhomogeneous opacities, like in granular dystrophy with an increase of glare and scatter, can lead to a great variety of the individual thresholds [8].

Cataract opacity could make interpreting the visual field indices more challenging, especially in patients with early glaucoma [9]. Cataract formation can increase intraocular straylight, arising from increased forward light scatter [10, 11]. This increase in straylight causes a shortening and widening of the point-spread function of the eye, resulting in reduced contrast sensitivity. Moderate-to-large increase in intraocular straylight significantly affects thresholds in SAP, and even frequency doubling technology, and Flicker-defined form perimetry [12]. Moss et al. showed that blue-on-yellow visual field is affected by posterior subcapsular opacity, and white-on-white visual field is affected by anterior cortical opacity [13]. Posterior subcapsular and cortical cataract opacity have been found to be more affected by intraocular straylight than nuclear cataract opacity [14].

Global measurements of visual field sensitivity, such as the mean deviation (MD) and total deviation map on the Humphrey visual field analyzer (HFA), can be affected by media opacities [15, 16]. Such depressions are typically diffuse on the total deviation map and correlate with the

T. Chauhan
Cornea, Cataract, and Refractive Surgery Services, Centre for Sight Eye Institute, New Delhi, India

M. Thulasidas (✉)
Comprehensive Ophthalmology Services, Centre for Sight Eye Institute, New Delhi, India

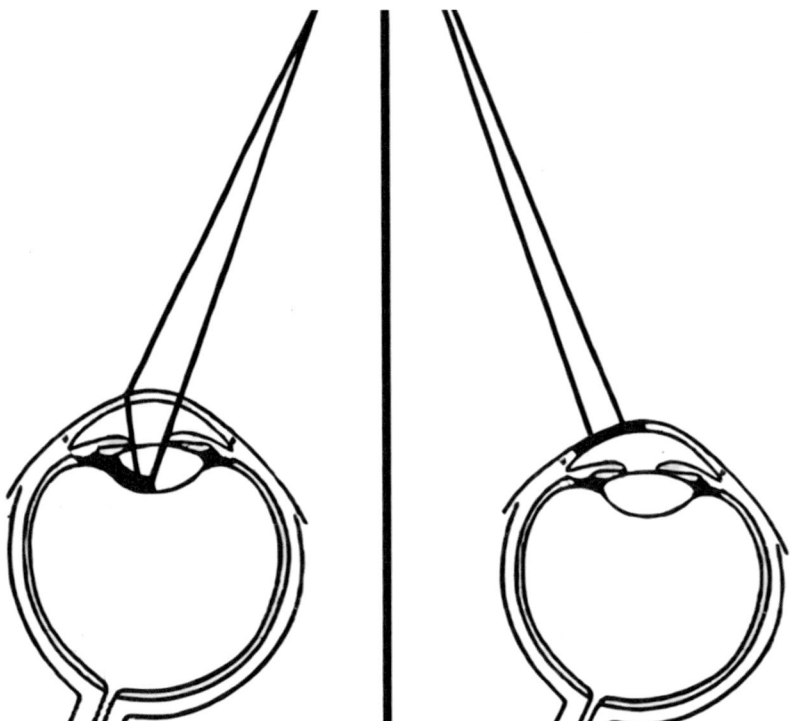

Fig. 12.1 Diagrammatic representation of a horizontal section of an eye with an opacity in the posterior layer of the lens resulting in loss of field of vision on the opposite side and an opacity in the cornea resulting in loss of visual field on the same side (Adapted from Lyne AJ, Phillips CI. Visual field defects due to opacities in the optical media. Br J Ophthalmol 1969;53:119–122)

location of the media opacity, although opacities that are sufficiently deep may also result in concurrent defects on the pattern deviation map [16]. Generalized reduction of sensitivity shows the homogenous nature of opacity [8]. Pupillary dilatation increases or decreases the area of scotoma depending on the distribution of opacity. A large opacity (more than the standard pupil size) prevents light rays from entering the eye through the opacity, increasing the area of scotoma after dilatation, whereas a small opacity allows light rays to enter the eye around the opacity, thereby reducing the defect [7].

The influence of cataract opacity on the visual field is well studied and reported in the literature [7–14]. Chen et al. and Chung et al. demonstrated that MD often improved significantly after cataract extraction in eyes with mild glaucoma [8, 9]. Chung et al. also found that posterior subcapsular opacity was associated with a significant change in MD after cataract extraction but not the PSD or visual field index values [9]. However, dense cataract can lead to focal depressions even in the pattern deviation map [16].

Figure 12.2 shows the visual field result of a patient with central posterior subcapsular opacity analyzed using the Swedish Interactive Threshold Algorithm (SITA) 24-2 program. The diffuse defects on the total deviation map were characteristic of generalized media opacity, while the focal depressions located primarily in the center of the pattern deviation map were mainly due to the relatively dense areas of posterior subcapsular opacity (Fig. 12.2a). After cataract extraction, no significant defects were observed in the total deviation and pattern deviation maps (Fig. 12.2b).

So far, little is known about the possible influence of the corneal opacity on the visual field of the eye. Phu et al. described a case of a 38-year-old woman with severe dry eye manifesting as confluent central corneal superficial punctuate epitheliopathy. Significant central total deviation defects with an accompanying MD value of −2.80 dB was observed. Some areas of punctate epitheliopathy were dense to result in pattern standard deviation (PSD) defects [16]. Contact lenses can also cause artifacts due to altered optical properties such as from multifocal lens

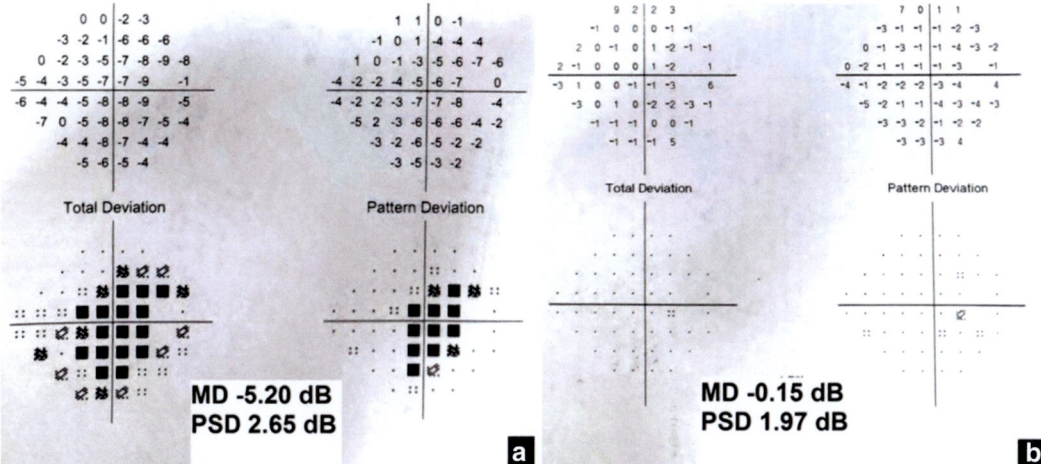

Fig. 12.2 Visual field of a patient with central posterior subcapsular opacity (**a**). Generalized media opacity on the total deviation map with dense regions resulting in focal depressions in the pattern deviation map (**b**). No significant defects in the total deviation and pattern deviation maps after cataract extraction

designs [17]. Tavolara, in 1959, described 22 cases of pterygium with a reduction of the isoptres proportionate to the extent of the lesion, which disappeared after the excision of the pterygium [18]. Blum, Gates, and James, in 1959, mentioned a nasal defect in the peripheral field due to the same condition which disappeared after the surgery [19].

In order to determine the effect of corneal opacity on the visual field, patients with nebulomacular corneal opacity were analyzed using the full threshold 24-2 program (stimulus III) on a single Humphrey® field analyzer 3 perimeter (Carl Zeiss Meditec AG, Jena, Germany). After performing the test in normal pupil state (3–4 mm), eyes were dilated with 1% tropicamide ophthalmic solution, and field tests were repeated to see the effect of pupillary dilatation on the visual field in patients with corneal opacity.

The visual field results of three patients (five eyes) with nebulo-macular corneal opacity involving the visual axis were evaluated. All eyes had a minimum corrected distance visual acuity of 6/9. There were significant central total deviation defects with accompanying higher MD value in all the eyes (Fig. 12.3a). Some regions of corneal opacity were dense enough to result in pattern deviation map defects (Fig. 12.4a); however, these focal defects were not numerous or dense enough to result in a significant PSD value. All eyes showed a generalized reduction of sensitivity. After pupillary dilatation, the total deviation defects and MD values worsened in three eyes (Fig. 12.3b) and improved in two eyes (Fig. 12.4b), compared to pre-dilatation results. None of the eyes showed a significant defect in the pattern deviation map after dilatation. Table 12.1 shows the patient data with MD and PSD values.

While modern technology has improved facets of visual field assessment using SAP, the primary psychophysical task of detecting incremental light stimuli has remained virtually unchanged since the 1970s. There are some recognized limitations of SAP, but it remains the clinical standard of assessing the visual field. Recent research has challenged the existing test paradigms. Preliminary results are promising in areas of research attempting to reconcile the structure–function relationship better, but more work is needed to produce a widespread paradigm shift in SAP [16].

A complete history taking and clinical examination of both anterior and posterior segment, asking ourselves questions regarding the interpretation and localization of defects (monocular/binocular, location, depth, completeness, and

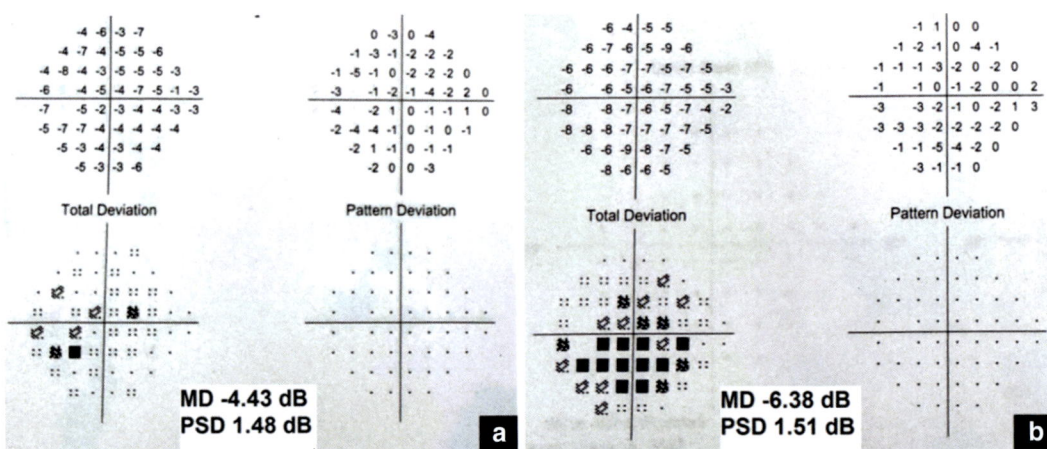

Fig. 12.3 Visual field of a patient with nebulo-macular corneal opacity (**a**). Total deviation defect with high MD value. (**b**) Total deviation defect and MD value worsened after pupil dilatation

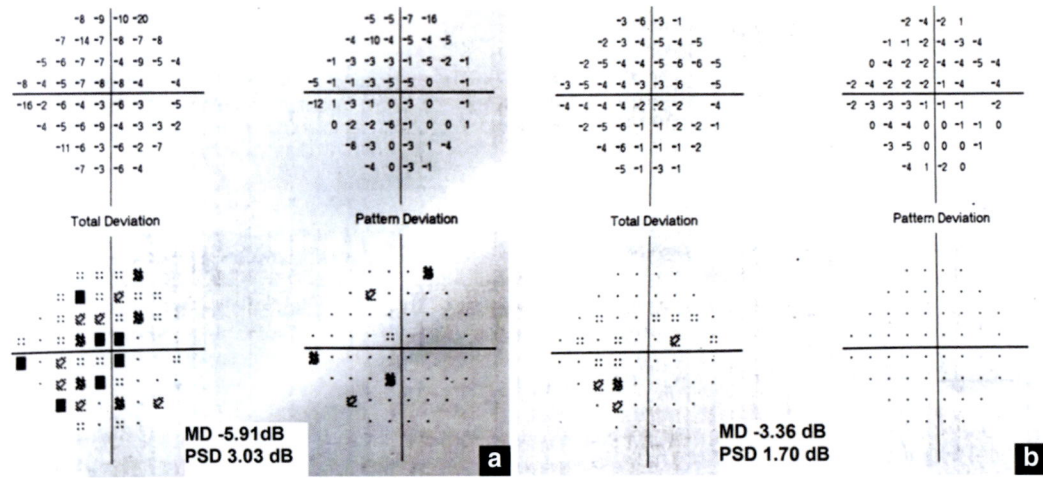

Fig. 12.4 Visual field of a patient with nebulo-macular corneal opacity (**a**). Total deviation defect with some dense regions resulting in depressions in the pattern deviation map. (**b**) Total deviation defect and MD value improved after pupil dilatation

Table 12.1 Data of patients with corneal opacity

S. No.	Corneal opacity characteristics	Corrected distance visual acuity	MD value (normal pupils) [dB]	PSD value (normal pupils) [dB]	MD value (dilated pupils) [dB]	PSD value (dilated pupils) [dB]
1	NMCO 2 × 2 mm	6/6p	−5.91	3.03	−3.36	1.7
2	NMCO 2 × 2 mm	6/9	−6.69	2.12	−5.43	1.72
3	NMCO 5 × 7 mm	6/9	−7.85	1.8	−9	1.69
4	NMCO 4 × 4 mm	6/9	−3.94	1.08	−6.55	1.33
5	NMCO 4 × 4 mm	6/9	−4.43	1.48	−6.38	1.51

NMCO nebulo-macular corneal opacity, *MD* mean deviation, *PSD* pattern standard deviation congruity of the defect), and most importantly, if the visual field does not match with the optic nerve head experience, we must look for other apparent causes.

Declaration of Competing Interest The authors have no financial disclosures.

Acknowledgments None.

References

1. Traquair HM. Clinical detection of early changes in the visual field. Trans Am Ophthalmol Soc. 1939;37:158–79.
2. Khuu SK, Kalloniatis M. Standard automated perimetry: determining spatial summation and its effect on contrast sensitivity across the visual field. Invest Ophthalmol Vis Sci. 2015;56:3565–76.
3. Heijl A, Patella VM. Essential perimetry - the field analyzer primer. Dublin, CA: Carl Zeiss Meditec; 2002.
4. Johnson CA, Wall M, Thompson HS. A history of perimetry and visual field testing. Optom Vis Sci. 2011;88:E8–E15.
5. Anderson AJ, Shuey NH, Wall M. Rapid confrontation screening for peripheral visual field defects and extinction. Clin Exp Optom. 2009;92:45–8.
6. Jampel HD, Singh K, Lin SC, et al. Assessment of visual function in glaucoma: a report by the American Academy of Ophthalmology. Ophthalmology. 2011;118:986–1002.
7. Lyne AJ, Phillips CI. Visual field defects due to opacities in the optical media. Br J Ophthalmol. 1969;53:119–22.
8. Greve E, Heijl A. Seventh international visual field symposium, Amsterdam, September 1986, vol. 1987. Dordrecht: M. Nijhoff/Dr. W. Junk Publishers. p. 64.
9. Chung HJ, Choi JH, Lee YC, Kim SY. Effect of cataract opacity type and glaucoma severity on visual field index. Optom Vis Sci. 2016;93:575–8.
10. Van den Berg TJ. Analysis of intraocular straylight, especially in relation to age. Optom Vis Sci. 1995;72:52–9.
11. De Waard PW, IJspeert JK, Van den Berg TJ, De Jong PT. Intraocular light scattering in age-related cataracts. Invest Ophthalmol Vis Sci. 1992;33:618–25.
12. Bergin C, Redmond T, Nathwani N, Verdon-Roe GM, Crabb DP, Anderson RS, Garway-Heath DF. The effect of induced intraocular straylight on perimetric tests. Invest Ophthalmol Vis Sci. 2011;52:3676–82.
13. Moss ID, Wild JM, Whitaker DJ. The influence of age-related cataract on blue-on-yellow perimetry. Invest Ophthalmol Vis Sci. 1995;36:764–73.
14. Bal T, Coeckelbergh T, Van Looveren J, Rozema JJ, Tassignon MJ. Influence of cataract morphology on straylight and contrast sensitivity and its relevance to fitness to drive. Ophthalmologica. 2011;225:105–11.
15. Heuer DK, Anderson DR, Feuer WJ, et al. The influence of decreased retinal illumination on automated perimetric threshold measurements. Am J Ophthalmol. 1989;108:643–50.
16. Phu J, Khuu SK, Yapp M, Assaad N, Hennessy MP, Kalloniatis M. The value of visual field testing in the era of advanced imaging: clinical and psychophysical perspectives. Clin Exp Optom. 2017;100:313–32.
17. Madrid-Costa D, Ruiz-Alcocer J, García-Lázaro S, et al. Effect of multizone refractive multifocal contact lenses on standard automated perimetry. Eye Contact Lens. 2012;38:278–1.
18. Tavolara L. Observations on the behavior of the visual field in patients with pterygium. Boll Ocul. 1959;38:442–54.
19. Blum FG Jr, Gates LK, James BR. How important are peripheral fields. AMA Arch Ophthalmol. 1959;61(1):1–8.

Visual Field Defects with Tilted and Torted Optic Discs

Sagarika Patyal

The tilted disc is a congenital anomaly of the optic nerve head, variously called situs inversus of papilla, nasal fundus ectasia syndrome, Fuch's coloboma, congenital optic crescents, conus, dysversion of optic nerve heads, and situs inversus [1, 2]. Disc tilt may also be acquired due to changes related with myopia progression [3]. Histological distinctions of the congenital anomaly from myopic tilted discs with peripapillary atrophy or crescents are difficult, and while the congenital anomaly is non progressive, tilted disc associated with myopia may progress [4].

The congenital tilted optic disc syndrome is clinically defined as an abnormality with inferonasal tilt of the optic disc, presence of inferior or inferonasal crescent, and an ectasia of the lower fundus or inferior staphyloma [5, 6]. Besides being tilted, the optic disc may also be rotated or torted, defined as the deviation of the long axis of the optic disc from the vertical meridian and appears oblique or horizontally oval due to its rotation on the z axis (anteroposteriorly directed axis) [7]. Both tilting and rotation of optic discs cause dilemmas in glaucoma diagnosis and progression.

On clinical examination, the tilted optic disc appears oval without simultaneous visibility of its margins. The superotemporal part of the optic disc appears elevated and its inferior or inferonasal part appears posteriorly displaced. Other features which may be seen are congenital conus, ectasia, thinning of choroid and retinal pigment epithelium of the inferior or inferonasal fundus, situs inversus of retinal vessels at the optic disc, myopic astigmatism, and visual field defects. The tilt lends it an oval appearance with an oblique orientation. Deviation of retinal vessels towards the crescent also enhances the tilted look of the optic disc [1].

The tilted disc syndrome is a nonhereditary condition, found bilaterally in 80% though rare unilateral cases have been reported, and is found equally in male and female population [8, 9]. Prevalence of tilted disc has been reported to range from 1.6% to 1.7% in Australian and Italian populations but the Tanjong Pagar study has reported a greater prevalence of 3.5% in an adult Chinese population [10–13].

Method of assessing tilt and torsion of optic disc: Disc ovality index is determined by the tilt ratio which is the ratio of the longest and shortest diameters (orthogonal to one another) of the optic disc and is considered its surrogate index [14, 15]. Disc tilt ratio is a continuous value, and different studies have used differing cut off values

S. Patyal (✉)
Centre for Sight, Dwarka, New Delhi, Delhi, India

for its identification [14–16]. The optic disc tilt is assessed by measuring the maximum, minimum, vertical, and horizontal diameters using optic disc color stereophotographs, after identifying the optic disc margins, defined as the inner border of the scleral ring, with a stereo viewer. Retinal photographs are exported to Adobe Photoshop, and the maximum and minimum diameters are marked [15]. Torsion of the optic disc, measured as degree of torsion, is the angle of deviation of the long axis of the disc from the vertical meridian, the latter being a vertical line perpendicular to the axis connecting the fovea to the center of the disc [13, 14]. A positive torsion value indicates an inferior torsion and a negative value indicates a superior torsion [14]. See Examples 1, 2, and 3.

Example 1 Disc ovality and disc torsion measured using the National Institutes of Health image analysis software (image) version 1.48 v, developed by Wayne Rasb and available at http://rsb.info.nih.gov/ij/index.html (in public domain) (picture courtesy: Dr. Gaurav Bharti)

Black line: longest diameter

Yellow line: Shortest diameter

Red line: The vertical meridian was identified as a vertical line 90° from a horizontal line connecting the fovea

Measured by Dr. Mithun Thulasidas, Fellow, Centre for Sight

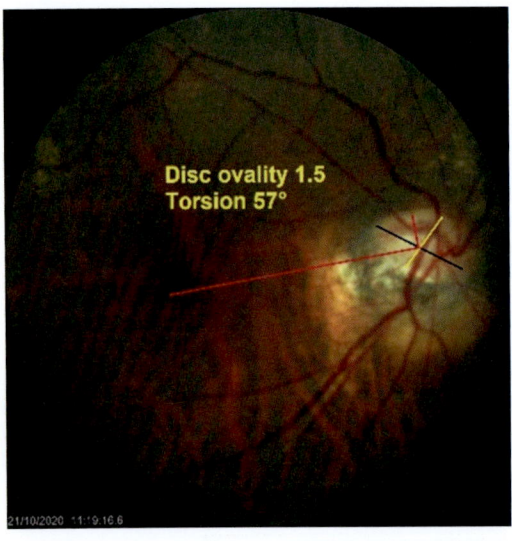

Example 2 Measurement of disc ovality and torsion in another eye (courtesy: Dr. Mithun Thulasidas).

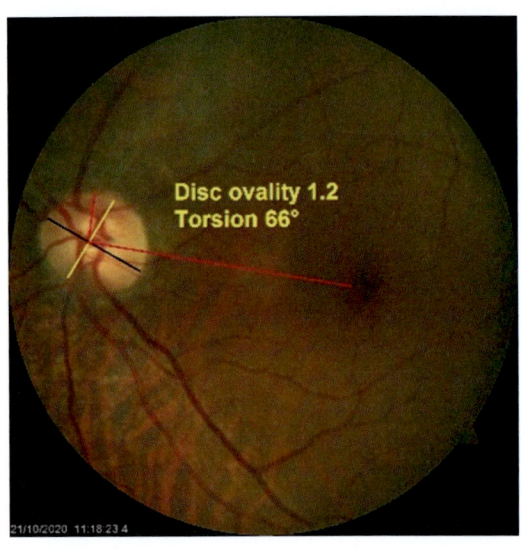

Example 3 Measurement of disc ovality and torsion (courtesy: Dr. Mithun Thulasidas).

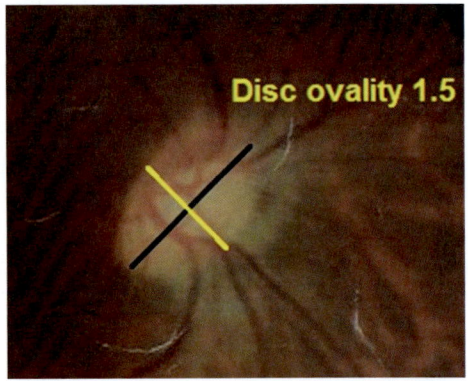

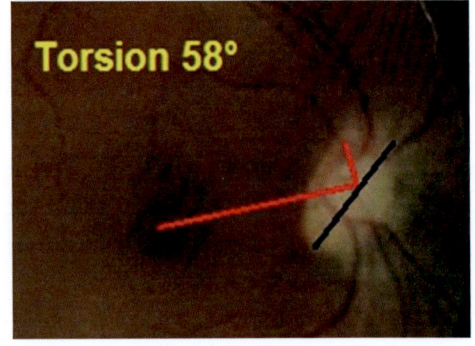

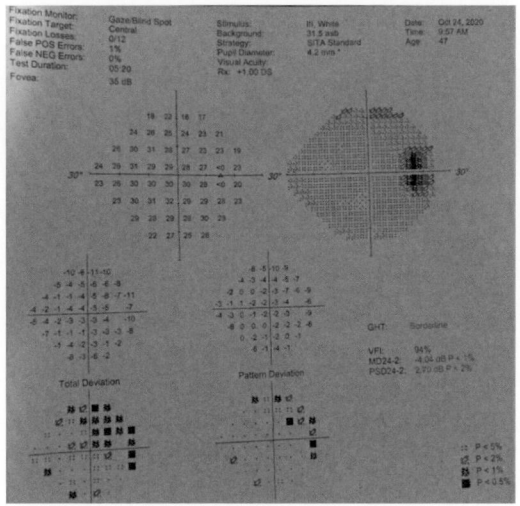

47 years old female on follow up after YAG laser iridotomy

Tilted disc of right eye only (ovality of 1.5, torsion of 58° with vision of 6/6 with -0.75 DS-0.75 DC at 140°

Visual field reveals supero-temporal visual defect.

Refractive errors generally associated with this condition are myopia and astigmatism. The Blue Mountain Eye study on urban adult Australians found 66.2% myopia in eyes with tilted discs compared to 12.4% eyes with normal disc appearance and a mean astigmatic error of 2.2 D in eyes with tilted discs compared to 0.7 D in eyes with normal optic disc appearance [10]. Corneal astigmatism, higher in tilted discs, has also been found to have its axis correlating with the longest optic disc diameter [17].

The congenital condition is due to incomplete or mal-closure of the optic fissure at 6 weeks gestation, and this colobomatous condition is typically found in the inferior and inferonasal area of the disc, peripapillary retina, retinal pigment epithelium, and choroid with deficiency of axons in the inferior and inferonasal aspect though there is lack of convincing evidence of the same [2, 4, 8]. It has also been hypothesized that optic disc tilt may result from hypoplasia of the optic nerve head [18]. Other abnormal features in this condition are moderate to severe hypoplasia, thinning of retinal, choroidal and scleral layers, focal hypopigmentation, ectasia of the posterior inferonasal wall of the globe, and oblique insertion of the optic nerve and retinal arteries [2]. The cause of tilt in high myopia, on the other hand, is due to axial elongation of the posterior pole with stretching of the temporal optic disc margin with tilting on the vertical axis resulting in a vertically oval disc. Vertically elongated discs are associated with open angle glaucoma with positive association of degree of tilt with severity of visual field damage in glaucoma [14, 16, 19]. Besides, disc tilt has been found to be an independent risk factor in bi-hemi-spheric retinal nerve fiber defects even after controlling for age, mean deviation, disc area, and axial length [20].

Optic disc assessment in glaucoma is integral for its diagnosis and progression and becomes difficult in tilted discs resulting in either over- or underdiagnosis and unnecessary treatment in many cases. Tilted discs, peripapillary atrophy, and myopia create problems due to field defects which mimic glaucomatous field defects and those due to chiasmal lesions. The commonest visual field defect seen in this condition is superotemporal depression, not respecting the midline (horizontal or vertical) (Examples 4 and 5), the vertex of which is turned towards the blind spot [18]; other defects which have been noted are: arcuate scotoma, blind spot enlargement, nasal contraction of the visual field [21–23]. Even altitudinal and mild depression in the sensitivity in all quadrants have been found in this condition [18]. Field defects are due to decreased number of axons in the area of retinal and choroidal thinning which decrease photosensitivity, and the oblique insertion of the papilla into the globe causes field defects mimicking chiasmal defects, the difference being extension of the field defect across the midline [1, 2]. Bilateral tilted disc syndrome may exhibit superior bitemporal depression akin to chiasmal compressive lesions. Quadrantanopsia like defects extending beyond the midline and altitudinal defects have also been reported in this condition. Visual field defects by automated perimetry have been found to be present in the central 30° [23].

Example 4 (courtesy Dr. Nirmala Sudhamala)

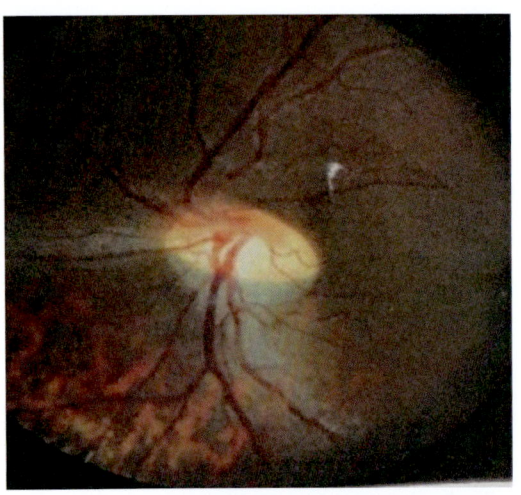

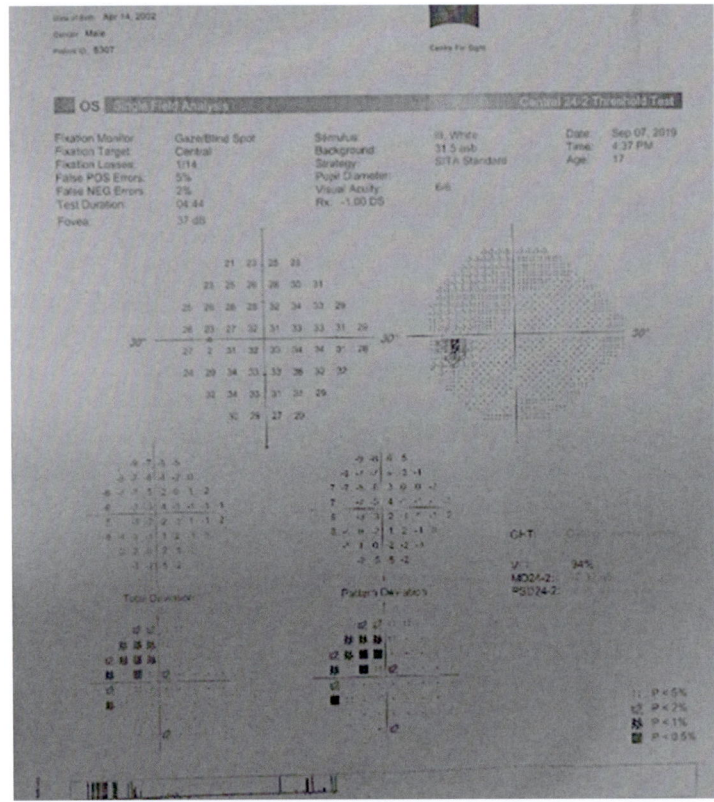

Unilateral horizontally tilted and rotated disc of the left eye with inferior thinning of nerve fibers with field defects in the superotemporal quadrant.

Example 5

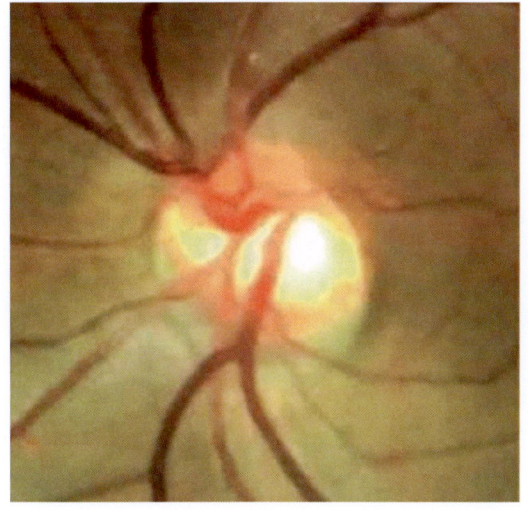

22 years old male with vision of the right eye 6/6 with −1.0 DC at 40°, the left eye vision of 6/9 with −6.0 DS with 0.5 DC at 90°. Horizontally tilted and torted left optic disc which was not associated with any field defect.

In myopic glaucoma, optic nerve head tilt and peripapillary atrophy indicate the location and direction of the visual field defect. Visual field defects have been found to be more localized in myopic open angle glaucoma with larger pattern standard deviation at baseline and final examination and more cases with one hemifield involvement than non-myopic eyes. There is still controversy about myopia being a risk factor for glaucoma progression but faster visual field progression has been found to be associated with inferiorly tilted discs in myopia [7].

Factors which help the clinician decide whether investigations like neuroimaging and treatment are required by the patient are clinical identification of conus and hypopigmentation of inferior and inferonasal fundus with associated superior bitemporal visual field defects not respecting the midline and nonprogressive visual field defects. Field defects are relative and may be eliminated with optical correction corresponding to the floor of the ectasia but in severe cases even myopic correction cannot improve the field defect [18]. Electroretinogram, electrooculogram, and vision-evoked potential also show abnormal results especially in areas of fundal hypoplasia, with visual-evoked potential showing abnormal latency in almost all cases [24].

Thus, the tilted discs may cause confusion in assessment and diagnosis of glaucoma especially when the latter is superimposed on it. Further misdiagnosis and unnecessary treatment may occur due to field defects which may mimic glaucoma.

References

1. Dorrell D. The tilted disc. Br J Ophthalmol. 1978;62(1):16–20.
2. Manfrè L, Vero S, Focarelli-Barone C, Lagalla R. Bitemporal pseudohemianopia related to the "tilted disk" syndrome: CT, MR, and fundoscopic findings. AJNR Am J Neuroradiol. 1999;20(9):1750–1.
3. Park KA, Park SE, Oh SY. Long-term changes in refractive error in children with myopic tilted optic disc compared to children without tilted optic disc. Invest Ophthalmol Vis Sci. 2013;54(13):7865–70.
4. Kim YC, Moon J, Park HL, et al. Three dimensional evaluation of posterior pole and optic nerve head in tilted disc. Sci Rep. 2018;8:1121.
5. Ribeiro-da-Silva J, Castanheira-Dinis A, Agoas V, Godinho-de-Matos J. Congenital optic disc deformities. A clinical approach. Ophthalmic Paediatr Genet. 1985;5:67–70.
6. Cohen SY, Quentel G, Guiberteau B, Delahaye-Mazza C, Gaudric A. Macular serous retinal detachment caused by subretinal leakage in tilted disc syndrome. Ophthalmology. 1998;105:1831–4.
7. Han JC, Lee EJ, Kim SH, Kee C. Visual field progression pattern associated with optic disc tilt morphology in myopic open-angle glaucoma. Am J Ophthalmol. 2016;169:33–45.

8. Sowka J, Aoun P. Tilted disc syndrome. Optom Vis Sci. 1999;76(9):618–23.
9. Ciftci S. Unilateral tilted disc and ipsilateral keratoconus in the same eye. BMJ Case Rep. 2011;2011:bcr0620103126.
10. Vongphanit J, Mitchell P, Wang JJ. Population prevalence of tilted optic disks and the relationship of this sign to refractive error. Am J Ophthalmol. 2002;133(5):679–85.
11. Riise D. The nasal fundus ectasia. Acta Ophthalmol Suppl. 1975;126(126):3–108.
12. Giuffrè G. Tilted disks and central retinal vein occlusion. Graefes Arch Clin Exp Ophthalmol. 1993;231(1):41–2.
13. How AC, Tan GS, Chan YH, Wong TT, Seah SK, Foster PJ, Aung T. Population prevalence of tilted and torted optic discs among an adult Chinese population in Singapore: the Tanjong Pagar Study. Arch Ophthalmol. 2009;127(7):894–9.
14. Park HY, Lee K, Park CK. Optic disc torsion direction predicts the location of glaucomatous damage in normal-tension glaucoma patients with myopia. Ophthalmology. 2012;119(9):1844–51.
15. Shoeibi N, Moghadas Sharif N, Daneshvar R, Ehsaei A. Visual field assessment in high myopia with and without tilted optic disc. Clin Exp Optom. 2017;100(6):690–4.
16. Tay E, Seah SK, Chan SP, et al. Optic disk ovality as an index of tilt and its relationship to myopia and perimetry. Am J Ophthalmol. 2005;139:247–52.
17. Jonas JB, Kling F, Gründler AE. Optic disc shape, corneal astigmatism, and amblyopia. Ophthalmology. 1997;104(11):1934–7.
18. Vuori ML, Mäntyjärvi M. Tilted disc syndrome may mimic false visual field deterioration. Acta Ophthalmol. 2008;86(6):622–5.
19. Hosseini H, Nassiri N, Azarbod P, et al. Measurement of the optic disc vertical tilt angle with spectral-domain optical coherence tomography and influencing factors. Am J Ophthalmol. 2013;156:737–44.
20. Choi JA, Park HY, Shin HY, Park CK. Optic disc characteristics in patients with glaucoma and combined superior and inferior retinal nerve fiber layer defects. JAMA Ophthalmol. 2014;132(9):1068–75.
21. Manor RS. Temporal field defects due to nasal tilting of discs. Ophthalmologica. 1974;168(4):269–81.
22. Berry H. Bitemporal of the visual fields due to an ocular cause. Br J Ophthalmol. 1963;47(7):441–4.
23. Brazitikos PD, Safran AB, Simona F, Zulauf M. Threshold perimetry in tilted disc syndrome. Arch Ophthalmol. 1990;108(12):1698–700.
24. Giuffrè G, Anastasi M. Electrofunctional features of the tilted disc syndrome. Doc Ophthalmol. 1986;62(3):223–30.

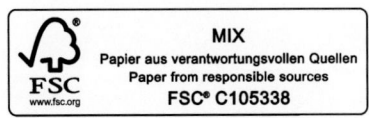

Printed by Books on Demand, Germany